The People's Pharmacy®

The
People's Pharmacy®

Completely New and Revised

Joe Graedon and Teresa Graedon, Ph.D.

ST. MARTIN'S PRESS
New York

Book design by Richard Oriolo

ISBN 0-312-14125-4

ATTENTION: IMPORTANT NOTE TO READERS

This book should not be used as a substitute for professional medical advice or care. The reader should consult a physician in matters relating to his or her health. In particular, the reader should consult his or her physician before acting on any of the information or advice contained in this book or undertaking any form of self-treatment.

Stopping a medication can be very dangerous. Every reader must consult with his or her physician before starting, stopping, or changing the dose of any medication. Any side effects should be reported promptly to the physician. The possibility of adverse effects should not cause the reader to overlook completely the benefits of medication. A reader concerned about adverse effects of medication should discuss with his or her doctor the benefits as well as the risks of taking the medication.

The information contained in this book regarding health and medications is the result of review by the authors of relevant medical and scientific literature. That literature at times reflects conflicting conclusions and opinions. The authors have expressed their views on many of those issues; the reader should understand that other experts may disagree.

The adverse reactions and drug interactions listed in Part V of this book (People's Pharmacy Guide to Popular Prescription Drugs) do not include every possible complication listed in the package insert or reported in the literature. In addition, information about drug effects remains incomplete, as new dangers are discovered all the time. And, the effects drugs can have vary from person to person. **As a result, the reader should not assume that because an adverse reaction or interaction is not mentioned in connection with a drug listed in this book, it cannot be caused by that drug.**

This Book Is Dedicated to:

The Memory of Sid Graedon
Who loved this book from day one and knew it would be successful long before we did. Thanks, Pop!

Phil Schwartz
Who keeps coming up with creative solutions to thorny problems

Hugh Tilson
Who opened our eyes wider than we ever imagined possible

Fred Eckel
Who has a dream of what pharmacy can truly be

People Everywhere
Who care about their health and want to protect themselves from drug misadventures

Acknowledgments

Charles Branton, who gives us help, encouragement, and valuable information.

George Brett, a friend, Internet visionary, computer wizard, and life saver.

Cliff Butler, an extraordinary pharmacist who always comes to our aid at the last minute.

Rob and Rose Capon, wonderful colleagues who have faith in our abilities, and have helped spread the health word around the world.

Virginia Cassell, a fabulous producer, who is well defined, enthusiastic, and always willing to stick her finger in the dike.

Fred Eckel, a pharmacist educator with a wonderful vision of what the future of pharmacy can be.

Dean Edell, who spurred us on and challenges us to keep trying harder.

Madeline Feinberg, a pharmacist who truly cares about older people.

Tom Ferguson, the guru of the medical self-care revolution and a soul mate, coauthor, colleague, and friend.

David Flockhart, a clinical pharmacologist with extraordinary wisdom about drug interactions and the limitations of the system. Thanks for sharing your expertise on grapefruit juice.

Teresa Gill, a patient attorney who held our hand through thick and thin.

Alena Graedon, a wonderful person, an excellent editor, and a great helper when we need you most. Thanks for being so patient and for hanging in there with us.

Tim Ives, a pharmacist who represents the best of his profession.

John McLachlan, a fabulous pharmacologist, a phenomenal friend, a superb director, and a fantastic researcher who is making this world a safer, better place.

Karen Mosely, who eases the burden, keeps us sane, and always has a smile.

Bill Pinna, who never gives up.

Ralph Scallion, a cardiologist with heart who is almost as well organized as we are.

Stephanie Shipper, who helps keep us on track with our values.

Brian Weiss, a wordsmith who has assisted in the evolution.

Michael Woyton, a fixer-upper, a fabulous editor, and Outbound soul mate.

Contents

Drugs That Can Lead to Bad Sunburn / **Bites, Stings, Rashes, and Itches / Fungus Infections:** Athlete's Foot / Jock Itch / **Cuts and Scratches / Pain Relief / Sniffles and Sneezes / Vitamins / Multipurpose Medicines / Recommended Reference Material**

Part V: People's Pharmacy Guide to Popular Prescription Drugs   321

Prologue

How It All Happened

How did *The People's Pharmacy* get started? It's a question we're frequently asked, so perhaps a few words of explanation are in order. First, there is no physical pharmacy, and, even if there were, we couldn't fill a prescription for love or money. We are not pharmacists and all we dispense is information.

In the spring of 1967 Joe was graduated from Pennsylvania State University and started work at the neuropharmacology laboratory of the New Jersey Neuropsychiatric Institute in Princeton. Research included the neurochemistry of mental illness, basic sleep physiology, and the investigation of various treatments for insomnia.

In 1969 he started graduate school in pharmacology at the University of Michigan in Ann Arbor. Pharmacology is a discipline that few people have actually heard of. It is quite different from the standard practice of pharmacy, and combines biochemistry, molecular biology, and physiology. This represents one of the basic disciplines in medical schools. Pharmacologists are involved in developing new drugs, testing old ones, unlocking secrets about how the human body works, and training health professionals to prescribe and dispense medications wisely.

While Joe was in graduate school in pharmacology, Terry was doing graduate work in anthropology. Her studies focused on nutrition and health in an ecological context. In 1972 she and Joe went to Oaxaca, Mexico, so that she could collect data on this topic for a doctoral dissertation in medical anthropology.

In Mexico Joe taught pharmacology in the medical school in the mornings and in the afternoons he started writing a book he had been thinking about—a book that turned out to be *The People's Pharmacy*. Family, friends, and neighbors had been asking him questions about their medicine—antibiotics, blood pressure pills, antidepressants—but they often didn't even know the names of the drugs they were taking. Here was a chance to empower people about an important aspect of their health.

To everyone's surprise, *The People's Pharmacy* went on to become a Number 1 bestseller on *The New York Times* list. The rest is history. Joe and Terry have gone on to write nine other books. This is the third edition of *The People's Pharmacy*. They also write "The People's Pharmacy" syndicated newspaper column (distributed by King Features to more than 100 papers around the country). They host *The People's Pharmacy* syndicated radio show, heard on more than 500 stations in the

U.S. and around the world through public radio, The Armed Forces Radio and Television Service, and the In Touch Radio Reading Service.

Through all their work Joe and Terry strive to help people become better informed about current health issues, especially as they relate to nutrition and medicine.

Part I

Overview

Introduction

Americans are spending more on medicine than ever before . . . and enjoying it less. Back in the early 1970s when we started writing the first edition of *The People's Pharmacy*, Americans shelled out roughly $11 billion each year for prescription drugs and another $2.6 billion for over-the-counter remedies.[1,2,3,4] An average prescription in the drugstore cost just over $4.[5] Prices rarely changed from year to year and when they did go up, the increase was so gradual most people didn't even notice. Medications were one of the best deals around, with increases well below the rate of inflation.

Over the last decade the pharmaceutical industry became the most profitable business in the world. Drug companies rake in roughly $60 billion annually, and that doesn't even take into account the pharmacist's markup and the extraordinary prices charged in hospitals (where an aspirin can cost $1 or more a pill). When you consider what consumers actually pay,[6] you can see that the yearly drug bill is out of control. Senator David Pryor took the industry to task: "Between 1980 and 1992, according to the Bureau of Labor Statistics, drug price inflation at the manufacturers' level was about 128 percent—about six times the overall rate of inflation, which was about 22 percent."[7]

Sticker Shock

The average prescription now costs more than $25.[8] We have watched with horror as the median price of the female hormone **Premarin** went from $7.75 for 100 pills in 1972 to $42.74 today.[9] **Valium** zoomed from $9.38 to $56.19, and the antibacterial drug **Flagyl** increased from $17 to over $142 for 100 pills.[10] It is not unusual for patients to experience sticker shock when they go to pick up their medicine.

Pharmacists have shared with us tragic stories of people breaking down in tears when they discover they can't afford to pay $79 for a ten-day supply of antibiotic for a sick child. Older people on fixed incomes are often hammered with monthly medication bills in the hundreds of dollars. Many are forced to skip pills to make ends meet. We have received letters from people forced to sell their homes to pay for doctors and for prescription drugs. Some of the new high-tech medicines for multiple sclerosis or cystic fibrosis can cost more than $10,000 a year.

The cost of over-the-counter remedies is also soaring. Annual sales are projected to increase from $12 billion in the early 1990s to more than $20 billion by the turn of the century. The self-care market is exploding as consumers opt for self-diagnosis and treatment. More and more prescription drugs are jumping the counter and becoming available without a physician's intervention. More than 400 over-the-counter products now being sold contain ingredients that were available only by prescription when the first edition of *The People's Pharmacy* was written.

Drug companies see their future in such prescription-to-over-the-counter switches. Sales often increase by double, triple or more when products can be sold directly to consumers on pharmacy shelves, in supermarkets, convenience stores, hotels, gas stations, airports, and almost everyplace else. Brands such as **Actifed, Advil, Afrin, Aleve** (by prescription as **Anaprox** and **Naprosyn**), **Benadryl, Cortaid, Dimetapp, Gyne-Lotrimin, Imodium A-D, Micatin, Motrin IB, Monistat 7, Nuprin, Sudafed,** and **Tinactin** have been incredibly successful. **Pepcid AC, Tagamet HB,** and **Zantac 75** are newcomers with lots of potential. We will undoubtedly see more and more prescription-to-OTC switches in the coming years. Candidates include such drugs as **Hismanal** and **Seldane** for allergies; **Feldene, Orudis,** and **Voltaren** for pain; and **Zovirax** for herpes.

The trouble is that although the Food and Drug Administration (FDA) is giving people more and more tools with which to play doctor, the agency is not providing them with adequate rules. Labels on OTC products are woefully inadequate. Most people assume that over-the-counter drugs are wimpy, hardly worth worrying about. Nothing could be further from the truth.

Drug Dangers

Although manufacturers of nonprescription products are not required to report adverse reactions to the Food and Drug Administration, there is growing awareness that OTC medications can produce serious harm or even death. Researchers at Emory University in Atlanta discovered that a surprisingly large number of patients who showed up at their hospital with bleeding stomach ulcers had taken OTC arthritis medicines (NSAIDs, known as nonsteroidal anti-inflammatory drugs, include aspirin or ibuprofen). They reported that "overall, 56% of our patients reported NSAID use during the week prior to admission."[11]

Bleeding or perforated ulcers are a potentially life-threatening situation. The Atlanta investigators concluded that these OTC pain relievers could represent "an important health hazard" and might well be "one of the most important precipitating factors for ulcer-related hemorrhage."[12] That is why it is so important for people to treat such nonprescription drugs with respect. While they may relieve pain and inflammation, they can also kill.

Don't assume, though, that just because a physician prescribes the medicine you take that you will be safe. Dr. James Fries is one of the country's leading arthritis experts. He notes that nonsteroidal anti-inflammatory drugs account for "more than 70,000 hospitalizations and 7,000 deaths annually in the United States."[13] Think of it this way: Estimates of the number of deaths from all illicit drugs combined (cocaine, heroin, marijuana, LSD) range from a low of 3,562 per year to a high of 10,710.[14,15] So almost as many people die each year from prescribed arthritis medicines as die from all illegal drugs. Older people are especially vulnerable. One report suggests that 73,000 die needlessly each year from adverse drug reactions and interactions.[16]

According to a 1995 study, "Medical therapy results in unintended injuries that have been estimated to affect 1.3 million people each year in the United States. Many of these injuries are unavoidable, but as many as two thirds may be secondary to errors in management."[17] In other words, the physicians prescribing, the pharmacists dispensing, or the nurses administering the medicine made mistakes that resulted in people being harmed.

Perhaps even more startling is the number of deaths from medication errors. Experts estimate that at least 125,000 people die annually because of prescription drug mistakes.[18] That is over ten times the number of deaths from illicit drugs. Yet politicians, bureaucrats, and health professionals continue to rant and rail about the war on drugs with barely a whisper about the other, far more devastating drug disaster happening to upstanding citizens. Too many people get the wrong drug, the wrong dose, and the wrong combination.

The National Council on Patient Information and Education (NCPIE) represents more than 350 professional health organizations, consumer groups, and government agencies (including the AMA, the American Pharmaceutical Association, and the FDA). It estimates that "half of the 1.6 billion prescriptions we take every year are taken incorrectly."[19] And roughly one third of the errors are very danger-ous, posing a "serious threat to the patient's health."[20] Some groups, like the National Pharmaceutical Council, believe the problem is worse—that as many as 90 percent of patients make mistakes with medicine.[21]

Although physicians often blame the victim ("ignorant" or "noncompliant patients" are terms we hear frequently), the truth is that health professionals don't always provide adequate or understandable information. Some years ago an FDA study uncovered the startling statistic that roughly one-third of those over 60 years of age received no counseling from either physicians or pharmacists.[22]

Even when an attempt is made to instruct patients, the information may be virtually useless. Walk behind any pharmacy counter and you are likely to see prescriptions written in illegible Latin code with instructions like *b.i.d.* (two times a day), *p.c.* (after meals), or *p.r.n.* (as needed). Most intelligent people would make mistakes with such ambiguous recommendations. "Twice a day" doesn't tell you if the medicine should be taken every twelve hours or just sometime in the morning and evening. There is rarely a reference to food or beverages (though the absorption of many medicines is affected by food or drinks). Does "after meals" mean immediately after eating or an hour later? And that old standby "as needed" is so broad it could mean anything—a dozen times a day or only when the pain is so bad you are ready to shoot yourself in the head. It's hardly any wonder mistakes are common.

Baby Boomers Beware

O lder people are the ones who suffer most. They are the ones that take the most medicine. But we're not talking about Granny. Aging baby boomers, on the verge of turning 50, are beginning to understand that their bodies aren't indestructible. Jogging can take a toll on ankles and knees. Hours at the computer keyboard can bring on carpal tunnel syndrome (a nerve condition of the wrist and hand). Hypertension, angina, anxiety, and depression are common.

These days it seems as if the whole world is on **Prozac** (fluoxetine) or one of its cousins (**Paxil** or **Zoloft**) for a "mood disorder" or a "personality problem." If you have a little stomach upset, how about some **Zantac** or **Tagamet**? Should sniffles and sneezes slow you down, swallow **Seldane**. When hot flashes start showing up, it's time for the **Premarin**. Feeling a little stressed out? Take **Xanax**.

What doctors may not mention, though, is that the more medicine people take, the more likely it is they will experience side effects or dangerous interactions. Richard P. Kusserow, Inspector General of the Department of Health and Human Services, dropped a bombshell on the medical community a few years ago. His 1989 government report detailed the "nation's other drug problem." It found that older people average 15.5 prescriptions per person per year. Roughly 250,000 "were hospitalized annually due to ADRs (adverse drug reactions)."[23] Other estimates place the number far higher.[24] Serious "mental impairment either caused or worsened by drugs" occurs in 163,000 people, and two million "are addicted or at risk of addiction to minor tranquilizers or sleeping pills because of using them daily for at least one year."[25]

Over the last 20 years researchers have tried to determine how many people of all ages are hospitalized because of adverse drug reactions. Some studies have indicated a low of 0.2 percent. Others report a high of 21.7 percent. A review of the collected data concluded that "Drug-induced hospitalizations account for approximately five percent of all admissions. . . . The true percentage may be much higher."[26]

Presumably the country's top drug cop (the Commissioner of the Food and Drug Administration) is in the best position to assess the size of the problem. He notes that "A recent review article[27] found that between 3% and 11% of hospital admissions could be attributed to adverse drug reactions."[28] Given that the American Hospital Association estimates that more than 33 million people are admitted annually, that would leave us with anywhere between 1,000,000 and 3,688,960 people who were hospitalized because of an adverse reaction to their medicine.[29]

It's easy to glaze over when such big numbers are bandied about. But the possibility that more than three million people are damaged and hospitalized because of their medicine is mind-boggling. Never forget that most of these folks were taking medicine to get better. When the cure becomes worse than the disease, there is something very wrong with the system. Adverse reactions can range from severe allergies and skin rashes to seizures, hallucinations, blood disorders, heart rhythm disturbances, and death. And doctors rarely warn patients in advance what dangers to be alert for.

Hospital Hazards

You might think that if you were admitted to a hospital you would no longer have to worry about drug problems. Presumably, the hordes of physicians, residents, pharmacists, nurses, and medical students who descend upon you will check every medication to make sure that you get better care than you would at home.

Even in the best of hospitals, however, adverse drug events are common. A study published in the *Journal of the American Medical Association* (July 5, 1995) uncovered shocking statistics at two of the nation's finest teaching hospitals. Medical students from all over the world vie to get accepted for residency at Brigham and Women's Hospital and Massachusetts General Hospital, both affiliated with Harvard Medical School. It is distressing that researchers found approximately 6.5 percent of hospitalized patients at these prestigious institutions experienced adverse drug events.[30]

This 1995 result is even more discouraging because about ten years earlier in-

vestigators found that 4 percent of the patients in New York State hospitals suffered an adverse event. Using the figures from this Medical Practice Study (MPS),
the authors of the more recent research drew the following comparisons:

> I f the numbers from New York are extrapolated to the country as a whole, over a million pa-
> tients are injured in hospitals each year, and approximately 180,000 die annually as a result
> of these injuries. Therefore, the iatrogenic [doctor-induced] injury rate dwarfs the annual au-
> tomobile accident mortality of 45,000 and accounts for more deaths than all other accidents
> combined. . . . The leading cause of medical injury in the MPS was use of drugs, accounting for
> 19.4 percent of these injuries.[31]

One might conclude from the new data that the situation is getting worse. The
physicians in Boston wrote: "We conclude that ADEs [adverse drug events] are a
major cause of iatrogenic injury, that many are preventable, and that for every preventable ADE there are almost three potential ADEs."[32] Frequent errors included
wrong dosing and preventable drug interactions. One of the most common causes
for such problems was found to be the inadequate "dissemination of drug knowledge, particularly to physicians."[33]

In his report, Inspector General Richard Kusserow chastised the medical community for allowing inadequate training in pharmacology and geriatrics. The FDA
Commissioner has also complained about "the limited training medical students
receive in clinical pharmacology . . . only 14% of them had required courses in core
skills and principles of therapeutic decision making and clinical pharmacology."[34]

So many new medications have come out in the last two decades that the average physician in his fifties probably didn't learn about more than a small fraction
of these compounds in medical school. Most drug information on new medicines
comes from salesmen representing pharmaceutical manufacturers, rather than
from formal education. A lack of understanding about drug dangers can lead to the
"illness-medication spiral," where adverse reactions "are diagnosed as new illnesses, leading to the prescribing of more and more drugs to treat symptoms and
toxicities caused by inappropriate drug therapy."[35,36]

The problems haven't gone away. If anything, the situation is worse today because physicians are overworked, inundated with paper, and overwhelmed by an
onslaught of new and more sophisticated pharmaceuticals. It is nearly impossible
to keep up with all the latest drug developments.

Advertising Assault

Pharmaceutical companies are doing their best to drum up business by scaring people. A few decades ago they dreamt up a malady called "the blahs." Naturally, they had developed a drug to relieve this problem. Nowadays promotional campaigns target "the worried well." The more hypochondriacs the drug companies can create, the more pills they can sell.

Slick advertisements for prescription medications are now aimed directly at consumers. Browse through almost any magazine these days and you might think you had picked up a medical journal by mistake. *Newsweek, Time, U.S. News & World Report, Smithsonian*, and *People* all carry prescription drug ads. They are aimed not at health professionals but at consumers. You will find ads for everything from **Rogaine** (to restore hair) to **Cardizem CD** (for heart problems or hypertension). Women are encouraged to ask for **Premarin** or **Estraderm** to prevent osteoporosis or menopausal symptoms.

Men are urged to "take the prostate test." If you flunk you are supposed to "Ask your doctor about **Hytrin**" for that enlarged prostate. Other ads have a detailed anatomical drawing of a man's bladder, prostate, and penis. Guys are warned that the prostate "problem will probably not get better by itself." So "Ask your doctor about the prescription medicine **Proscar**." People with arthritis or allergies are told to "Ask your doctor" about **Daypro** for pain and swelling or **Claritin** to relieve nasal symptoms.

Now, keep in mind that you can't buy any of these medicines off the shelf in your neighborhood drugstore. The ads suggest that it would be a good idea for people to contact their physician for a prescription. Presumably doctors respond to prodding. Drug companies are nothing if not pragmatic. Given the millions of dollars being spent on these ad campaigns, they must be working. People are asking, cajoling, and otherwise demanding prescriptions for drugs they saw on TV or read about in ads.

We have nothing against these advertisements per se. We encourage an active dialogue between patients and physicians about new treatment options. But these promotional campaigns have not impressed us with their balance or objectivity. Side effects and risks are de-emphasized. If you want to learn more you have to flip the page and decipher the fine print and doctorspeak. Our biggest fear is that the avalanche of ads appearing in consumer publications will lead to unrealistic expectations and will reinforce Americans' tendency to believe there is a pill for every ill.

Good News

By now you are probably feeling nervous if not downright depressed. Drug prices have skyrocketed. Adverse drug reactions are a greater cause for concern than ever given the proliferation of new and potent medications. Doctors are overwhelmed and have a hard time keeping up with the flood of drug information. We could easily understand feelings of pessimism, and yet there is also cause for celebration.

There have been extraordinary drug advances since we initiated *The People's Pharmacy*. Back in the 1970s there were relatively few medications for high blood pressure, and the ones that were prescribed often caused a variety of unpleasant side effects. It was just accepted that the trade-off for control of hypertension would be dizziness, drowsiness, diarrhea, depression, stomach upset, or impotence, to name some common complications.

Today it is possible to manage high blood pressure with few if any adverse effects. And researchers have discovered unexpected benefits of some of these drugs. ACE inhibitors such as **Capoten** (captopril) and **Vasotec** (enalapril) appear useful for people with heart failure, and help stave off kidney complications of diabetes.

Schizophrenia

There have been extraordinary advances in so many areas over the last decade or two it is hard to know where to start. Some of the most important have involved the brain. Treatment of mental problems has taken a leap forward. Until recently all we had for schizophrenia were major tranquilizers such as **Haldol** (haloperidol), **Mellaril** (thioridazine), **Stelazine** (trifluoperazine), and **Thorazine** (chlorpromazine). These drugs could make people feel totally spaced out, or make them feel agitated. Drowsiness, dizziness, weakness, jitteriness, slurred speech, and uncontrollable muscle twitching were common side effects. It's no wonder patients were unhappy with these medications.

We now have several advances in the treatment of this devastating condition. **Risperdal** (risperidone) and **Clozaril** (clozapine) are not cures for schizophrenia, but they seem better tolerated than traditional drugs and have helped patients cope more effectively with their disordered thinking. They are far less likely to cause the uncontrollable muscle movements (tardive dyskinesia) that characterize older antipsychotic drugs.

Depression and OCD

Although physicians have been prescribing antidepressants for decades, most of these medications leave much to be desired. They could take away the blues, but they rarely helped people feel really happy. We often heard complaints about weight gain, sluggishness, constipation, forgetfulness, fatigue, and a general blah feeling.

Now there is a veritable smorgasbord of new medications to choose from, including **Prozac** (fluoxetine), **Paxil** (paroxetine), **Wellbutrin** (bupropion), **Zoloft** (sertraline), and **Effexor** (venlafaxine), with more on the way. These drugs have made an extraordinary difference for millions of people, many of whom feel they not only relieve depression, but also help improve self-esteem and emotional resiliency.

Those with OCD (obsessive-compulsive disorder) also benefit from these new drugs. It is estimated that four to seven million individuals are affected by persistent, unwanted thoughts or repetitive actions. Some are compelled to wash their hands constantly, pull out hair, or check repeatedly to make sure the door is locked. Drugs such as **Prozac, Anafranil** (clomipramine), or **Luvox** (fluvoxamine) help many people overcome the chemical imbalance that leads to intrusive thoughts or uncontrollable rituals.

Alzheimer's Disease

The first drug against Alzheimer's disease was approved several years ago. While clearly not a cure, **Cognex** (tacrine) has helped some regain a piece of their personality. Although it brings only temporary respite, this drug is the first step in slowing the progression of a condition that affects four million older people.

Some patients appear to do better than others while on **Cognex**. There are reports that they may even regain some memory function and improve activities of daily living such as dressing and eating. Perhaps the insights gained from this medication will lead to better treatments in the future. Preliminary research suggests that anti-inflammatory drugs delay the onset of this disease or perhaps even help improve outcome.

Epilepsy

For the first time in decades we have seen a dramatic improvement in the treatment of seizure disorders. Three new drugs, **Felbatol** (felbamate), **Lamictal** (lamotrigine), and **Neurontin** (gabapentin), offer people with epilepsy new hope.

Although many of the older medicines such as **Dilantin** (phenytoin), phenobarbital, **Tegretol** (carbamazepine), and **Depakene** (valproic acid) are effective, they can produce a number of unpleasant side effects.

The new antiseizure drugs will be a godsend for patients (estimated at 500,000) who have had difficulty controlling their condition with traditional medications. Drugs such as **Neurontin** and **Lamictal** are much less likely to interact with other medications than previous epilepsy medicine. This will be especially welcome for women on birth control pills. In addition, their side-effect profile appears to be quite favorable.

Migraines

People who suffer from really bad headaches can tell you that life sometimes seems barely worth living when you are having an attack. One woman confided that she kept a loaded pistol just in case the pain became unbearable. And men who experience cluster headaches have been known to hurt themselves in an attempt to stop the agony inside their heads.

Imitrex (sumatriptan) has made an important difference for people in pain. The majority of migraine victims can stop an attack in its tracks. After self-injecting **Imitrex**, most patients experience dramatic relief within one hour or less. Oral **Imitrex** offers convenience *and* effectiveness.

Insomnia

People who had trouble getting a decent night's sleep once had to rely on barbiturates. But these drugs were habit-forming and in overdose could lead to unintended suicide.

Then came benzodiazepines. Drugs such as **Valium** (diazepam), **Librium** (chlordiazepoxide), **Dalmane** (flurazepam), **Restoril** (temazepam), and **Halcion** (triazolam) were very popular in the 1970s and 1980s. The trouble was that these drugs were also capable of creating dependence, and sudden withdrawal could lead to unpleasant symptoms including rebound insomnia, anxiety, and panic attacks.

Ambien (zolpidem) is a different kind of sleeping pill. It appears less likely to modify the normal sleep cycle and seems unlikely to lead to physical dependence or withdrawal. There is also exciting new research on a natural brain biochemical called melatonin. This substance may ultimately produce the most natural kind of sleep with the fewest side effects. While not yet approved by the FDA, there is hope that further research will lead to a safe and effective formulation.

Allergies and Asthma

It used to be that if you wanted relief from sniffles, sneezes, and stuffiness you had to put up with drowsiness. Antihistamines were the mainstay in allergy treatment, but drugs such as **Actifed, Benadryl, Chlor-Trimeton,** or **Dimetapp** could space you out. For some people, driving, working, or even thinking was hazardous.

Then along came the nonsedating antihistamines. Drugs such as **Seldane** (terfenadine), **Hismanal** (astemizole), and **Claritin** (loratadine) offered improvement of allergy symptoms without drowsiness. For many allergy sufferers these medications were enough by themselves. Others who were miserable from August through October found that the addition of a cell stabilizer such as **Nasalcrom** (cromolyn) or steroid nasal sprays such as **Beconase** (beclomethasone), **Flonase** (fluticasone), **Nasalide** (flunisolide), and **Rhinocort** (budesonide) could get them through allergy season intact.

Asthma treatment has also undergone a mini-revolution. Traditional treatment involved bronchodilators as the first line. Oral medicine containing ephedrine that could stimulate the heart or make urination difficult has pretty much faded from the radar screen. Such drugs as theophylline (**Slo-bid, Theo-Dur**) or albuterol (**Ventolin, Proventil**) were often prescribed for daily use. Nowadays pulmonary experts believe that asthmatics do best when the underlying inflammation is controlled with inhaled steroids such as **Beclovent** (beclomethasone), **AeroBid** (flunisolide), and **Serevent** (salmeterol), or with anti-inflammatory agents such as **Intal** (cromolyn). Bronchodilators are more often reserved for symptomatic treatment rather than prevention.

Ulcers and Heartburn

For decades doctors had a motto: "No acid—no ulcer." Patients who complained of indigestion or experienced ulcer pain were admonished to eat bland food and glug gallons of chalk in the form of calcium carbonate or aluminum and magnesium (**Maalox** or **Mylanta**).

Then came acid suppressers. Drugs such as **Tagamet** (cimetidine), **Zantac** (ranitidine), **Axid** (nizatidine), **Pepcid** (famotidine), and **Prilosec** (omeprazole) have become the most successful compounds in the history of the pharmaceutical industry. Annual earnings exceed $5 billion, with **Zantac** pulling in more than $3 billion all by itself. These compounds became popular because they were no-muss, no-fuss drugs. Pop a pill and your stomach felt better. Many of these compounds are now available in lower doses without a prescription. **Pepcid AC** was first, soon followed by **Tagamet HB.** This represents a dramatic advance in self-care. And a new prescription drug for severe heartburn called **Propulsid** (cisapride) is modernizing the treatment of this common condition.

An extraordinary shift in our understanding and treatment of ulcers has taken place over the last decade. The discovery that many ulcers as well as gastritis and stomach cancers are caused by an infectious agent has led to "triple therapy." Doctors can now cure most ulcers caused by the bug *Helicobacter pylori* within a week or two. By combining antibacterial agents such as metronidazole, amoxicillin, and **Pepto-Bismol**, the recurrence rate has dropped dramatically.

Prostate Problems

Men with enlarged prostates used to have one option . . . the Roto-Rooter job. That is the euphemistic name for TURP (transurethral resection of the prostate). Physicians would insert a device into the urethra and up through the penis, then electrically cauterize the overgrown prostate tissue. Nowadays urologists tend to prescribe medicine while they watch and wait. For many men that is all that is necessary. Drugs such as **Hytrin** (terazosin) and **Cardura** (doxazosin) relax the muscles that can make urination difficult, and **Proscar** (finasteride) may actually shrink the enlarged gland. There is even some hope that **Proscar** may reduce the risk of prostate cancer.

New Drugs on the Horizon

There is lots more good news. Antiviral drugs were once considered impractical if not impossible. Now we have **Zovirax** (acyclovir), an exceptionally safe medicine with a proven track record against herpes, shingles, and chicken pox. This drug is being considered for OTC status. A related compound, **Naltrex** (valaciclovir), looks promising against shingles. Amantadine (**Symmetrel**) and rimantadine (**Flumadine**) have proven beneficial against type A influenza. We have no doubt that there will be more and better antiviral agents in the future—perhaps even against the common cold. **Pulmozyme** (DNase) is a real breakthrough for people with cystic fibrosis. It helps break up mucus in the lungs and might be beneficial for other lung conditions as well. Better allergy and asthma compounds are also being developed.

Osteoporosis may affect as many as one out of three older women. Exciting new treatments are now on the horizon. **Fosamax** (alendronate) represents a welcome development. **Didrocal** (etidronate) may be another option in that class. **Evista** (raloxifene) has impressed some investigators, and we are tracking it especially carefully. We also anticipate the arrival of **Miacalcin** (calcitonin), a nasal spray that can literally help fight osteoporosis by rebuilding bone.

Arthritis patients may also have something to celebrate. They are eagerly awaiting word on high-tech chicken soup. Preliminary research on solubilized chicken collagen has shown impressive power against the inflammation of rheumatoid arthritis. **Calcipotriene** is a chemical cousin of vitamin D_3. It appears to offer another way to treat psoriasis. **Soriatane** (acitretin) represents another option for this difficult skin condition.

Newer medications for anxiety, Alzheimer's, Parkinson's disease, depression, migraines, and schizophrenia are being actively pursued by a number of major drug companies. **Gepirone**, for example, is nearing the end of the approval process for treatment of both nervousness and depression and may offer advantages over some existing antianxiety agents. **Accolate** represents a whole new approach to asthma therapy.

We also anticipate substantial improvement in glaucoma therapy over the next several years. Current treatment focuses on reducing fluid flow into the eye in order to get pressure down. But Dr. David Epstein, chairman of the ophthalmology program at Duke University Medical Center, states that "We know unequivocally that for all forms of glaucoma, it is not a disease of excess formation of fluid, it is a disease of impaired drainage."[37] Others have described the problem as a "plugged-up filter."[38] Dr. Epstein believes that an old-fashioned diuretic, ethacrynic acid, may be able to clean out the "tissue sludge" that clogs the eye's filtering system, reduce pressure, and improve outcome for glaucoma patients. The medicine is being developed under the brand name **Tekron** (Telor Ophthalmic Pharmaceuticals in Woburn, Massachusetts) as once-a-day eyedrops.

Diabetics may also have good news soon. Improved understanding of this common condition is leading to better therapies. Complications such as kidney disease and eye problems may be diminished. Vitamin E, for example, appears to be a worthwhile addition for many patients. Researchers are looking carefully at other mineral and vitamin supplements as well. And new drugs are on the horizon.

How to Use This Book

By now you must understand our dilemma. We are excited about many of the new drugs in the pharmaceutical pipeline. At the same time, we are concerned about drug-induced adverse reactions. Although doctors swear to "first, do no harm," they risk breaking that principle tenet of the Hippocratic oath every time they write a prescription. All drugs can cause harm. And millions are hospitalized each year because of their medicine. Balancing benefits against risks is like walking a tightrope.

Our most precious possession is our health. Money in the bank and health insurance can't protect us from drug dangers. Knowledge, caution, communication, and assertiveness are critical ingredients if you want to be a careful health consumer. Our goal is to give you some of the tools you'll need to make informed decisions. You will have to take personal responsibility for using this information wisely.

This book is not meant to replace a visit to the doctor or to enable you to second-guess your physician. You MUST establish good communication with all your health providers, especially your pharmacist. Drugs save lives and ease suffering. They can improve life and prolong it. They can also produce permanent injury, and sometimes drugs kill. It's your body and you are, after all, the final inspector.

In the following chapters you will read about how the Food and Drug Administration has let us all down and how doctors often don't know when there is inadequate information about risks. We will provide checklists for asking crucial questions, and resources for finding some of the answers. You will learn how to expand your medical library so you can have your own up-to-date references. If you're into computers and modems, we will teach you how to access electronic bulletin boards and on-line help systems.

There will be lots of news you can use about over-the-counter drugs and home remedies. We will try to provide you with practical information on treatments for everyday maladies such as dandruff, headache, heartburn, motion sickness, bad breath, bug bites, and dry skin. We will warn you about the dangers of mixing medicines. Certain combinations can lead to unpredictable reactions that can be hazardous if not life-threatening.

Throughout this book we will try to give you balanced information on the medicines your physicians are prescribing for allergies, asthma, high blood pressure, anxiety, insomnia, depression, and many more common conditions. There will be lots of tips on how to save money on medicine. There is a trade-off between the latest and greatest drug developments that are pricey, and old-fashioned treatments that are affordable but may make you feel lousy. We will do our best to balance these competing forces. At the end of the book you will find a humongous guide that lists drug data on some of the most commonly prescribed medicines. You will learn about the best way to swallow these pills, the most common side effects, and important interactions to watch out for.

But before you read another page, please consider several important caveats. There is no way we could list every drug detail or danger. Even the *Physicians' Desk Reference* (your doctor's drug bible) does not contain every piece of critical information, and that oversized reference book has more than 2,600 pages of fine print. There are also many questions that neither the regulators, the manufacturers, nor the doctors can answer. In fact there is rarely one final Truth about anything medical. Ask a dozen doctors about a particular medicine or therapy and you are likely to get a dozen different answers and recommendations. Estrogen replacement therapy, for example, has its champions and its critics. Each person is different, and what is right for one individual might be a disaster for someone else. This book is about empowerment and about how to forge an active partnership with your physician and pharmacist. We hope you will use the information you learn here in good health.

References

1. Muller, Charlotte. "The Overmedicated Society: Forces in the Marketplace for Medical Care." *Science* 1972; 176:488–492.
2. Rucker, Donald T. "Drug Use Data, Sources, and Limitations." *JAMA* 1971; 230:888–890.
3. Marketing Emphasis. "76 Drug, Cosmetic, and Toiletry Expenditures." *Product Marketing* 1977; July/August: 43–51.
4. Silverman, M., and P. R. Lee. *Pills, Profits and Politics*. Berkeley: University of California Press, 1974.
5. "For the 1st Time, 7 Generic Drugs Climb to The Top 50." *Pharmacy Times* 1972; 38(4):30–35.
6. Pharmaceutical Manufacturers Association. "PMA Annual Survey Report: Trends in U.S. Pharmaceutical Sales and R&D." Washington, D.C., 1993.
7. Statement of Senator David Pryor on release of Staff Report of the Senate Aging Committee: "Earning a Failing Grade: A Report Card on 1992 Drug Manufacturer Price Inflation." February 3, 1993.
8. "What are Pharmacists Dispensing Most Often?" *Pharmacy Times* 1993; April: 29–44.
9. Derived from *Prescription Drug Pricing: An Almost Total Absence of Competition* (Washington, D.C.: Consumers Federation of America), September 1972. As cited in *Pills, Profits, and Politics* by Dr. Milton Silverman and Dr. Philip R. Lee. Current prices as of 1994 chain-store survey.
10. Ibid.
11. Wilcox, C. Mel, et al. "Striking Prevalence of Over-the-Counter Nonsteroidal Anti-inflammatory Drug Use in Patients With Upper Gastrointestinal Hemorrhage." *Arch. Intern. Med.* 1994, 154:42–46.
12. Ibid.
13. Fries, James F. "NSAID Gastropathy: Epidemiology." *J. Musculoskeletal Med.* February 1991.
14. Nadelmann, Ethan A. "Drug Prohibition in the United States: Cost, Consequences, and Alternatives." *Science* 1989; 245:939–946.
15. "Substance Abuse: The Nation's Number One Health Problem." Prepared by the Institute for Health Policy, Brandeis University, for The Robert Wood Johnson Foundation, Princeton, New Jersey, October 1993.
16. Masterson, Mike, and Chuck Cook. "Drugs' Link in Deaths Often Undetected." *The Arizona Republic* 1988; June 28: 1–13.
17. Leape, Lucian L., et al. "Systems Analysis of Adverse Drug Events." *JAMA* 1995; 274:35–43.
18. Clepper, Irene. "Noncompliance: The Invisible Epidemic." *Drug Topics* 1992; 136(16):44–65.
19. Gebhart, Fred. "R.Phs. Needed to Overcome 'Consumer Fear' of Medicines." *Drug Topics* 1991; 135(12):14–16.
20. "Misused or Unused Prescriptions May Cost Your Health Plan Plenty." *Business & Health* 1992; 10:17–19.

21. Clepper, op. cit.

22. Starr, Cynthia. *Drug Topics* 1987; 131:22–24.

23. Kusserow, Richard P. Inspector General's Report, Department of Health and Human Services, February 15, 1989.

24. Masterson, op. cit.

25. Ibid.

26. Einarson, Thomas R. "Drug-Related Hospital Admissions." *Ann. Pharmacotherapy* 1993; 27:832–840.

27. Beard, K. "Adverse Reactions as a Cause of Hospital Admissions in the Aged." *Drugs and Aging* 1992; 2:356–367.

28. Kessler, David A. "Introducing MEDWatch: A New Approach to Reporting Medication and Device Adverse Effects and Product Problems." *JAMA* 1993; 269:2765–2768.

29. American Hospital Association, Personal Communication, March 22, 1994, based on *The American Hospital Association Hospital Statistics Edition*, 1993–1994.

30. Bates, David W., et al. "Incidence of Adverse Drug Events and Potential Adverse Drug Events: Implications for Prevention." *JAMA* 1995; 274:29–34.

31. Ibid.

32. Ibid.

33. Leape, op. cit.

34. Kessler, op. cit.

35. American Hospital Association, op. cit.

36. Carruthers, S. G. "Clinical Pharmacology of Aging," in *Fundamentals of Geriatric Medicine*. New York: Raven Press, 1983.

37. Cotton, Paul. "Focus in Glaucoma May Change from Keeping Fluid Out to Letting Fluid Out." *JAMA* 1993; 269:2711.

38. Ibid.

2

You're on Your Own: What You Need to Know About the Drug Approval Process

FDA Failures

Who's guarding the henhouse? Most people believe that the Food and Drug Administration (FDA) is protecting them from dangerous drugs and medical devices. In our opinion, this watchdog is more like a pussycat. First, you must understand that the agency does virtually no testing of its own. The FDA relies on drug company data to determine both effectiveness and safety. If that sounds suspiciously like the fox has the upper hand, we won't argue.

Clinical drug testing is big business. Yet it is carried out almost like a cottage industry. Doctors around the country are paid by pharmaceutical manufacturers to give new medicines to volunteers. Subjects are recruited through newspaper ads or radio commercials (with toll-free 800 numbers to call) and often compensated to participate in clinical trials that generally last anywhere from several days up to several months. These human guinea pigs help determine whether experimental compounds are effective (better than placebo) and safe enough for widespread human use.

The trouble is that safety is a relative concept. People assume that when the FDA gives its seal of approval, a new drug is safe and effective. Wrong, WRONG, **WRONG!** We said it in the first edition and repeat with more emphasis today—*there is no such thing as a safe drug!* Every medication can cause side effects in some people. Often those side effects are trivial—a stuffy nose or a little diarrhea—but other times they can be crippling or even lethal. Frequently, medication misadventures are invisible because they create an indirect domino effect. Drug-induced dizziness, for example, can lead to a fall, which in turn can cause a devastating hip fracture, which commonly causes death from other complications, especially in the elderly.

Suppose, for a moment, that the Consumer Product Safety Commission tested 1,000 toasters from one manufacturer. In this hypothetical test, 600 of them worked great, 200 worked erratically, 100 didn't do anything, not even warm the slices, while the other 100 caused a variety of problems ranging from minor cases of burned toast to life-threatening electrical shocks. There would be righteous indignation and no Seal of Approval for such a bread burner. Yet drugs are routinely approved that are effective for only 60 percent of the patients who take them in clinical trials. And it is common for prescription medications to gain FDA support with a 10 percent incidence of adverse effects, or more. Even death (which we can think of as the ultimate adverse effect) is a risk that the FDA considers acceptable for a surprisingly large number of drugs.

Kelly Garbus, a staff writer for *The Kansas City Star*, was researching an article on a new migraine medicine called **Imitrex** (sumatriptan). She was concerned about the unexpected death of a seemingly healthy 41-year-old Kansas City woman 90 minutes after getting an injection of this medicine. Although Kelly got very little cooperation from the FDA, she did obtain vast amounts of raw material under the Freedom of Information Act. On May 3, 1994, Kelly Garbus wrote an article based on a memo she inadvertently stumbled across in the FDA files:

A top U.S. Food and Drug Administration official predicted in a memo two years ago that a now widely used migraine drug was almost "certain" to cause deaths.

But one day later, the FDA approved the marketing of Imitrex—known generically as sumatriptan—after concluding that the drug's benefits outweighed its risks.

Transcripts of an FDA advisory committee meeting also suggest the agency wrestled with approval of sumatriptan, which some medical experts now fear may cause heart attacks in certain migraine sufferers.

In a memo dated December 28, 1992, Paul Leber, chief of the FDA's Division of Neuropharmacological Drug Products, wrote: "What counts more? The rights of millions of otherwise healthy migraineurs to have access to an effective and, for them, safe treatment, or the rights of those who may be inadvertently injured by its marketing?

"If there are to be potent drugs like sumatriptan . . . society must be willing to tolerate the injury they will cause to some proportion of those who use them."[1]

After reading the article by Kelly Garbus in *The Kansas City Star*, we contacted the Food and Drug Administration to obtain the tantalizing memo from Dr. Paul Leber to Dr. Robert Temple, Director of the FDA's Office of Drug Evaluation I. Our Freedom of Information Act request Number F95-00866 produced the closest thing to a smoking gun we have ever seen from the agency. Here are some selected quotes:

Used appropriately, Imitrex is reasonably safe; used in the patient with pre-existing cardiovascular disease, however, it may be dangerous, even deadly. . . .

The division's recommendation to approve the Imitrex NDA [New Drug Application] reflects a risk benefit assessment which, in common with all such determinations, turns as much on personal values and implicitly held private assumptions as it does on evidence and reason. . . .

In sum, a case can be made that, from the viewpoint of the public health, the benefit accruing to the population of migraineurs is outweighed by the injury and fatalities that Imitrex's marketing seems certain to cause.[2]

Dr. Leber had advanced this argument solely for the sake of thorough consideration of every angle and titled it "Alternative Perceptions of Imitrex's Risks and Benefits." We were stunned to see such candor, however. The acknowledgment that this drug is likely to kill some patients and that the decision to approve was based more on "personal values and sentiments" than on "evidence and reason" is astonishing.

One does not have to be a pharmacologist to realize that the FDA is playing Russian roulette with the American public. Millions of people have undiagnosed heart disease. The FDA knows they are at risk from **Imitrex**. The agency knows that millions of migraine victims will benefit from this marvelous drug, but some will almost assuredly suffer serious, if not life-threatening, reactions. It's a gamble Dr. Paul Leber appears willing to take.

The really shocking story is that everybody but the consumer understands this dangerous game. The drug manufacturers know even the best of their medicines always cause problems for at least some people; the FDA knows it; and your doctor knows it. The hitch is, the FDA talks to the drug companies; the drug companies talk to the doctor; and, more often than not, the doctor doesn't talk to you, at least not about drug side effects. So guess who's left holding the bag?

How can the FDA go on approving drugs that cause problems or don't work? The answer is simple. The feds understand, as you should too, that people are different. What cures Alfred can make Bertha sicker than a dog, and Charlotte may get neither sick nor better taking the identical drug. Often there is no way to predict in advance who will benefit and who will be hurt. In other words, it is a giant guessing game and you are the guinea pig.

Here is the crux of the problem. Although the law states all medicines must be proved "safe" and "effective," these words are so broad and ambiguous that drug approval entails a giant judgment call. Theoretically the scales are tipped in favor of benefit and away from risk, but there are NO money-back guarantees.

Traditionally, experimental drugs have been tested on a relatively small number of people who did not represent a slice of real life. Women, children, and older people were usually excluded. According to the Commissioner of the Food and Drug Administration, "A new drug application, for example, typically includes safety data on several hundred to several thousand patients. If an adverse event occurs in perhaps one in 5,000 or even one in 1,000 users, it could be missed in clinical trials but pose a serious safety problem when released to the market."[3]

A few thousand subjects may seem like a lot, but you'd be amazed at how many complications slip through the cracks. The General Accounting Office (GAO) is an investigative arm of Congress. When it looked into the question of how many drugs are found to have serious side effects after marketing, the FDA was rocked to its foundation.

The GAO report "found that more than half of the new drugs approved for marketing in this country have some severe or fatal side effects not found in testing, or not reported until years after the medications have been widely used."[4] When these adverse reactions were finally uncovered they led to important labeling changes or outright withdrawal of the drugs from the market. The "system" really can't assess the safety of long-term drug exposure.

The Congressional investigators have pointed out that lives could be saved if the FDA monitored drugs more carefully after marketing and reported complications promptly to physicians and patients. But to this day the agency falls short on several counts. It has no organized, scientific method of tracking adverse drug reactions and interactions. When problems are uncovered, there is no efficient way to alert people to dangers or controversies. After the bureaucrats have cleared a medication for marketing it's a pharmacy free-for-all. If any unexpected reactions crop up, doctors are supposed to report them "voluntarily" to the drug company, which then has to file a report with the FDA.

But how is a doctor supposed to know if a peculiar symptom—or worse yet, a really ordinary one, such as headache, hair loss, arthritis, or forgetfulness—is due to the medicine unless there's already a warning in the prescribing information? A patient may or may not make the connection between the problem and the medicine. If he or she doesn't, the doctor may never even hear about it. And even if, somehow, the patient figures out that the reaction is related to the drug and convinces the doctor, there's still the problem of filling out the forms and sending them to the company or the FDA. In some cases, a doctor may not want to admit that he or she prescribed a medicine that may have done the patient harm.

FDA Commissioner David Kessler has stated the problem candidly: "Unfortunately, many health professionals do not think to report adverse events that might be associated with medications or devices to the Food and Drug Administration or to the manufacturer . . . this may be due to the limited training medical students receive in clinical pharmacology and therapeutics. . . . Another factor inhibiting physician reporting is that it is not an ingrained practice—it is not in the culture of U.S. medicine to notify the FDA about adverse events or product problems."[5] Most damning of all is the admission by Dr. Kessler that "Only about 1% of serious events are reported to the FDA, according to one study."[6,7] That means that 99 out of 100 severe adverse reactions go unreported!

Let's face it, there's no incentive for physicians to report adverse drug reactions. It takes precious time and it might get the doctor into hot water with a patient. Physicians worried about the risk of a lawsuit might adopt the motto, "See no evil, hear no evil, speak no evil." Consequently, this voluntary reporting system is inherently flawed. At best it represents the unscientific tip of a huge, invisible iceberg. At worst, it provides misleading, inaccurate, and confusing information to federal bureaucrats who don't seem to know what to do with it, even when it arrives at their doorstep.

Silicone Scandal

When reports do manage to make it to the FDA, there are major hurdles to overcome. It appears to us that the feds are often more concerned with protecting their bureaucratic backsides than safeguarding the public health. Take silicone. More than two million women had breast implants over a period of three decades. There were no well-controlled long-term studies to determine safety. It was just assumed that silicone was inert and would not cause adverse effects.

Despite reports that silicone could occasionally migrate out of implants and spread throughout a woman's body, no action was taken. The FDA apparently did not request tests or probe deeply into company records. Although doctors had been reporting cases of autoimmune and connective-tissue diseases such as scleroderma, lupus, Raynaud's phenomenon, and arthritis since the 1960s,[8] the FDA ignored the problem. Even as evidence accumulated and media attention grew, the FDA vacillated. In August 1991 the agency released a statement that "there is no conclusive evidence at present that women with breast implants have an increased risk of developing arthritis-like disease or other auto-immune diseases. . . . "[9]

But in 1992, after revelations from court cases and pressure from consumer groups and legislators, the FDA called for research and issued a moratorium on silicone-gel breast implants. The agency seemed more interested in blaming the silicone industry than confronting its own lack of action all those years.

At the time of this writing there is still no sound scientific evidence to prove silicone is safe . . . or hazardous. One epidemiological study conducted by researchers at the Mayo Clinic compared 749 women who had received breast implants with 1,498 community controls who had no implants. They found no relationship between connective-tissue diseases such as arthritis, lupus, or other inflammatory conditions, and silicone implants.[10] That may be somewhat reassuring, but millions of women are still left to wonder whether they will someday experience serious complications.

We may have to wait years before the final answer is in. Meanwhile, articles have started cropping up that demonstrate silicone is not inert. Once scientists started searching, they found that silicone was sometimes associated with "atypical immunologic reactions."[11,12,13] What that means remains unclear.

Manufacturers of silicone, afraid of large lawsuits and litigation expenses, have agreed to settle with thousands of patients who believe they might have been injured. The sum set aside—roughly $4 billion. This could be one of the greatest boondoggles of all time, in large measure because the FDA did not do its job.

Other Scary Screwups

The silicone scandal represents only one symptom of a system that screwed up. There are lots of examples to choose from. Temporomandibular joint (TMJ) syndrome can cause clicking of the jaw, earaches, headaches, and facial pain. Physicians have been arguing for years about how best to deal with a perceived misalignment of the lower jaw. Some favor watchful waiting while others have aggressively promoted surgery. During the 1980s many oral surgeons inserted a synthetic jaw implant made by a company called Vitek, Inc.

More than 25,000 of these "interpositional implants" were inserted into unsuspecting patients. Then the truth came out. An article in the *Wall Street Journal* (August 31, 1993) revealed the personal suffering and anguish some people must now live through:

Robyn Ruggles is weeping. "This isn't my face," she says. "I used to be real pretty." Eight oral-surgery operations have left her disfigured, without jaw joints, her mouth permanently agape. She can't bite into a sandwich. She can't purse her lips for a kiss.

And alone at night, she can hardly bear the muscle spasms and the pain. "It never goes away; it's God-awful pain," says the onetime nurse, who lives in Cuyahoga Falls, Ohio. "I have to pretend it's something else to hold onto my sanity."[14]

The problem is that the surgical implants failed, often at an alarming rate. Apparently a "fundamental flaw doomed the tiny implant: It simply couldn't withstand the wear and tear of the lower jaw sliding on its Teflon surface. In some cases, it disintegrated within a few months."[15] Patients like Robyn Ruggles have been left with severe damage to facial bones, muscles, and nerves. The pain can be excruciating.

The FDA approved the Vitek implant in 1983 with little pre-market testing. There were no animal experiments or human trials, just "mechanical simulation" on a machine. By the mid-1980s reports were coming in that many patients were in serious trouble. Then product liability and malpractice suits started surfacing. But not surprisingly, the FDA was slow to pick up on the problems. There were no comprehensive inspections of the plant where Vitek was made until after the product had been pulled off the market in 1988, and the agency didn't issue a safety alert until 1990.

The FDA also approved **Orcolon,** in 1991, despite red flags. This eye gel, used during cataract surgery, could apparently raise pressure within the eye to dangerous levels and increase the risk of blindness.[16] (**Orcolon** was eventually withdrawn from the market.) Add to that FDA debacle the Bjork-Shiley heart valve—"blamed for more than 300 deaths," and "15 fatal cases of anaphylactic shock apparently triggered by latex tips on enema devices."[17] Whether it was silicone breast implants, lasers, infant breathing monitors, radiation therapy machines, cardiac catheters or resuscitators, the level of FDA oversight has been characterized as "too little, too late."

Halcion Headache

For years **Halcion** (triazolam) was the best selling sleeping pill in the world. (At its peak, approximately 11 million prescriptions were dispensed annually.)[18] It is a fast-acting benzodiazepine, somewhat similar to such drugs as **Xanax** (alprazolam) and **Valium** (diazepam). **Halcion** is a little different, though, because its effects come on very quickly and last for a much shorter period of time. From a theoretical perspective this would make **Halcion** ideal as a sleeping pill, since an insomniac wants something that goes to work rapidly and won't cause a morning "hangover."

In 1977 **Halcion** was first approved for marketing in the Netherlands. Reports of bizarre side effects (paranoia, depression, anxiety, hallucinations, and aggression) led Dutch regulators to bar higher doses of the drug in 1980, after which Upjohn withdrew it from the Dutch market. Nevertheless, Upjohn, the manufacturer, was given the green light by the U.S. Food and Drug Administration (at a lower dose—0.5 mg) in 1982. Despite extraordinary success in the marketplace, questions about safety began to surface.

The spontaneous reporting system at the FDA was accumulating some intriguing statistics. Compared to two well-established sleeping pills, **Dalmane** (flurazepam) and **Restoril** (temazepam), **Halcion** was apparently producing far more side effects (8 to 30 times more adverse reaction reports). People were complaining about forgetfulness and amnesia, aggressiveness, confusion, rebound insomnia, agitation, personality changes, daytime anxiety, panic attacks, hallucinations, and other psychological problems.

Equally disconcerting were questions about pivotal studies conducted in the 1970s to determine safety and efficacy. One private physician hired by Upjohn to do clinical investigations, Dr. Samuel I. Feurst, apparently falsified data.[19,20]

Despite serious questions about incomplete and inaccurate data, "transcription errors" by Upjohn, and their own internal reports of a higher incidence of adverse reactions linked to **Halcion**, federal officials chose to downplay the controversy. An FDA internal report stated that Upjohn "engaged in an ongoing pattern of misconduct with **Halcion**," but no penalties or official actions were taken against the company.[21] Even after regulatory agencies in five countries (including England, Norway, and Finland) banned **Halcion**, FDA authorities defended the drug. And a fraud investigation was cut short by agency insiders.[22]

Dr. Anthony Kales is one of our heroes. He is chairman of psychiatry at Pennsylvania State University Medical School and one of the country's leading sleep researchers. His conclusion: "This is a very dangerous drug. No other benzodiazepine has such a narrow margin of safety. The only justification for keeping it on the market is to ensure the company's profitability. From a public-health standpoint, there is no reason at all."[23] You'll have to forgive us if we come away from this whole messy affair with the impression that FDA officials seem more intent on protecting the reputation of Upjohn than alerting the public to problems.

Unanswered Questions

A lthough authorities at the FDA like to think they are doing a fabulous job protecting the public, the agency has really let us down. For one thing, the feds rarely monitor drug company trials. The limited on-site inspections that were carried out between 1977 and 1994 "found that 56% of sites had problems with patient consent forms, 22% could not adequately account for the drugs they were dispensing, 29% did not strictly adhere to the protocol, 23% had inadequate and inaccurate records . . . and 3% had a significant fraction of records missing."[24]

The problem is far worse when it comes to long-term follow-up. In preapproval tests, subjects may be exposed to a new drug for a few weeks. In the real world patients take medicines for months and years. They often have underlying medical problems that were never addressed in the early experiments, and quite commonly must take more than one medicine at a time. FDA Commissioner Kessler admits that "patients taking marketed drugs in conjunction with other drugs may experience interactions not revealed during the premarketing phase."[25,26] Since we have already established that there is no organized, scientific system for following drugs once they are cleared for marketing, most Americans are on their own.

Premarin Problems

There are a lot of questions the FDA can't answer and, frankly, that scares us. For example, the number one, most-prescribed drug in America is **Premarin,** which has experienced a roller-coaster ride of popularity. This mixture of natural estrogens, "derived from pregnant mares' urine,"[27] is one of the oldest (approved for marketing on May 8, 1942) and most successful drugs in history. In 1974 **Premarin** was riding high—number five on the doctors' hit parade, just behind **Darvon** and **Librium.**[28] Women took **Premarin** to relieve the hot flashes and other symptoms associated with menopause. Some physicians touted its usefulness against nervousness and aging. There was even a popular book titled *Feminine Forever* that encouraged use of estrogen.

But then reports started to surface linking drugs such as **Premarin** to cancer of the uterine lining (endometrial carcinoma). We sounded an early alarm in the first edition of *The People's Pharmacy*. Eventually an epidemic of cancer cases was discovered, articles appeared in medical journals, and prescriptions started to fall. By the early 1980s **Premarin** had lost a lot of its luster, falling to 25th on the hit parade. Then researchers discovered that if progesterone (usually in the form of **Provera**) were given with **Premarin**, the combination could still relieve hot flashes, but with little risk of uterine cancer.

Investigators found that estrogen replacement therapy could help prevent osteoporosis and heart disease, and once again prescriptions soared. Between 1990 and 1993 sales practically doubled from $379 million to more than $700 million annually.[29] Today, **Premarin** is queen of the mountain—the most frequently dispensed drug in America. The company proudly proclaims that "30,000,000,000 **Premarin** tablets have been dispensed without a single recall since introduction."[30]

In the May 1995 issue of *Med Ad News*, an industry insiders' publication, **Premarin** was heralded as "Brand of the Year," with worldwide sales of $853 million.[31] This "award" was granted because such long-running success (greater than 50 years) is unprecedented. At last count 6 million women were taking **Premarin**, with a potential market of 50 million once the baby boomers reach menopause.

The trouble is that the FDA can't tell us at this time whether estrogen, alone or in combination with progesterone or testosterone, increases the risk of breast cancer. This is one of the most controversial issues in medicine. The research is contradictory. Some studies point to a problem while other data downplay the danger.

The most comprehensive overview to date of all the relevant research "estimated that the risk of breast cancer after 10 years of estrogen use increased by at least 15% and up to 29%."[32] And this may have been the most conservative interpretation by epidemiologists at the Centers for Disease Control (CDC). Their conclusion in July 1994: "We do believe that the consistency and biologic plausibility of our results are cause to invest in basic and epidemiologic research to answer the question: does long-term estrogen use increase risk of breast cancer?"[33]

Roughly one year later this issue was revisited. The lead article in the *New England Journal of Medicine* (June 15, 1995) detailed results of the Nurses Health Study. Researchers at Harvard Medical School have followed nearly 122,000 nurses since 1976 to see how their diet, lifestyle, and medications affect their health. These investigators found that women using hormone replacement therapy (estrogen and progesterone) after menopause had about 30 to 40 percent more breast cancer than women who never took hormones.[34] This article stimulated a cover story in *Time* magazine entitled "Estrogen: Every Woman's Dilemma."[35]

One month later women were further confused by headlines on a report in the *Journal of the American Medical Association* (July 12, 1995). A different group of researchers found no connection between postmenopausal hormone therapy and the risk of breast cancer.[36] This study included far fewer women (537 breast cancer patients and 492 controls). The contradictory results from these two reputable research groups did nothing to resolve the dilemma.

Here is a drug that has been on the market for more than 50 years. More than 30 billion pills have been dispensed to tens of millions of women. Breast cancer now strikes one in eight and is a leading killer of women. That physicians and patients still do not have a clear answer to this crucial question after so many years is nothing short of scandalous!

Prozac Predicament

When **Prozac** (fluoxetine) first arrived on the scene, we were delighted. It represented an entirely new class of drugs that seemed to relieve depression without causing the unpleasant side effects (weight gain, dry mouth, constipation, dizziness, sluggishness, etc.) of traditional tricyclic medications.

Early reports were encouraging. People told us that **Prozac** changed their lives. For many, the green-and-white capsules improved outlook, eliminated obsessive thoughts, instilled confidence, and chased away the blues. Others reported that this drug helped create a feeling of optimism that had been missing for years.

It looked like **Prozac** was a fabulous advance in treating depression, not to mention obsessive compulsive disorder (OCD) and perhaps even overweight.

Prozac took off. Its first year on the market this antidepressant earned $125 million—a very good showing for a new drug. The second year (1989) sales zoomed to $350 million. By 1993 sales had hit $1.2 billion, making it the blockbuster of mind medicine. **Valium** in its heyday never even approached this level of popularity. It is estimated that about a million prescriptions are written for **Prozac** each month.[37]

But while **Prozac** was still picking up steam, we got a puzzling phone call. An ophthalmologist contacted us about the unexpected death of his daughter in 1988. He was convinced that **Prozac** had somehow led her to commit suicide. It seemed implausible to us. We did a computerized search of the literature and found no connection between **Prozac** and suicide. Assuming that the woman had been depressed, and that people in that situation sometimes commit suicide, we tried to comfort this grieving physician and reassure him that her medicine couldn't have contributed to the tragedy.

Months later we stumbled upon a new article in the *American Journal of Psychiatry* that offered a different perspective. Psychiatrists associated with Harvard Medical School reported that six patients developed an "intense violent suicidal preoccupation after 2–7 weeks of fluoxetine [**Prozac**] treatment."[38]

We immediately contacted the ophthalmologist and his wife to get more details. We learned that their 40-year-old daughter had had an eating disorder. Although at that time **Prozac** was approved only for depression, her physician thought it might help improve her eating habits. One month later she hung herself, even though according to her parents there had been no signs of depression or suicidal tendencies.

We were to hear similar stories over the next several years. People who had not been suicidal suddenly took their lives in gruesome ways. Some people told us they heard voices urging them to harm themselves. Others hallucinated scenes of violence. Readers of our syndicated newspaper column sent us poignant letters:

I believe that Prozac may be implicated in my daughter's death by self-immolation. I suspect that the drug intensified her anxiety to an unbearable degree and provoked self-injurious and highly dangerous behavior not present before she started taking the drug (in January 1989).

Beginning in April of 1989, I was unable to leave her by herself. She was terrified by violent obsessive thoughts of killing herself. I feel these symptoms, which emerged several months after she began treatment with Prozac, were substantially different from those observed through 1988 and that there may be more than coincidence involved.

I don't know whether any of the doctors who treated her chose to report her case to the company or the Food and Drug Administration.

The Food and Drug Administration received lots of similar stories. Hundreds of cases of violent or self-destructive behavior were reported, and additional articles appeared in the medical literature.[39,40,41,42] But these reports were viewed as anecdotes with virtually no scientific merit. The manufacturer, Eli Lilly, reviewed its own databases and concluded that there was no association between **Prozac** and violent, suicidal, or aggressive behavior.[43,44]

After reviewing the controversy the FDA concluded that "there is no way to know whether to attribute the reported suicides and deaths to the underlying disease, intervening life events or drug therapy." Tucked away in the package insert is a heading: "Postintroduction Reports." Along with more than a dozen other reactions you will find "suicidal ideation" and "violent behavior," though the point is made that such adverse events "may have no causal relationship with the drug."[45]

Where does all this leave consumers? At the time of this writing, the consensus among psychiatrists seems to be that **Prozac** is not a problem. It can cause anxiety, nervousness, insomnia, tremor, restlessness, nausea, headache, diarrhea, loss of appetite, rash, sweating, sexual dysfunction, and a number of other unpleasant side effects. During premarketing studies roughly 15 percent of test subjects dropped out because of adverse reactions to **Prozac**. Nevertheless, many people find it a lifesaver.

In our opinion **Prozac** is neither a good drug nor a bad drug. Like all medications it has benefits and risks. There is no way to predict in advance who will do well and who will find that this medication causes unacceptable side effects. What truly disturbs us is that the FDA appears to have neither the desire nor the ability to answer questions about the possibility that this drug can cause suicide or violence. Most psychiatrists respond to our queries about the **Prozac** predicament with the same reflex answer that we originally employed—depressed people commit suicide. But if drugs cause the very same side effects they are supposed to prevent, the system has a hard time responding.

Cardiac Arrest

One of the greatest scandals in American medicine involves drugs prescribed to control irregular heart rhythms. It is probably the most serious example of an FDA system failure. Medications that were supposed to ward off sudden death actually ended up causing the very problem they were supposed to prevent. If it hadn't been for a government study (CAST) sponsored by the National Heart, Lung, and Blood Institute, this tragedy might never have been discovered. Neither the pharmaceutical industry nor the FDA would likely have figured out that the cure was worse than the disease.

Cardiologists have long known that ventricular "arrhythmias" (serious electrical abnormalities in heart rhythm) are a major cause of sudden death each year. People with clogged coronary arteries are vulnerable to these disturbances, as are those who have suffered prior heart attacks. Instead of beating in a rhythmic fashion, the heart looks like a bag filled with writhing worms. No blood gets pumped and death comes within minutes unless the normal rhythm is restored promptly. Physicians assumed that if you could suppress premature ventricular contractions (PVCs), especially after heart attacks, you would prevent ventricular fibrillation and save lives.

In November 1985 the FDA approved **Tambocor** (flecainide) for treatment of heart rhythm disturbances. A leading cardiologist hailed it as a "major advance in antiarrhythmic drugs in terms of efficacy, safety and patient compliance."[46] **Enkaid** (encainide) followed a year later in December 1986.

One outside expert for the Food and Drug Administration, Dr. Raymond Woosley, raised a concern before these new drugs were marketed: "We know that they will kill some people. We only hope that they are going to be used in situations where they would save more than they kill."[47] This warning was largely ignored.

Cardiologists quickly embraced these two new compounds, believing they would be more effective and better tolerated than existing antiarrhythmic agents. They were widely prescribed to patients with extra ventricular beats. By April 1989 at least 200,000 patients were taking **Enkaid** and **Tambocor**.

But then something extraordinary happened. The CAST (Cardiac Arrhythmia Suppression Trial) was halted prematurely because people taking these medications were dying faster than was expected. The patients who received inactive placebos were living longer than the patients taking the drugs.

Physicians and patients were stunned. Years after approval, investigators had discovered that these heart medications were hurting more patients than they were helping. The results rocked the cardiology community and the FDA. An editorial in the *New England Journal of Medicine* told the story.

> The preliminary results . . . have astounded most observers and challenge much of the conventional wisdom about antiarrhythmic drugs and some of the arrhythmias they have been used to treat. Although many issues remain unresolved, CAST has determined beyond question that the use of encainide and flecainide . . . to treat asymptomatic or minimally symptomatic ventricular arrhythmias in patients after myocardial infarction [heart attack] is associated with a substantial increase in the sudden-death rate and total mortality.[48]

A lot of cardiologists were astonished when the results of the CAST study were published and it was discovered that the drugs tripled the risk of dying. Others weren't so surprised. A number of heart specialists confided to us that they had suspected antiarrhythmic drugs for years. Paradoxically, most of these medications actually cause more dangerous heart rhythms than they cure. In doctorspeak, they are "pro-arrhythmic." While covering up premature contractions, these drugs may set the heart up for far more hazardous complications, such as the ventricular fibrillation they were supposed to prevent. This was a dark secret that has not been widely shared outside the cardiology community.

Think of it like this. You're driving your car on a long trip and develop a small leak in the radiator. Although it's not very serious you decide to add a chemical that is advertised to stop up the leak in the radiator. It seems to work because you no longer have to add any antifreeze. You congratulate yourself on a quick fix. But before you know it, the engine overheats, burns out, and you are stuck in the middle of nowhere. What you couldn't see was that the chemical jammed up the proper flow of liquid in the radiator and ended up causing more harm than good. If you complain to the garage where you bought the chemical, they might well tell you that the engine was probably in bad shape and would have died anyway.

When an older person with a history of heart trouble drops dead, no one thinks to blame the medicine. They just assume that the patient died in spite of the treatment. What CAST proved was that antiarrhythmic drugs like **Enkaid** and **Tambocor** were, in many cases, worse than nothing at all.[49]

The total death toll from this incident remains a mystery. Reports at the time suggested that up to 3,000 patients had died prematurely.[50] But within a short period of time the issue faded from public awareness and the FDA put this sordid chapter behind it. When Thomas Moore's fascinating book, *Deadly Medicine*, was published in 1995 he suggested that the true extent of the tragedy was much greater. The television show *20/20* covered the controversy:

Timothy Johnson, M.D.: "By taking the death rate from the CAST trial and applying it to the hundreds of thousands of people taking all the drugs in this class during the two years of the CAST trial, Moore comes up with an estimate as high as 50,000 deaths during that two-year period."

Tom Moore: "It depends on the assumptions you use and how you do the calculations. What we can be sure of is that so many people died that it is the worst medical drug disaster in the history of the United States."

Timothy Johnson: "I asked Salem Yusif, an internationally recognized expert on heart drug studies, about these numbers."

Salem Yusif, M.D.: "My guess would be a number in the region of ten to twenty thousand deaths a year. Now even that is a large number."

Timothy Johnson: "It is a stunning number when you think of comparing that to plane crashes."

Salem Yusif: "Absolutely."

Timothy Johnson: "But you're quite confident as an expert in numbers that using reasonable assumptions that we're talking about tens of thousands, not 50,000 but at least tens of thousands?"

Salem Yusif: "Yes, I'm comfortable that it's likely that about tens of thousands of people would be prematurely killed by the use of these drugs."[51]

Whether this was the greatest drug disaster in U.S. history, or just a striking signal of an inherent flaw in the system, there is little doubt that the FDA dropped the ball and too many died. Later testing of yet another antiarrhythmic drug called **Ethmozine** (moricizine), prescribed to control mild premature ventricular contractions, revealed that it too "is not only ineffective but also harmful."[52]

Enkaid, **Ethmozine**, and **Tambocor** aren't the only drugs that are used to control irregular heart rhythms. Many physicians still prescribe a number of antiarrhythmic agents for mild preventricular contractions. But some of this country's leading cardiologists, especially those who participated in the CAST investigation, point out that such patients should probably not be receiving these drugs until they are proven beneficial.[53,54] At the time of this writing no such research has been published.

If it hadn't been for the CAST studies and their shocking results, it is entirely likely that hundreds of thousands, maybe millions, of heart patients would continue to be exposed to medicine that could have killed them prematurely. Although **Ethmozine** and **Tambocor** are still being prescribed for patients with life-threatening heart problems, there are strong warnings on the package inserts. One can't help but wonder though, if some of the other untested heart drugs (such as quinidine) might not also have the potential to increase the risk of dangerous heart rhythm disturbances.[55] That the Food and Drug Administration has seemingly tried to distance itself from this controversy is, in our opinion, a black mark on the agency.

One might be tempted to assume that this sad story was an isolated event. In truth, many of the drugs on the market today were approved by the FDA based on incomplete data. The faulty logic lies in the assumption that surrogate markers (such as suppression of premature ventricular contractions) are beneficial. This has led to the approval of dozens of drugs to lower blood pressure and cholesterol without actual proof that they improve and prolong life. Many experts worry that studies that rely solely on surrogate markers may come to conclusions that are "misleading or unreliable."[56]

Calcium Channel Blocker Controversy

One such issue that recently emerged directly affects millions of people. Two articles appeared in the medical literature that challenged the safety and ultimate effectiveness of calcium channel blockers. These drugs became extremely popular during the 1980s for heart and blood pressure problems.

Calcium channel blockers appeared to produce fewer side effects than beta blockers (which may cause depression, fatigue, sexual dysfunction or elevated cholesterol levels). Because they seemed so well tolerated, physicians began prescribing these medications in huge quantities to patients with hypertension and angina. The most frequently prescribed products included nifedipine (**Adalat** and **Procardia**), verapamil (**Calan, Isoptin, Verelan**) and diltiazem (**Cardizem, Dilacor XR, Tiazac**).

At the time of this writing, Wall Street analysts estimate that combined sales for calcium channel blockers amount to $8 billion annually. Six million Americans rely on these drugs daily. Nifedipine, the most popular drug in the class, earned over $1 billion all by itself; over 26 million prescriptions were written in the U.S. during 1994.

But are these drugs safe? The FDA approved calcium channel blockers based on their ability to lower blood pressure and relieve chest pain. There is no doubt that they accomplish these goals. The FDA assumed, as did most physicians, that these "surrogate markers" were all that mattered. But during almost 20 years of use, the most fundamental question remained unanswered: Do these drugs improve and prolong life?

An article in the *Journal of the American Medical Association* (Aug. 23–30, 1995) addressed this problem and stunned the medical community with its findings. Dr. Bruce M. Psaty and Dr. Curt D. Furberg and their colleagues reported that "In this study of hypertensive patients, the use of short-acting calcium channel blockers, especially in high doses, was associated with an increased risk of myocardial infarction [heart attack]." These investigators found a 60 percent elevation in heart attack when they compared calcium channel blockers with diuretic therapy.

Two weeks later, a meta-analysis of 16 other studies appeared in the journal *Circulation* (vol. 92, no. 5, September 1, 1995). The authors concluded:

In patients with coronary disease, the use of short-acting nifedipine in moderate to high doses causes an increase in total mortality. . . . Long-term safety data are lacking for most calcium antagonists. . . . Thus, there is no clinical trial evidence that any of the three main groups of calcium antagonists improves survival in coronary patients. . . .

> The mortality data from randomized clinical trials of short-acting nifedipine are alarming. The twofold to threefold increase in all-cause mortality associated with high doses is similar to that reported for encainide and flecainide in the Cardiac Arrhythmia Suppression Trial. . . .

Few physicians and fewer patients realize that some of the most frequently prescribed drugs in the world "lack adequate documentation of long-term safety." That doesn't mean these are bad drugs. And certainly no one should stop taking calcium channel blockers without careful medical supervision. Uncontrolled hypertension is hazardous. But we are dismayed that millions of people are taking medicines that have not been proven effective for the desired goals, reducing illness and death. It could be many more years before the drug companies and the FDA can establish the true benefit (or risk) of these medications.

Unfinished Business

The darkest secrets in medicine these days are the unanswered questions the FDA seems to be ignoring. Not surprisingly, pharmaceutical companies are not rushing to resolve these dilemmas either. This leaves physicians, pharmacists, and patients in the lurch.

Open the *Physicians' Desk Reference* and turn to **Flagyl** (metronidazole). You will find it is a powerful antibacterial medication that is used for a variety of infections, especially vaginal *Trichomonas*. It is also extremely effective against amoebic dysentery and more recently has become a key player in something called "triple therapy" for ulcers. Doctors give it in combination with **Pepto-Bismol** and amoxicillin (or tetracycline) to kill *Helicobacter pylori*, a bacterium thought to be responsible.

Flagyl has been prescribed for decades and is a valuable medicine. But the first thing you see when you locate it in the *PDR* is a scary little box with a black border.

WARNING

Metronidazole has been shown to be carcinogenic in mice and rats (see *Precautions*). Unnecessary use of the drug should be avoided. Its use should be reserved for the conditions described in the *Indications and Usage* section.

Read further and you discover that this drug has been linked to cancer in half a dozen animal studies. Of course these were generally long-term investigations, probably at high doses. What does this mean for people? How should physicians or patients interpret this data? Is there a risk worth worrying about after a few weeks of treatment? How about a few months? Is it likely we will have an answer to these questions anytime soon? Please do not hold your breath. The FDA has left us holding the bag yet again.

Flagyl isn't the only drug with a black-box warning. **Aldactone** (spironolactone) is a diuretic that has become popular for treating hirsutism—a condition of unsightly facial hair in women. It too comes with a warning. It is described as a "tumorigen" in rats, and the FDA cautions doctors that, "Unnecessary use of this drug should be avoided."

What does that mean? Would any physician intentionally prescribe a drug for an unnecessary use? What about hirsutism? Excessive hair growth in an older woman can be incredibly distressing, yet it is unclear if long-term exposure represents an unacceptable risk of cancer. Will the FDA help resolve these questions, or will it continue to hide behind a boxed warning with its head in the bureaucratic bog?

There are so many other unanswered questions that we couldn't possibly list them all, and new ones crop up almost daily. Concern has been raised about the cancer-causing potential of such cholesterol-lowering drugs as **Lopid** (gemfibrozil), **Mevacor** (lovastatin), **Pravachol** (pravastatin), and **Zocor** (simvastatin).[57] Studies in rodents show carcinogenicity, but no one knows what implications this has for humans. Similarly, a study of mice found a possible risk of liver tumors associated with **Ritalin** (methylphenidate), which is frequently prescribed for years at a time to treat attention deficit disorder. A commmon ingredient in laxatives, phenolphthalein (found as of January 1996 in **Correctol tablets, Ex-Lax,** etc.), is "clearly carcinogenic" in test animals.[58] The FDA doesn't seem to know what to do with this information. Nor do physicians, leaving the rest of us in the lurch.

One of the most common questions we are asked is, "What are the long-term side effects of taking my medicine?" No matter what the drug, the FDA can rarely, if ever, answer such queries. For example, does exposure to aluminum in certain antacids for long periods of time increase the risk of neurotoxicity? The FDA can't tell us.

Keep in mind that when a drug is newly approved (and for at least a year or so afterwards) it's essentially still being tested for safety and effectiveness! Think about the consequences of taking a medication when it first comes on the market. If you're over sixty, female, suffer from chronic illnesses, or take other medications, it's entirely possible that nobody quite like you has ever swallowed the drug before! In effect, you're taking part in an uncompleted experiment.

Are the Benefits Worth the Risks?

By now we're sure you'll agree that taking medicine is, or should be, a carefully considered balancing act. Everyone—physician, pharmacist, nurse, and patient—must weigh risks and benefits. There are no good drugs or bad drugs. Every medication, prescription and OTC, has risks but so does being sick. Every drug has (or is supposed to have) benefits. When the benefits outweigh the risks you've got something worth taking. But remember: Since you will be the person swallowing that pill or potion, YOU should make the final decision.

To make that decision wisely you will need information from your physician and pharmacist. According to the American Medical Association, "A physician must obtain the consent of his patient before he can render any form of treatment."[59] Consent in this context means INFORMED consent. You must know the most common side effects and the most serious ones, even if they are rare. You have to be told about controversies surrounding any given medication. And you should be advised about other drugs that should be avoided in order to prevent dangerous interactions.

Now, you also know the emperor wears no clothes. In other words, the Food and Drug Administration is not an all-knowing, all-wise institution that has all the answers. Safety and effectiveness are relative terms. Serious adverse reactions may not turn up for months or even years. Effectiveness sometimes is far less than originally anticipated. The prescribing information that your physician relies on this year may be different next year as new dangers are revealed.

Finally, have you ever wondered what the ℞ symbol stands for on every prescription you get from your doctor? Thanks to Dr. Gordon Muir, who sent us a photocopy from his twentieth edition of *Dilling's Clinical Pharmacology*, we were able to track down the following:

Before a drug is mentioned [on a prescription] it is commonly preceded by the sign ℞ which stands for *Recipe*—meaning "*Take thou*"—recalling that in writing a prescription the doctor is in fact addressing the pharmacist and asking him to take the drugs listed and compound them in suitable fashion. The stroke across the tail of the letter R is said to have been introduced as an invocation to Jupiter to make the medicine effective.[60]

We trust that these days we no longer need to pray to Jupiter to get our medicines to work. But it is worth remembering what the origins of the ℞ on each prescription stand for and that nothing works for everyone every single time.

We hope this book will help you be more informed and inquisitive about medications. That should mean you will ask a LOT of questions the next time the doctor starts to reach for a prescription pad or the next time you start to reach for a remedy on the shelf of the local pharmacy. Never forget that there is no such thing as a 100-percent-safe drug.

References

1. Garbus, Kelly. "Does Drug's Risk Outweigh Benefit?" *The Kansas City Star* 1994; May 3: A1–A9.
2. Freedom of Information Act request File Number F95-00866, from Bernice Carter, Freedom of Information Officer, Center for Drug Evaluation and Research, January 23, 1995: Memorandum N20-070, December 28, 1992, from Paul Leber, M.D., Director, Division of Neuropharmacological Drug Products, to Robert Temple, M.D., Director, Office of Drug Evaluation I.
3. Kessler, David A. "Introducing MEDWatch: A New Approach to Reporting Medication and Device Adverse Effects and Product Problems." *JAMA* 1993; 269:2765–2768.
4. Hilts, Philip J. "Dangers of Some New Drugs Go Undetected, Study Says." *New York Times* 1990; May 27:10.
5. Kessler, op. cit.
6. Scott, H. D., et al. "Rhode Island Physicians' Recognition and Reporting of Adverse Drug Reactions." *R.I. Med. J.* 1987; 70:311–316.
7. Kessler, op. cit.
8. Germain, B. F. "Silicone Breast Implants and Rheumatic Disease." *Bull. Rheum. Dis.* 1991; 41:1–5.
9. FDA Backgrounder, August 1991.
10. Gabriel, Sherine E., et al. "Risk of Connective-Tissue Diseases and Other Disorders After Breast Implantation." *N. Engl. J. Med.* 1994; 330:1697–1702.
11. Bridges, Alan J., et al. "A Clinical and Immunologic Evaluation of Women with Silicone Breast Implants and Symptoms of Rheumatic Disease." *Ann. Int. Med.* 1993; 118:929–936.
12. Hochberg, Marc C. "Editorials: Cosmetic Surgical Procedures and Connective Tissue Disease: The Cleopatra Syndrome Revisited." *Ann. Int. Med.* 1993; 118:981–983.
13. Press, Raymond I., et al. "Antinuclear Autoantibodies in Women with Silicone Breast Implants." *Lancet* 1992; 340:1304–1307.
14. Ingersoll, Bruce and Rose Gutfeld. "Implants in Jaw Joint Fail, Leaving Patients In Pain and Disfigured." *The Wall Street Journal* 1993; 222(43):1–4.
15. Ibid.
16. Ingersoll, Bruce. "Amid Lax Regulation, Medical Devices Flood a Vulnerable Market." *The Wall Street Journal* 1992; March 24:1–6.
17. Ibid.

18. Gladwell, Malcolm. "There May Be Nothing Unsafe in the Numbers About Halcion." *Washington Post* 1992; June 15:A3.

19. Cowley, Geoffrey. "More Halcion Headaches." *Newsweek* 1994; March 7:50–52.

20. Kolata, Gina. "Maker of Sleeping Pill Hid Data on Side Effect, Researchers Say." *New York Times* 1992; January 20:A1–A9.

21. Cowley, Geoffrey. "Halcion: A Damaging Report." *Newsweek* 1994; May 2:6.

22. Cowley, op. cit.

23. Cowley, Geoffrey, et al. "Sweet Dreams or Nightmare?" *Newsweek* 1991; August 19:44–51.

24. Cohen, Jon. "Clinical Trial Monitoring: Hit or Miss?" *Science* 1994; 264:1534–1537.

25. Peck, C. C., et al. "Understanding Consequences of Concurrent Therapies." *JAMA* 1993; 269:1550–1552.

26. Kessler, op. cit.

27. Package insert for Premarin from Wyeth–Ayerst Laboratories.

28. "The Top 200 Drugs." *Pharmacy Times* 1975; 41:39–46.

29. Ruriani, Deborah Catalano. "Estrogen Therapy Gains Respect." *Med Ad News* 1994; 13(4):16–46.

30. Premarin advertising in *Drug Topics* 1994; 138(3):45–47.

31. Hawryluk, Markian. "The Unbeatable Brand: Premarin Topples the Odds Against Off-Patent Success." *Med Ad News* 1995; 14:19.

32. Steinberg, Karen K., et al. "Breast Cancer Risk and Duration of Estrogen Use: The Role of Study Design in Meta-Analysis." *Epidemiology* 1994; 5:415–421.

33. Ibid.

34. Colditz, Graham A., et al. "The Use of Estrogens and Progestins and the Risk of Breast Cancer in Postmenopausal Women." *N. Engl. J. Med.* 1995; 332:1589–1593.

35. Wallis, Claudia. "The Estrogen Dilemma." *Time* 1995; 145(26):46–53.

36. Stanford, Janet L., et al. "Combined Estrogen and Progestin Hormone Replacement Therapy in Relation to Risk of Breast Cancer in Middle-aged Women." *JAMA* 1995; 274:137–143.

37. Begley, Sharon, et al. "Beyond Prozac." *Newsweek* 1994; February 7:37–43.

38. Teicher, Martin H., et al. "Emergency of Intense Suicidal Preoccupation During Fluoxetine Treatment." *Am. J. Psychiatry* 1990; 147:207–210.

39. Teicher, Martin H., et al. "Antidepressant Drugs and the Emergence of Suicidal Tendencies." *Drug Saf.* 1993; 8(3):186–212.

40. Hamilton, M. S., and L. A. Opler. "Akathisia, Suicidality, and Fluoxetine." Comment in *J. Clin. Psychiatry* 1993; 54:280.

41. Hawthorne, M. E., and J. H. Lacey. "Severe Disturbance Occurring During Treatment for Depression of a Bulimic Patient with Fluoxetine." *J. Affect. Disord.* 1992; 26:205–207.

42. Hamilton, M. S. and L. A. Opler. "Akathisia, Suicidality, and Fluoxetine." *J. Clin. Psychiatry* 1992; 53:401–406.

43. Heiligenstein, J. H., et al. "Fluoxetine Not Associated with Increased Aggression in Controlled Clinical Trials." *Int. Clin. Psychopharmacol.* 1993; 8:277–280.

44. Goldstein, D. J., et al. "Analyses of Suicidality in Double-Blind, Placebo-Controlled Trials of Pharmacotherapy for Weight Reduction." *J.. Clin. Psychiatry* 1993; 54:309–316.

45. *Physicians' Desk Reference*, 48th ed. Montvale, N.J.: Medical Economics Data Production Company, 1994; pp. 877–880, "Prozac."

46. Moore, Thomas J. *Deadly Medicine: Why Tens of Thousands of Heart Patients Died in America's Worst Drug Disaster.* New York: Simon & Schuster, 1995; p. 18.

47. Ibid; p. 129.

48. Ruskin, Jeremy N. "The Cardiac Arrhythmia Suppression Trial (CAST)." *N. Engl. J. Med.* 1989; 321:386–388.

49. Echt, Debra S., et al., "Mortality and Morbidity in Patients Receiving Encainide, Flecainide, or Placebo: The Cardiac Arrhythmia Suppression Trial." *N. Engl. J. Med.* 1991; 324:781–788.

50. "3,000 May Have Died Early from Heartbeat Control Drugs." AP wire story as published in *The Durham Sun;* 1989: 100(126):1.

51. Timothy Johnson on ABC's *20/20,* March 10, 1995.

52. The Cardiac Arrhythmia Suppression Trial II Investigators, "Effect of the Antiarrhythmic Agent Moricizine on Survival After Myocardial Infarction." *N. Engl. J. Med.* 1992; 327:227–233.

53. Ibid.

54. Epstein, Andrew E., et al. "Mortality Following Ventricular Arrhythmia Suppression by Encainide, Flecainide, and Moricizine After Myocardial Infarction: The Original Design Concept of the Cardiac Arrhythmia Suppression Trial (CAST)." *JAMA* 1993; 270:2451–2455.

55. Teo, Koon K., et al. "Effects of Prophylactic Antiarrhythmic Drug Therapy in Acute Myocardial Infarction: An Overview of Results from Randomized Controlled Trials." *JAMA* 1993; 270:1589–1596.

56. Nowak, Rachel. "Problems in Clinical Trials Go Far Beyond Misconduct." *Science* 1994; 264:1538–1541.

57. Newman, Thomas B., and Stephen B. Hulley. "Carcinogenicity of Lipid-Lowering Drugs." *JAMA* 1996; 275:55–60.

58. NIEHS (National Institute of Environmental Health Sciences). Press release: "NTP Technical Report on the Toxicology and Carcinogenesis Studies of Phenolphthalein." Research Triangle Park, North Carolina: December 6, 1995.

59. Simonaitis, Joseph E. "Photographs of Patients." *JAMA* 1974; 229:844.

60. Alstead, Stanley. Chapter 1 Introduction, in *Dilling's Clinical Pharmacology*, 20th ed. London: Cassell, 1960, p. 7.

3

Protecting Yourself

I t would be great if there were a medicine that always worked for everyone and never had any side effects. Since there are no such drugs, though, there can only be safe patients. Those are the ones who are concerned and informed enough to ask the right questions every time about what they're being given, why they're taking it, which precautions to take, and what the known adverse effects are.

So who's going to make certain that what you get is as safe as possible? Ultimately, you. And you'd better be prepared to do your job almost every time you go to the doctor. This also applies if you take a child or an older person to see a physician. They may not be able to speak up for themselves.

One study conducted more than a decade ago by the National Center for Health Statistics found that drugs were prescribed or dispensed at 62 percent of office visits.[1] These days it is possible that the percentage is even higher. That means almost every time you visit a physician the treatment will involve medication. Learning to be a savvy drug consumer isn't just desirable—it's a matter of life and death.

Drug safety depends on communication. Remember, the FDA talks to the drug company, the drug company talks to the doctor, and the doctor is supposed to talk to you. All too often that vital last step may be incomplete. In two surveys conducted by the FDA, 70 percent of the people polled said their doctors didn't inform them of precautions for and possible side effects of drugs, and only 2 to 4 percent of the people took the initiative and asked questions about their prescriptions.[2]

What were the other 98 percent doing? Many were trying to be "good" patients. Often physicians prefer people who are considered "compliant"—those who rarely ask difficult questions and always swallow their pills dutifully. The doctor may let you know directly and indirectly (through body language) that too many queries are unwelcome. But if you don't insist on having your questions answered fully, you are courting disaster. It's your responsibility to make sure you understand your treatment. Only by becoming a persistent and well-informed patient will you be the safest possible drug consumer. Good communication and a working partnership with your doctor are just as important as all the medications and fancy high-tech equipment thrown at you—perhaps even more so.

What Your Doctor Doesn't Know

There is no way your physician can know everything about all the medicines he or she prescribes. No one person is capable of retaining that much information. Theoretically, the doctor prescribing a drug is supposed to have thoroughly researched that medication by reviewing the scientific literature and poring over all the labeling information cleared by the FDA and supplied by the drug company. Each prescription drug container comes with a detailed "package insert." This same material is also found in the book often referred to as the doctor's bible—the *Physicians' Desk Reference (PDR)*.

Once a physician has absorbed all the clinical pharmacology, instructions, warnings, precautions, contraindications, drug interactions, and adverse reactions, it is expected that the pertinent details will be relayed to the ailing patient. But in the real world quite the opposite often takes place. Doctors usually try to put the drugs they prescribe in the best possible light. They do this partly to retain their own sanity.

Keep in mind that the Hippocratic oath contains a key concept—*primum non nocere* (often translated to mean "first, do no harm"). The only problem with this wonderful idea is that every drug has the potential to harm someone. Since it is not easy to predict in advance who will be vulnerable, a physician risks breaking this solemn oath with each prescription he writes. To avoid feeling guilty, many doctors try to put a positive spin on the medicine and downplay its risks both to themselves and to their patients.

Some physicians may also feel that most of the side effects are relatively infrequent, and that telling you about them will just tend to plant a seed of suggestion that could sprout into an annoying phone call in the middle of the night. Let's face it, if your doctor told you that a medicine he was prescribing for your indigestion could cause sexual dysfunction, mental confusion, disorientation, and depression, you might have doubts about his judgment. Yet one of the best-selling drugs of all time—**Tagamet** (cimetidine)—can, in certain circumstances, cause such complications.

While most people don't experience side effects from **Tagamet**, it is impossible to predict in advance exactly who will be susceptible to such reactions. This is the crux of all drug-prescribing problems. Even a rare complication can be devastating if it happens to you or someone you love. Take **Floxin** (ofloxacin), for example. This is an antibiotic that its manufacturer (Ortho) claims "has been used by over 100 million people worldwide and has been shown to be safe and effective when used in accordance with product labeling recommendations."[3] Yet some people taking this drug experience side effects including insomnia, visual disturbances, confusion, dizziness, hallucinations, seizures, breathing difficulties, and even cardiac arrest.

In a moving account published in *The Washington Post Magazine*, journalist Stephen Fried described what happened to his wife, Diane, after taking **Floxin:**

> It started out with just one pill. My wife's gynecologist had given her samples of a new antibiotic to treat a minor urinary tract infection. The doctor told her to take this wonder drug twice a day for three days. When I left for work the next morning, I said goodbye to Diane as she took the first pale yellow, oval tablet with breakfast. Six hours later I was bringing her, delirious, to the emergency room. Her life hasn't been the same since.
>
> In the first hours after Diane took the pill, her left arm went numb and her vision became cloudy. She got lost in her home office, and when she found her desk, she couldn't figure out how to turn off the computer she writes on every day. When she went to lie down, she started shaking uncontrollably and then saw white. She felt like she was dying.[4]

Diane survived, but was left with "aggressive insomnia, visual distortions and aphasia: She would get halfway through a sentence and not be able to get the rest of the words out."[5] Doctors rarely warn people about these kinds of complications because they are considered extremely rare and not worth worrying about. But because no one can know for sure whether you will suffer side effects from a particular drug, you must be informed in advance of the earliest danger signs.

Then again, the doctor may not know what all the side effects and interactions are. Think about this. When was the last time you saw a doctor look in a book to check on the adverse reactions and interactions while prescribing a drug? You've probably never seen it happen, any more than you've seen the pilot of a 747 reading the operating handbook right before takeoff. The 747 pilot, however, DOES use a checklist during every phase of the flight, to make certain that no routine but critical step has been omitted.

Your doctor, on the other hand, probably attempts the impossible feat of trying to remember everything there is to know about dozens or even hundreds of drugs he prescribes. Even if the busy doctor did take the time once to analyze carefully and critically the scientific literature and read the complete, detailed labeling with all the warnings on interactions and side effects, is it reasonable to expect him to remember everything weeks, months, or years later? And never forget that drug information is a constantly moving target. New discoveries about complications and interactions appear with alarming frequency, but may take years to get into the *PDR*. Only a physician who is conscientious and vigilant will be able to protect you from drug dangers.

Making a List: Checking It Twice!

T hink of yourself as the copilot of your life flight®. Let's assume your physician is a great captain. He or she is still going to need your assistance in completing the trip safely. Your job (and this is one assignment you can't afford not to accept) is to go down the checklist and make sure all the crucial questions have been answered. Here's our list:

1. Where are we going? This may seem fundamental, but you'd be amazed how often we are asked, "Why am I taking this medicine?" The ultimate goal of the treatment should be specified. And we're not interested in intermediate stops. We are looking for the final destination. Lowering cholesterol in itself may not be enough. The real goal is to reduce the risk of premature death from heart attack. Years ago a cholesterol-lowering drug called **Atromid-S** (clofibrate) was very popular. Then researchers found that the drug was not prolonging life and in fact seemed to be responsible for more deaths than the inactive placebo that it was compared to. Make sure you know what the final goal of drug therapy is all about and how to determine if you are achieving it.

2. Is there a nondrug approach or treatment that will achieve the same result? Many physicians make an assumption that people have a hard time changing. That may be true for some folks, but no one should make assumptions about you. Let your doctor know if you would like to try nondrug approaches and ask if any are appropriate. Often there are ways to bring down blood pressure and cholesterol without resorting to pills. The same holds true for anxiety, insomnia, and many other ailments.

3. What is this stuff? Find out exactly what the medicine is and how it works. Make sure you know the brand name and/or the generic name. What are the anticipated benefits and how will you know if it is working? Learn for how long you are supposed to swallow the medicine—a week, a month, or the rest of your life.

4. Can you read the prescription? Do not accept an illegible prescription. Doctors' handwriting has apparently gotten so bad that the American Medical Association (AMA) recently felt compelled to admonish physicians to practice their penmanship.[6] The AMA board of trustees noted that prescription errors "are not rare events," and are a major contributor to adverse reactions in hospitals.

While you're at it, reject those Latin codes, too. We have polled pharmacists and are shocked to learn that most prescriptions are still being written using Latin abbreviations such as *b.i.d.* (twice a day), *h.s.* (at bedtime), or *p.c.* (after meals). These are absolutely unacceptable! The standard textbook of pharmacology that virtually every medical student must read is *Goodman and Gilman's The Pharmacological Basis of Therapeutics*. It is the gold standard of pharmacology references. For many years this book has stated unequivocally that:

Abbreviations should be avoided since their use frequently results in error. . . . The directions to the patient should always be written in English. The use of Latin abbreviations serves no useful purpose. . . . Expressions such as "take as directed" and "take as necessary" are never satisfactory and should be avoided. If the drug is to be taken at a specific time of day or if it is to be taken three or four times a day, the exact time or times should be specified on the label; patients are often confused by directions such as "every 8 hours."[7]

Any physician who ignores such explicit recommendations to write clearly and avoid Latin is taking a risk with your life. Be nice, but politely refuse to accept any prescription that is unreadable, ambiguous, or incomplete. If assertiveness is not your style, you can ask the nurse privately to print or type the prescription information in complete English on a separate piece of paper. We have also provided a checklist at the end of this chapter that we encourage you to photocopy and hand to your doctor to fill out with your prescription. When all else fails, turn to page 52 for a handy guide to doctorspeak. It will tell you the meaning of such abbreviations as *gtt.*, *P.O.*, and *q.i.d.*

5. Do you have the prescription in your possession? Whenever you can, discourage phone-in prescriptions. Once upon a time doctors made house calls and dispensed their own medicines. Few mistakes were possible. Then the norm was to hand the patient a prescription to be filled in the local drugstore. Nowadays it is very common for a physician to phone in your prescription so it will be waiting when you reach the pharmacy. On the surface this might seem like a tremendous convenience. No one wants to wait while a prescription is being filled.

Oh yes you do. Mistakes are made in drugstores. Ask any pharmacist with integrity and you will learn that errors happen. Sometimes it's because the doctor's handwriting is so unreadable that it is misinterpreted. That is why it can be worthwhile to make a photocopy of your prescription before giving it to the pharmacist. One woman did that very thing with her husband's prescription written for clonidine 0.2 mg. When the medicine came from the pharmacy it was marked with the label quinidine 200 mg. Instead of blood pressure pills he had received heart medicine. It could have been a lethal mistake. The photocopy caught the error.

Phoned prescriptions pose an even greater risk. You'd be amazed how many drugs sound alike. **Mellaril** (a major tranquilizer) could be confused for **Elavil** (an antidepressant). Then there's **Xanax** vs. **Zantac, Temaril** vs. **Tepanil, Anturane** vs. **Artane,** or **Trimox** vs. **Tylox**. There are dozens of such sound-alike drugs. Keep in mind that often a nurse or receptionist has to interpret the doctor's handwriting and call in the prescription. The possibility for error is too great! Carry that little piece of paper to your pharmacist personally.

6. How, when, and with what should I take this medication? You need specific instructions with each prescription. Reject instructions like "before meals" or "three times a day." There is no room for ambiguity with medicine. Get the details. Your prescription should say something like "Take on an empty stomach at 9 A.M. and 4 P.M." You need to know if your pills should be taken with meals or swallowed on an empty stomach. Find out if a medicine that needs to be taken four times a day calls for you to get up in the middle of the night for the last dose. If timing or food do not matter, that is important information too. No one wants to go to extra trouble trying to schedule medicine precisely if it doesn't make any difference. And you need to find out if there are certain foods or beverages that don't mix well with your pills. This is vital and often lifesaving information.

7. What about side effects? Every medicine can cause some adverse reactions for someone. You must never leave your doctor's office without knowing what the most common and most serious complications can be. And DO NOT rely on memory. Get it down on paper. Some adverse reactions don't show up for weeks or months. If you try to remember what your physician said that long ago you are taking too big a risk.

An alternative would be to ask the doctor if you can record his words of wisdom. That way you get to listen in a relaxed atmosphere at home where the message can sink in and can be replayed if anything is confusing. Some physicians may find a recording device threatening. Fear of legal action can be very scary. In reality, though, a recording is the doctor's best protection against litigation. First, it is verbatim truth, so people can't play the guessing game of "he said—she said." Everyone's memory can be flawed, including the doctor's, so a tape will tell you what was actually said.

8. Are any of the side effects life-threatening, and what should I do if I experience them? Some drugs may produce such serious reactions in a few individuals that quick response is critical. Find out if there are any symptoms that should trigger an immediate call to the physician or a trip to the emergency room. For example, the popular heart and blood pressure medicine **Vasotec** (enalapril) occasionally causes swelling of the face, lips, tongue, and throat. If allowed to progress, the airways can become so swollen and tight that susceptible patients may not be able to breathe. Patients must be alerted to this rare, but potentially fatal, reaction so they can seek emergency treatment at the first signs of trouble.

9. Are there any interactions that may be dangerous? This is often the weakest link in the chain of communication. No physician or pharmacist can possibly remember all of the medications that can form dangerous combinations. Make sure that your health-care providers know absolutely everything else you are taking, including vitamins or over-the-counter medicines. Don't forget herbals or other alternative remedies. Then ask them to check a reference to see if any of the combinations you are taking could prove hazardous.

10. How should I store my medicine? Your physician may not have a clue as to how to answer this question so it might be better asked of your pharmacist. Everyone has read instructions to "Store in a cool dry place," just as everyone has ignored those instructions. If you don't believe us, go look in your bathroom cabinet. If you have medicine in there, think about what it's like inside that cabinet each morning as you take your shower and the mirror fogs with steam. "Cool dry place." Not on your life. Researchers have found that crucial antiseizure medicine such as **Tegretol** (carbamazepine) can quickly lose one-third of its potency when stored under conditons similar to the bathroom medicine cabinet. Light and heat can be just as detrimental.

Doctors have long noted with some wonder the highly variable response of patients to nitroglycerin, a heart medicine that dilates blood vessels and relieves chest pain (angina). The mystery was solved with a study that proved packaging and storing of nitroglycerin were the most important factors in the uneven response One three-month-old bottle had lost 84 percent of its original oomph. The label stuffed inside the bottle had absorbed most of the drug the patient was supposed to get! The plastic vial in which the tablets were stored also absorbed some of the drug, and the cotton filler plug got a phenomenal one-third of the active ingredient . . . in just one week of storage!

Reformulation of most nitroglycerin tablets has improved the situation but nitroglycerin still requires careful handling. It should be dispensed and kept in the manufacturer's original glass container with a screw-on cap. It must be kept tightly sealed, without cotton, in a dry location. NEVER store nitroglycerin in a plastic pillbox or other storage device. Many modern medicines are even more complex and require careful handling and storage. Never leave your prescription in a hot or cold car and be wary of mail-order services during the summer or winter when the delivery vehicle may be exposed to extremes in temperature.

11. When should I discard my prescription? This question is for your pharmacist. Never leave the drugstore without an expiration date on the prescription label. When your pharmacist receives a shipment of medicines it always has an expiration date stamped on it. That is so he can throw it out or return it to the manufacturer if it is not dispensed within the specified time limit.

When you buy a nonprescription drug off the shelf it has an expiration date on the package. This is because the Food and Drug Administration has ruled that all drugs are subject to deterioration and have to meet appropriate standards and "at the time of use the label of all such drugs shall have suitable expiration dates which relate to stability tests performed on the product." Unfortunately, at the time of this writing, there is still no federal law requiring pharmacists to put a discard date on your prescription. This is a mystery to us, in light of the fact that the FDA feels it is crucial for all over-the-counter medicines to have an expiration date on the label.

Manufacturers are required by law to test their drugs under various storage conditions and to determine how long they will last. The expiration date therefore is pretty much the manufacturer's guarantee of the potency of the drug. Of course the medication doesn't just magically disintegrate on the appointed day. On the other hand, after that time nobody, especially not the manufacturer, is making any promises that you'll be getting what you should out of the pills you're taking. That is why it is so important to make sure your pharmacist has included a discard date on your prescription.

Your Safety Net

L ife carries risks. No matter how carefully you drive, there is always the possibility that someone else will ignore a stop sign or run a red light and hit your car. You can reduce the danger by wearing your seat belt, remaining vigilant, and driving defensively. The pilot of a 747 jet knows that there are backup safety devices to cover most contingencies. If one engine goes out he knows how to fly the plane with what is left. For your safety, you need to build backup and redundancy into your drug information system. Remember, think of yourself as the copilot of your life flight, carrying a clipboard with the critical checklist. After your physician has answered the questions on the list you will find on pages 50–51, give your pharmacist a blank copy and have him fill it out, too. Compare the answers. If you see conflicting information, that could indicate areas of uncertainty and should be followed up further.

You are the one who cares most about what happens to you or someone you love. You may want to do some of your own checking at home or in the library. At the back of this book you will find basic information about some of the most commonly prescribed drugs. Use it to balance what you get from your physician or pharmacist. When in doubt never hesitate to contact these health professionals for clarification. For even more detailed drug information here is a list of references we have found helpful over the years. Some, such as *The Pill Book,* are affordable, understandable, and readily available in most bookstores. Others, such as *Drug Interaction Facts,* are expensive, written for health-care providers, and can usually be found only in medical libraries or medical bookstores. We have been delighted to observe and participate in a self-care revolution that strives to empower people to become better informed.

Drug Information Resources*

1. *The Pill Book.* Harold M. Silverman, Pharm. D., ed-in-chief. New York: Bantam.
2. *Drug Facts and Comparisons.* Bernie R. Olin, ed.-in-chief. St. Louis: Facts and Comparisons (A Wolters Kluwer Company).
3. *Physicians GenRx: The Complete Drug Reference.* Philip L. Denniston, Jr., ed-in-chief. Smithtown, NY: Physicians GenRx.
4. *Physicians' Desk Reference.* Montvale, NJ: Medical Economics Data Production Company.
5. *Drug Interaction Facts.* David S. Tatro, ed. St. Louis: Facts and Comparisons (A Wolters Kluwer Company).
6. *Professional's Guide to Patient Drug Facts.* Bernie R. Olin, ed.-in-chief. St. Louis: Facts and Comparisons (A Wolters Kluwer Company).
7. *Handbook of Nonprescription Drugs.* Laura C. Lawson, managing ed. Washington, D.C.: American Pharmaceutical Association.
8. *The Complete Drug Reference.* United States Pharmacopeia. Yonkers, NY: Consumer Reports Books.
9. *Goodman and Gilman's The Pharmacological Basis of Therapeutics.* Alfred Goodman Gilman, Theodore W. Rall, Alan S. Nies, Palmer Taylor, eds. New York: Pergamon.
10. *The People's Guide to Deadly Drug Interactions.* Joe Graedon and Teresa Graedon, Ph.D. New York: St. Martin's Press.

*Always obtain the latest edition of any of these resource books as drug labels and reported side effects are constantly being updated.

Drugs relieve suffering and save lives. They can also harm or even kill. Your physician may be happy prescribing a medicine that can cause side effects in 15 percent of patients. That may or may not be acceptable to you. By taking an active role in your health care you can tip the balance in favor of a successful therapeutic outcome. Over the years we have met a number of informed laymen who knew more about their medical problems and treatments than their physicians because they cared enough to do a lot of reading and research. You don't have to go that far, but the more you know, the better able you will be to protect yourself, your family, and your friends.

To report an adverse reaction to the FDA, have your physician call 800-FDA-1088. He will reach one of those maddening phone message machines, but it is possible to request a MEDWatch reporting form. You could request one yourself, and if your physician doesn't wish to assist you, it is possible to complete the paperwork and submit it yourself. Only by informing the FDA of serious adverse events will the system begin to improve.

People's Pharmacy Checklist

Dear Doctor/Pharmacist,
To assist me in taking my medicine properly, please help me with the answers to these questions:

1. What is the name of the medicine?　　brand: _____

　　　　　　　　　　　　　　　　　　　　generic: _____

2. What is the dose? _____

3. Why am I taking this medicine? _____

_____

4. What time(s) should I take this medicine? _____ am _____ am

pm　　　　　　pm　　　　　　pm　　　　　　pm

5. Should I take this medicine with food? _____

at least one hour before or two hours after eating? _____

6. Are there any special foods I should avoid? _____

_____

7. Are there any precautions or warnings I should know about? _____

_____

8. Are there any contraindications that would make this drug inappropriate?

_____

_____

9. Which other medicines should I avoid? _____

_____

10. What side effects are common with my medicine? _____

_____

_____

11. Are there any symptoms that are so serious you would want to know about

them immediately? _____

_____

12. When and how should I stop this medicine, if ever? _____

_____

Photocopy this checklist and take it to your health care provider

Common Latin Abbreviations

Abbreviation	Latin	Translation
ad lib	ad libitum	freely, as needed
a.c.	ante cibos	before meals
b.i.d.	bis in die	twice daily
caps	capsula	capsule
gtt.	gutta	drop
h.s.	hora somni	at bedtime
p.c.	post cibos	after meals
P.O.	per os	by mouth
p.r.n.	pro re náta	according to circumstances (as needed)
q.4h.	quaque 4 hora	every 4 hours
q.i.d.	quater in die	4 times a day
Sig.	Signa	write on label
t.i.d.	ter in die	3 times a day
UD	ut dictum	as directed

Reading a Prescription

On the next page are two actual prescriptions that pharmacists sent in to the journal *Pharmacy Times*.[8,9] Even if you know how to interpret the Latin abbreviations, it won't do you much good if you can't understand the chicken scratching that describes the medication. If you cannot read your doctor's scrawl, ask the nurse to print or type it out in English.

Erythromycin 250 mg #24
Sig.: One q.i.d.

Elixir Pyribenzamine Expectorant
with Ephedrine 3 oz.
Sig.: One teaspoonful q. 4 h. for cough

Using the Computer for Access
to Health Information

L et's face it, we live in an electronic age in which information is being transmitted at ever-increasing speeds. Once upon a time (only about a decade or two ago) we relied on books and journals for most of our knowledge. A trip to the medical library was essential to track down the latest discoveries. We loved holding the books or magazines in our hands and slowly flipping pages, sometimes turning up unexpected treasures of pharmaceutical folklore. But it was hard to examine more than an infinitesimal fraction of the collected wisdom.

Today, it is possible to search online, full-text databases using a computer and a modem. That means that from our office we can access most of the world's most relevant medical journals, download any article in seconds, and store it electronically in our computer system or print out hard copy. We can search thousands of books, newspapers, magazines, and journals in the time it took you to read this paragraph.

Let's say we want to look up the latest on **Ritalin** and other treatments for attention deficit hyperactivity disorder (ADHD). We dial up Dialog or BRS Colleague (acquired by Ovid Technologies), two of our preferred electronic information services. Within seconds our computer is linked to Medline, produced by the National Library of Medicine. Or we might go straight to Dialog's "Health Periodical Database" or *New England Journal of Medicine* for full text access. A fast search might turn up dozens of relevant articles, which we can narrow down to the most current and complete. Within minutes our printer can be spitting out the most up-to-date research on a constantly evolving and controversial topic.

PaperChase is another online information service that provides access to Medline and Cancerlit (a database of the National Cancer Institute), as well as several other valuable resources. Although we have not used PaperChase, it might well be the most user friendly of the bunch. The Quick Guide is far less intimidating and more understandable than most other manuals we have seen. PaperChase was developed by staff at Boston's Beth Israel Hospital. They are committed to making medical information readily accessible to professionals and laymen.

To use a database service such as Dialog, BRS (Ovid Technologies), or Paper-Chase requires some familiarity with searching techniques. A different approach would be to access one of the online services. America Online, CompuServe, and Prodigy offer a variety of excellent health resources that are very user friendly. CompuServe provides *"Consumer Reports'* Complete Drug Reference," "Health-Net," syndicated columns, and a superb search tool called "Health Database Plus."

Another option would be to turn to the Internet. Trying to describe this vast electronic "information superhighway" is almost impossible. Tens of millions of people all around the world are linked through their computers. We can send instant electronic mail to our friends in New Zealand or browse through a medical library in Sweden. There are databases, special-interest "newsgroups," bulletin boards, and dozens of other information options. We are particularly fond of newsgroups, such as "sci.med.pharmacy," that allow pharmacists, physicians, pharmacologists, and interested laymen to trade information. Drug questions are asked and answered electronically.

We highly recommend a book by our friend and colleague, Tom Ferguson, M.D. His latest effort is titled *HEALTH ONLINE: How to Go Online to Find Health Information, Support Forums, and Self-Help Communities in Cyberspace* (Addison-Wesley). This wonderful book will guide you onto the "information highway" at your own speed. Even if you are mystified by bytes and bauds, this book will get you started.

If computers leave you cold, there are organizations that will do the searching for you. For a fee it is possible to get up-to-date computer printouts on a wide variety of medical and pharmaceutical topics. Planetree Health Resource Center in San Francisco will run a computer search for you and mail the results.

Electronic Databases/Information Services

BRS/OVID Online
333 Seventh Avenue
New York, NY 10001
(800) 950-2035
(212) 563-3006
FAX (212) 563-3784

DIALOG Information Services
Knight-Ridder
240 El Camino Real
Mountain View, CA 94040
(800) 334-2564

PaperChase
350 Longwood Avenue
Boston, MA 02115
(800) 722-2075
(617) 278-3900
FAX (617) 277-9792

Online Services and Internet Access:

America Online (AOL)
Starter Kit available at:
(800) 827-6364

CompuServe
(800) 848-8199

DELPHI
To join:
(800) 695-4005

Planetree Health Resource Center
(will run computer searches for you)
2040 Webster Street
San Francisco, CA 94115
(415) 923-3680
or
(415) 923-3681
FAX (415) 673-7650

References

1. "Psychotropic Drug Study Notes Prescribing Habits." *Medical World News* 1983; September 12:139.
2. "The Doctor Isn't Talking; The Patient Isn't Asking." *Medical World News* 1983; September 12:47.
3. Fried, Stephen. "Floxin Follow-Up." *Philadelphia* 1993; June:15–19.
4. Fried, Stephen. "Prescription for Disaster." *The Washington Post Magazine* 1994; April 3:13–29.
5. Ibid.
6. Associated Press. "AMA: Doctors' Sloppy Writing Spells Danger for Patients." *The Herald Sun* 1994; June 14:A10.
7. Benet, Leslie R. "Principles of Prescription Order Writing and Patient Compliance Instructions." Gilman, A.G., T. W. Wall, A. S. Nies, and P. Taylor, eds. *Goodman and Gilman's The Pharmacological Basis of Therapeutics*, 8th ed. New York: Pergamon Press, 1990, p. 1642.
8. "Can You Read These Rxs?" *Pharmacy Times* 1977; 43(2):9, 86.
9. Ibid.; 43(3):78,98.

Part II

Over-the-Counter (OTC) Drugs and Home Remedies

Snake Oil or Self-Care?

Are OTC Remedies Really Safe and Effective?

O ver the last two decades there has been a quiet, almost silent pharmacy revolution in the over-the-counter (OTC) drug market. Hundreds of chemical ingredients and thousands of products have slowly disappeared from pharmacy shelves. Old standbys such as terpin hydrate (a cough medicine) have disappeared without a trace. Familiar brands such as **Contac** and **Kaopectate** have been reformulated. Hundreds of new products have appeared, many once available only by prescription.

What's been happening? The wheels of the federal bureacracy turn slowly, but they do turn. The Food and Drug Administration has gradually begun to implement a law that Congress passed in 1962. At that time our legislators made a small change in the Federal Food, Drug and Cosmetic (FD&C) Act. Up until then, drugs were required to be proved safe—that's all, just safe—before they were allowed to be put on the shelf.

Given those standards, all sorts of things were put into bottles, tubes, tubs, and vials. And as far as manufacturers were concerned, anyone who could be convinced to pay for the privilege to swallow, sip, or smear on their concoctions was fair game. And that included some of the biggest and most respectable drug companies in America.

The former Smith Kline & French company (now SmithKline Beecham) once marketed a hot seller called **Red Raven Water,** which was supposed to be a "sure-fire cure for hangover!"[1] Another historical winner for the company was a strychnine and alcohol concoction called **Eskay's Neuro Phosphates,** which was supposed to help those who were overworked, "constitutionally delicate," aged, or convalescing. Once upon a time Eli Lilly promoted its **Pil Damiana** as a "powerful, permanent and determined aphrodisiac."[2] More recently scam artists have sold quick-weight-loss remedies, hair restorers, memory boosters, wrinkle erasers, and arthritis cures.

In 1962 the FD&C Act was amended to say that OTC drugs had to be both safe *and* effective. That may not seem like it's asking much from the companies that are making billions of dollars a year on the products, but you should have heard the howling. A lot of manufacturers were not eager to step forward and prove their products really did anything. Maybe they feared it would be an exercise in futility.

At first the FDA didn't appear much more anxious to know the truth than the drug makers were to tell it. It took our faithful watchdog agency four years just to round up a panel of experts from the National Academy of Sciences (NAS) to check out a sample of OTC drugs. Three years later, in 1969, the FDA received a bombshell. The NAS experts found that only about 25 percent of the ingredients in the OTC products could actually live up to their claims. There was no scientific proof of effectiveness for the rest.

You can probably imagine the FDA's reaction to that. Consumers were plunking down billions of dollars every year on popular brand-name concoctions monitored by the agency. Then along comes a super-prestigious panel to say that three-fourths of the ingredients in those products might not live up to expectations. This definitely called for a closer look, and that's what we got . . . eventually.

In 1972, ten years after the NAS study, the Food and Drug Administration finally began its official Over-the-Counter Drug Review. For the first time in history the feds hoped to find out which drugs actually worked and which didn't.

Seventeen expert panels were recruited to examine in detail 700 or so ingredients found in roughly 300,000 products. How, you might ask, could there be so few active compounds in so many different brands? The answer is duplication. Take antacids, for example. The FDA estimates that there are more than 8,000 different products on the market, but only a handful of active ingredients—things such as calcium carbonate, aluminum and magnesium hydroxide, and sodium bicarbonate. Hundreds of cough and cold remedies often contain the same combinations of antihistamines and decongestants repeated over and over. Only the brand names, shape, and color of the pills differ.

The experts studied everything from hemorrhoidal preparations, vaginal sprays, and athlete's foot remedies to cough medicine, deodorants, and dandruff shampoos. They even looked into aphrodisiacs.

It's a big job, the FDA said, so please be patient. It will take us three to five years. We should have been so lucky. Eleven years later, in late 1983, the shocking story was beginning to unfold. Close scrutiny by the expert panels revealed that only one-third of the ingredients in OTC products were both safe and effective! That's a little better than the results of the original NAS study, but still not much to be proud of.

In a public statement the FDA hastened to point out that the results didn't mean that only one-third of all OTC products were safe and effective. It didn't? No, the FDA told us, because "Most popular products have safe and effective ingredients even if they sometimes contain other ingredients that are ineffective or have not yet been shown to be effective."[3] See, if you put one good thing in with three useless things and claim the whole mess works, that's not really so bad, is it? This is called "FDA Math."

Besides, hope springs eternal. The panels classified ingredients into three categories. Category I contained compounds for which there was valid scientific evidence of safety and effectiveness. These things do what they say they do and are worth paying for if you need them.

Category II was for things that were either unsafe or ineffective. In spite of searching high and low the panels couldn't find any evidence to justify these products.

Then there was Category III, for which "Available data were insufficient." This might be thought of as the dog-pound category, where hot potatoes, controversial cases, pet projects, and other such things got deposited in the hope they'd be picked up before someone got around to putting them to sleep. In a word, Category III became a wastebasket for drugs that lacked decent data. Rather than throw them out altogether, they passed into regulatory limbo to wait for new research to be completed.

This administrative dodge didn't go unchallenged. The Health Research Group (a Ralph Nader affiliate) sued the FDA. They pointed out that the 1962 law didn't say anything about "maybe" safe and effective. It said that a drug was either safe and effective or it wasn't to be on the market. Period. End of discussion. The federal judge—Judge John Sirica, of Watergate fame—apparently agreed and ordered the FDA to banish Category III.

The agency acted with its usual dispatch—it took two years to get the regulations in line with the law. Even then they fudged, since the rule allows the companies to keep these questionable substances on the shelf while testing continues. This gives the manufacturer further opportunity to come up with supporting data, and the American consumer further opportunity to come up with money for a drug that could eventually be jerked off the market when all the administrative games have been played.

It's been a long-running road show. By the 1990s all the panels had filed their reports. "Proposed Monographs" had been printed, "Tentative Final Monographs" had mostly been reviewed, and "OTC wrap-up regulations" had required removal of 415 ingredients because they were judged either ineffective or unsafe, or because they lacked sufficient data to permit continued sale. Once the dust began to settle the feds reached a now-familiar conclusion that "About one-third of the ingredients were judged to be safe and effective for their intended use."[4]

But there is still some pondering, commenting, and reviewing going on because we await the ultimate "Final Monographs," which will have the force of regulation. After three decades of paper shuffling, data analysis, drug company whining, and bureaucratic bungling, we are finally reaching the end of the tunnel. In our opinion, the time consumed in accomplishing the whole OTC Review has been an insult. By the way, the FDA has estimated that the job will really, truly be done around the year 2000. Stay tuned, but please don't hold your breath. It wouldn't be the first time the agency was late.

The good news is that over the last several decades we have seen changes in OTC products. Doubtless some effective brands have been removed because no one could figure out how to prove they worked. People swear to us that terpin hydrate was a great cough medicine and they miss it dearly, but it's gone for good.

The FDA has been hassling the maker of **Preparation H** because it has had a hard time proving that one of the original ingredients (live yeast cell derivative) is a "wound-healing agent in the anorectal area."[5] Never mind that a physician at the Alta Bates Burn Center in Berkeley, California, has shown that it was able to accelerate "wound-healing beyond its normal rate" in other parts of the body.[6] The feds want unequivocal "anorectal" relief. Imagine trying to design an experiment, or worse yet, do the testing, to prove *that* claim.

The company (Whitehall—a division of American Home Products) couldn't convince the FDA, so it reformulated our old favorite. Instead of live yeast cell derivative, it put in some boring stuff found in certain other mundane hemorrhoidal creams. That's a pity. We have heard from dozens of readers that **Preparation H** was good for dry cracked skin, itching at the site of surgical scars, bed sores, eczema, and mild burns. One person even insisted that it was a great salve for a tree that had been damaged by a lawn mower. And women on the West Coast have been smearing it on their faces for years in an attempt to reverse wrinkles.

Preparation H notwithstanding, we feel that you can have greater confidence when buying over-the-counter products today than ever before. A lot of old-timey, marginal products have been eliminated. And quite a few new sleazy and otherwise fraudulent ones have also disappeared. Lest you get complacent, though, there are some serious hazards just lying in wait for the unsuspecting consumer.

When Are OTC Remedies Harmful?

Most folks tend to think of OTC remedies as innocuous, mild nostrums that have received the FDA's seal of approval. After all, the 1938 Federal Food, Drug and Cosmetic Act mandated that drugs have to be proven safe to be marketed. Ah, and there's the rub—that pesky little word "safe." What does it mean?

Anyone who thinks OTC compounds come without side effects would be taking a mighty risk. Even after decades of review, Tentative Final Monographs, Final Monographs, rules, and regulations, there are no guarantees that OTC medications are safe. We cannot say this too many times: Every drug has the potential to cause some side effects for someone.

We probably wouldn't be overly concerned about this issue except for the fact that most OTC labels are often woefully inadequate. They usually overlook important side effects and the potential for interaction with other drugs. Look up **Motrin** in the *Physicians' Desk Reference,* for an example. You will find more than two pages of tiny print loaded with detailed information about contraindications, warnings, precautions, adverse reactions, overdosage, and lots more. If you then check the small print on your OTC bottle of ibuprofen (**Advil, Motrin IB, Nuprin**, etc.), you will find only a tiny fraction of the important data transmitted to physicians. There is virtually nothing about drug interactions or side effects (including nausea, heartburn, ringing in the ears, blurred vision, rash, depression, or dizziness). More alarming is the fact that there are no words about really life-threatening reactions such as bleeding or perforated ulcers, severe liver disease, jaundice, hepatitis, or kidney damage. There have been fatalities associated with ibuprofen, but this detail is not mentioned on the OTC label. We don't understand why the FDA gives you the tools to play doctor, but not the know-how.

Companies may cover their derrieres with one of those wonderfully ambiguous phrases: "If you experience any symptoms which are unusual or seem unrelated to the condition for which you took ibuprofen, consult a doctor before taking any more of it." What a useless warning! If someone doesn't realize that blurred vision, dizziness, depression, or kidney problems could be related to ibuprofen, they might not think to mention such symptoms to a physician.

Perhaps even worse, the feds have not had an organized system for monitoring adverse reactions associated with OTC drugs. On February 27, 1992, the General Accounting Office dropped a bombshell. This investigative arm of Congress submitted a stinging report of FDA oversight.[7]

Manufacturers of nonprescription drugs have not been required to report adverse effects to the FDA or evaluate serious complications the way prescription drug companies do. Remember that although that system is terribly flawed because it relies on voluntary reporting by physicians, at least it allows for some follow-up. Until now that has been virtually lacking from nonprescription remedies. At the time of this writing the FDA is promising a proposal for OTC adverse-reaction reporting . . . sometime soon. Based on past performance we aren't about to hold our breath.

The Big Switch: ℞ to OTC

The most important reason to be informed and vigilant about OTC drugs is the fact that these are powerful medicines. Over the last several decades some of the hottest drugstore products have evolved from medications that were once available only by prescription. These compounds do not magically lose their side effects when they jump the counter. Whether it's ibuprofen (**Advil, Excedrin IB, Medipren, Motrin,** etc.) or naproxen (**Aleve**), diphenhydramine (**Benadryl**) or oxymetazoline (**Afrin**), these drugs have the capacity to cause problems for some people.

Please understand. We love the extraordinary opportunity for informed self-care that these medicines represent. Overall, we are very pleased to see more effective medicines available without prescription and we welcome the news that more switches are on the way. The difficulty lies in the inadequacy of information that is provided to consumers. We also fear that many people will assume that just because these drugs are sold OTC, they can safely pop them down without worry.

We only wish the U.S. followed the Canadian and Australian model, in which many such medicines are available behind the counter with the pharmacist's supervision. In other words, you don't need a prescription but you do have to chat with the pharmacist before you can purchase ibuprofen. Since the forces of greed aren't likely to give in to reason, the system isn't likely to change anytime soon. Please make sure you have done your homework before swallowing any OTC product. Throughout this book you will find information about a variety of powerful OTC medications.

The following list is a partial compilation of some formerly prescription drugs that we can now find on pharmacy shelves. Even a product that we take for granted, such as **Tylenol,** was once available only by prescription. Introduced in 1955 as a prescription elixir to treat children's fevers, **Tylenol** didn't go OTC until 1960.[8] Interestingly, this popular pain reliever was a slow starter. Americans loved aspirin and it took some time for them to adapt to the upstart analgesic.

Products That Have Gone from Rx to OTC Status

Brand Name	Generic
ACT	fluoride
Actidil	triprolidine
Actifed	triprolidine; pseudoephedrine
Advil	ibuprofen
Afrin	oxymetazoline
Afrin Tablets	pseudoephedrine
Aleve	naproxen
Allerest 12 Hour	chlorpheniramine; phenylpropanolamine
Antiminth	pyrantel
Anusol HC-1	hydrocortisone
Bayer Select Pain Relief	ibuprofen
Benadryl	diphenhydramine
Bronkaid Caplets	ephedrine
Caldecort Light	hydrocortisone
Cheracol Sinus	dexbrompheniramine; pseudoephedrine
Chlor-Trimeton	chlorpheniramine
Cortaid	hydrocortisone
Cortizone	hydrocortisone
Dimetapp	brompheniramine; phenylpropanolamine
Dristan 12 Hour Nasal	oxymetazoline

Brand Name	Generic
Drixoral Cold & Flu	acetaminophen; dexbrompheniramine, pseudoephedrine
Duration	oxymetazoline
Efidac/24	pseudoephedrine
Excedrin P.M.	acetaminophen; diphenhydramine
Extra Strength Tylenol PM	acetaminophen; diphenhydramine
Femcare Vaginal Cream	clotrimazole
Fluorigard	fluoride
Gyne-Lotrimin	clotrimezole
Haltran	ibuprofen
Imodium	loperamide
Listermint w/Fluoride	fluoride
Lotrimin AF	clotrimazole
Maalox Anti-Diarrheal	loperamide
Micatin	miconazole
Midol 200	ibuprofen
Monistat 7	miconazole nitrate
Motrin IB	ibuprofen
Mycelex OTC Cream	clotrimazole
Mycelex-7 Vaginal Cream	clotrimazole
Neo-Synephrine	phenylephrine

Brand Name	Generic
Neo-Synephrine 12 Hr	oxymetazoline
Nix	permethrin
Nizoral Shampoo	ketoconazole
Nuprin	ibuprofen
Nytol Tablets	diphenhydramine
Otrivin	xylometazoline
Pamprin IB	ibuprofen
Pepcid AC	famotidine
Pepto Diarrhea Control	loperamide
Pin-Rid	pyrantel
Pin-X Pinworm	pyrantel
Primatene Tablets	ephedrine; theophylline
Robitussin Cold & Cough	guaifenesin; dextromethorphan; pseudoephedrine
Sinex	phenylephrine
Sinex Long-Acting	oxymetazoline
Sominex Caplets/Tabs	diphenhydramine
Sucrets Maximum Strength	dyclonine
Sudafed	pseudoephedrine
Tagamet HB	cimetidine
Tavist	clemastine

Brand Name	Generic
Tavist-D	clemastine; phenylpropanolamine
Tinactin	tolnaftate
Tylenol	acetaminophen
Unisom	doxylamine
Vicks NyQuil	acetaminophen; pseudoephedrine; dextromethorphan; doxylamine
Zantac 75	ranitidine

We haven't seen the end of ℞-to-OTC switching. Drug companies are drooling over the opportunities for the future. Highly successful prescription ulcer compounds such as **Pepcid, Tagamet,** and **Zantac** have been approved for OTC sale. The herpes drug **Zovirax** is under consideration. Just some of the other possibilities include the antismoking patch **Nicoderm**, allergy drugs **Nasalcrom** and **Seldane**, the acne cream **Retin-A**, arthritis medicines such as **Dolobid, Feldene, Nalfon, Orudis,** and **Voltaren**, and the antibaldness drug **Rogaine**. We suspect this is a bandwagon that will continue to pick up steam.

Beware Brand Names

There is one fascinating dilemma that ℞-to-OTC switching and reformulation creates. A letter to the editor of the *Annals of Internal Medicine* notes that: "There is a new hazard in over-the-counter medication. Apparently, drug companies can change the ingredients of a brand-name product without any notice to the consumer."[9]

The FDA in its infinite wisdom realized that reformulation posed a real danger to the consumer. People who depend on a favorite OTC remedy may eventually take it for granted. They may scan the brand name quickly and are unlikely to read the ingredients on the label or check for precautions, interactions, or side effects. For example, a woman who used **Midol PMS** for menstrual cramps would be getting acetaminophen, pamabron, and pyrilamine, ingredients unlikely to upset her stomach. But **Midol IB** or **Midol 200** contain ibuprofen, a drug that can cause heartburn and may interact with prescription drugs.

On March 27, 1974, the FDA proposed a regulation that would have required drug companies to change a brand name if there was a fundamental change "in the indications for use or active ingredients of the drug product."[10] How wonderfully logical. Too bad the idea was never implemented. No doubt the pharmaceutical industry complained bitterly. After all, the drug companies spend gazillions of dollars on the care and feeding of brand names. With little fanfare the FDA officially withdrew their proposal on December 30, 1991.

What this means is that you had better know what's in your OTC medicine. Most people don't have a clue as to the ingredients in those highly advertised products they swallow, smear, and insert so enthusiastically. **Anusol**, for example, is a popular hemorrhoidal suppository. It has been reformulated and now contains an ingredient that might interact with certain antidepressants or blood pressure medicines. We wonder how many people will bother to check out something they have been safely using for decades.

There's another problem with names. In the last decade we have seen brand-name pollution in the pharmacy. Once it was possible to keep track of what was what. Take **Tylenol,** for example. It contained one ingredient—acetaminophen—and represented the primary OTC alternative to aspirin. Now look at what's available:

- **Tylenol** (acetaminophen) **Children's Chewable Tablets, Elixir, and Suspension Liquid**

- **Children's Tylenol Cold Multi Symptom Chewable Tablets and Liquid**

- **Children's Tylenol Cold Plus Cough Multi Symptom Liquid**

- **Tylenol Hot Medication, Cold & Flu Packets**

- **Tylenol Cold Medication, Effervescent Tablets**

- **Tylenol Cold Medication No Drowsiness Formula Caplets and Gelcaps**

- **Tylenol Cold Night Time Medication Liquid**

- **Tylenol Extra Strength** (acetaminophen) **Adult Liquid Pain Reliever**

- **Tylenol Extra Strength** (acetaminophen) **Gelcaps, Caplets, Tablets**

- **Tylenol Extra Strength Headache Plus Pain Reliever with Antacid Caplets**

- **Tylenol Infants' Drops and Infants' Suspension Drops**

- **Tylenol Junior Strength** (acetaminophen) **Coated Caplets and Chewable Tablets**

- **Tylenol Maximum Strength Allergy Sinus Medication Gelcaps and Caplets**

- **Tylenol Maximum Strength Cough Medication**
- **Tylenol Maximum Strength Cough Medication with Decongestant**
- **Tylenol Maximum Strength Flu Medication**
- **Tylenol Multi Symptom Cold Medication Caplets and Tablets**
- **Tylenol Maximum Strength, Sinus Medication Gelcaps, Caplets, and Tablets**
- **Tylenol No Drowsiness Cold & Flu Hot Medication Packets**
- **Tylenol Regular Strength** (acetaminophen) **Caplets and Tablets**
- **Tylenol PM Extra Strength Pain Reliever/Sleep Aid Gelcaps, Caplets, and Tablets**

We'd be amazed if the average **Tylenol** user—or his physician or even his pharmacist—could tell you what's in these products without checking the labels carefully. People relate to brand names, which is why there has been such a proliferation of products. But could you tell us the ingredients in **Tylenol Hot Medication Cold & Flu Packets**? For your edification here is the list: acetaminophen 650 mg, chlorpheniramine maleate 4 mg, pseudoephedrine hydrochloride 60 mg, and dextromethorphan hydrobromide 30 mg. Totally confused? Not surprising.

Pharmacy shelves are now cluttered with a dizzying array of popular brands. At last count we found ten different **Actifed** products, seven formulations of **Afrin**, and eight variations of **Alka-Seltzer**.

And let's not forget the greatest marketing coup of the decade—"**Bayer Select**." Just a few years ago **Bayer** was synonymous with aspirin. Now there are a bunch of nonaspirin **Bayer** products targeted at specific symptoms. There is **Bayer Select Chest Cold, Bayer Select Head Cold, Bayer Select Head & Chest Cold, Bayer Select Flu Relief, Bayer Select Headache Pain Relief Formula, Bayer Select Menstrual Multi-Symptom Formula**, and **Bayer Select Night Time Pain Relief Formula**. Are we getting out of control?

How Drug-Company Competition Can Affect Your Cold

Most people probably think that the shelves of their local pharmacy are filled with helpful products, put there by companies that care about their health. Instead, try and think of it as war. The aisles are the trenches and the fight is for your hard-earned dollars. The weapons are advertising, marketing know-how, and money. Especially money. The shelves are the battlefields. The more branded products a company can put out, the more shelf space it captures. More shelf space equals more sales. If a drug company could promote 57 varieties of its leading cold or cough remedy, we suspect they would give it a go.

Our modern-day pharmaceutical hypesters are happy serving the sizzle instead of the steak. They would probably still sell you snake oil if they could get away with it. Let's examine cold remedies, a billion-dollar market for an ailment for which there is no cure. Cold remedies offer only symptomatic relief, but that hasn't stopped drug companies from marketing more than 800 cold-relief products.[11,12]

Antihistamines are one of the most common ingredients in OTC remedies. Check all the big sellers—**Actifed, Alka-Seltzer Plus, Benadryl, Contac, Dimetane, Dimetapp, Drixoral, NyQuil, Sudafed Plus, TheraFlu**, and **Tylenol Multi-Symptom Cold Medication**—and you will find antihistamines included in the formulas. But experts have testified before Congress that antihistamines "cause cold sufferers more harm than good and should be banned from the products."[13]

Please don't get us wrong. Antihistamines can be helpful against allergy symptoms. There is, however, real doubt that they do anything for the common cold. A comprehensive review of most clinical trials carried out between 1950 and 1991 was published in the *Journal of the American Medical Association* (May 5, 1993). The authors found that "Over-the-counter cold medications form a common part of every-day medical therapy. The data on their effectiveness are limited and weak, especially for children."[14] Antihistamines seemed most questionable.

Consumer Reports on Health leaves little doubt about its position: "Consumers Union's medical consultants believe that antihistamines have no place in cold remedies."[15]

If it was just a case of doubtful efficacy, we wouldn't belabor you with this issue. Believe it or not, we have mellowed with age. Once we ranted and railed against shotgun, multisymptom cold remedies. We're still opposed to this "everything but the kitchen sink" kind of therapy, but we're also pragmatic enough to realize that people are gulping down **NyQuil** in huge quantities whether we like it or not. What concerns us, though, is that antihistamine-containing cold remedies can have side effects.

According to a report in *The Wall Street Journal*, Leslie Hendeles, professor of pharmacy and pediatrics at the University of Florida, testified, "These products are not only a waste of money, but they can also place the cold sufferer or innocent child in harm's way." Additionally, Dr. Hendeles cited studies dating back to the mid-1970s that show that antihistamines are no more effective against cold symptoms than placebos.[16]

The problem with OTC antihistamines is that they often make adults drowsy, while they can have the opposite effect on children. This means that any grown-up who tries to drive to work or do anything productive is taking a mighty risk. Children, on the other hand, have different nervous systems from adults and may be stimulated by the same medicine that puts Mom to sleep.

We have received numerous reports from parents who gave little Sam or Suzie a cold remedy at bedtime so they wouldn't sniffle and sneeze all night long. But instead of going to sleep the youngsters became hyper. This paradoxical effect of antihistamines is well known to health professionals but not always obvious on the labels. There have also been rare reports of bizarre "visual hallucinations or psychosis" in children who have taken antihistamines.[17]

So what do we recommend for the common cold? KIS (Keep It Simple)! Treat each individual symptom as it occurs instead of using a shotgun remedy from the onset. Most colds go through an evolution. You may start with sniffles or a scratchy throat, so try a salt-water gargle (half a teaspoon of salt in an eight-ounce glass of warm water).

A bad sore throat should be cultured to make sure it isn't strep. If you feel compelled to relieve the pain, any OTC analgesic (aspirin, acetaminophen, ibuprofen, naproxen) should work. But try to keep this aspect of therapy short. Australian researchers have suggested that the pain relievers in most cold remedies may be counterproductive. They found that aspirin, acetaminophen, and ibuprofen lowered immune response by reducing antibody titers and actually "increased nasal symptoms."[18] Once again we are reminded that many multisymptom cold remedies may be irrational.

Although the studies on it are controversial and conflicting, we still like vitamin C. One of the country's leading cold researchers, Dr. Elliot Dick at the University of Wisconsin, found that vitamin C reduced symptoms and made people feel better. At a cost of less than 2 cents for a 500-mg tablet, this could be one of the least expensive and most effective treatments on the market. We can't make a dosage recommendation, but we personally take 500 mg three or four times a day when we have a cold.

Should your nose become too stuffy for words, a simple decongestant might make you feel better. Assuming you have no medical problems that would conflict (such as high blood pressure, heart disease, diabetes, enlarged prostate, or thyroid disease), we have found pseudoephedrine (**Efidac/24, Novafed, Sudafed**, generic house brands, etc.) to be a reasonably effective symptomatic treatment for congestion.

If you get a cough we would first encourage you to tough it out. This is the body's natural way of dealing with irritation and mucus. On the other hand, if it is a dry hack that is unproductive (doesn't bring up mucus) and is keeping you awake at night, a cough supressant might help. Again, simplicity is in order. We would recommend plain codeine (15 mg) every four to six hours. This is a very effective cough medicine, should be quite cheap, and is especially good at night because there is also some sedative effect. Unfortunately, codeine is considered a narcotic and won't be available over the counter in every state.

The alternative is dextromethorphan. It works, but in our opinion tastes yucky. You will find plain dextromethorphan in **Benylin DM, Children's Hold, Delsym, Drixoral Cough Liquid Caps, Hold DM, Pertussin CS, Robitussin Cough Calmers, Robitussin Pediatric, St. Joseph Cough Suppressant, Suppress, Trocal,** and **Vicks Formula 44**.

Long-Term Consequences

One of the biggest problems with over-the-counter medicines is that no one knows the consequences of taking them on a long-term basis. Most labels carry a standard warning about restricting use to a short period of time, but we fear that caution is often overlooked.

A friend of ours (who happens to be a physician) ended up in the emergency room with a life-threatening bleeding ulcer after taking three or four aspirins a day for months. Many other people treat pain relievers such as ibuprofen (**Advil, Motrin IB, Nuprin**, etc.) or naproxen (**Aleve**) just as casually. But they too can cause serious harm to the digestive tract and other organs if taken for extended periods of time without supervision.

Perhaps more disturbing are the products that lend themselves to regular use. Nasal sprays work so well that some folks use them beyond the three-day limit. That can lead to addiction. We have received hundreds of letters from people who could not stop using their nasal sprays. Some slept with a spray bottle of **Afrin** under the pillow. Others made sure they had extras in the car and at work. One fellow admitted he had been relying on nose drops nonstop for almost 20 years. Getting off can be a real struggle.

People who suffer insomnia may get into the habit of taking an OTC sleeping pill nightly, just in case they have trouble. But no one knows the long-term consequences. A disturbing report from the National Center for Toxicological Research linked doxylamine (an antihistamine found in the sleeping pill **Unisom** and the cold remedy **NyQuil**) to liver toxicity and tumors in mice and rats.[19] On June 14, 1991, an outside panel of experts recommended that the FDA warn consumers about this connection.[20] In an extraordinary burst of speed, the agency sent a letter on July 19th to the Nonprescription Drug Manufacturers Association (a drug-industry trade organization) asking them to start thinking about warning language.

This must have turned into a hot potato for the FDA. Over the next two years no labeling change occurred, although FDA staffers apparently developed language along the lines of "Use of this product may be hazardous to your health. This product contains doxylamine succinate which has been determined to produce tumors in laboratory animals."[21]

On June 28, 1993, a new FDA advisory committee met to decide what to do about the tumor warning. A contingent of drug industry heavyweights argued that the animal data was not significant for humans.[22] Even though animal studies have long been the standard approach for evaluating long-term dangers, the FDA committee must have sided with the drug industry perspective because it ultimately concluded that no warning label was necessary.

Presumably such a warning might be frightening and discourage some sales in this lucrative market. The consumer representative on the FDA advisory committee objected, on the grounds that withholding information was a "disservice and patronizing" and that "To say the warning might scare people is also to say that people don't have the intelligence to seek the type of information that they need and they deserve."[23] The result of the debate was that the same FDA committee that said no warning was necessary recommended that consumers be alerted to the tumor data.

Guidelines for Smart OTC Use

For the most part the snake oil of yesteryear is now gone. OTC medicines are far more powerful than ever before and the science behind them is stronger. There are still lingering doubts about things such as antihistamines in cold remedies, but, overall, consumers can have more confidence that the products they buy will live up to the claims.

Safety, on the other hand, can never be taken for granted. Nonprescription drugs can cause serious side effects or even death. Bleeding ulcers, for example, can be a life-threatening situation. A recent study uncovered a strong link between this condition and the use of over-the-counter pain relievers such as aspirin and ibuprofen. In fact, this striking association was more frequent with OTC compounds than with prescription anti-inflammatory arthritis medicines.[24]

If you are going to self-diagnose and self-medicate by using OTC remedies, you had best do your homework. If your OTC remedy was formerly a prescription drug, you can look it up in the *Physicians' Desk Reference, The Pill Book,* or at the back of this book. Talk to your pharmacist, who can usually make excellent recommendations and advise you about side effects and interactions. Here are some additional guidelines that may help make your self-treatment safer.

- **Be Conservative.** Remember the Hippocratic oath: Doctors must swear to first do no harm. Treat your body with the same respect. Pharmaceutical companies may promise a pill for every ill, but not every ache or pain deserves a drug. Tincture of time can be a marvelous healer.

- **Know Your Limits.** Just as every car repair isn't a do-it-yourself project, lots of body ills will be beyond the reach of any OTC medicine. If you're in doubt, get professional assistance. Anything that doesn't get better quickly should be taken to the doctor, and so should anything that continues to get worse in spite of your treatment.

- **Start Slow—Go Low.** Stepped care is an important concept in medicine. Start with the lowest effective dose of the safest medicine available. Beware the "lottle" principle that maintains if a little is good a lottle must be better. Too many people think that a handful of pills will work faster and be more effective than the recommended dose. Not true. Two aspirin will still solve a lot of problems, and more might be dangerous.

- **Beware of Mixtures.** There is a tremendous tendency on the part of OTC drug makers to whip up complicated combinations of things. Marketing mavens want to be different, or appear to be different, from a competitor. They love the "shotgun" approach. Instead of killing the fly with a swatter, they prefer to pull the trigger and blow away the fly and the barn door he's sitting on. But the more ingredients in a compound the greater the risk of side effects or interactions. In general it is best to treat your problem with a single effective ingredient whenever possible.

- **Shop Comparatively.** Once you know what drug you need, look for the lowest-price equivalent. This will frequently mean a generic or house brand, rather than the product you saw advertised on a clever TV commercial the night before. Savings can be spectacular. If the generic ingredients are too hard to pronounce or remember, ask the pharmacist to point out the least costly product.

- **Read Labels.** Most people seem to hate reading instructions for anything. "Plug it in and start her up!" is the battle cry. Please resist the urge to pop those pills without checking the directions, precautions, dosage, and warnings.

In the next chapter we will provide you with some basic news you can use about OTC medications. You will learn the do's and don'ts for some popular drug-store items. Always keep in mind that these are pharmacological agents with the same capacity for good and bad as their prescription-only relatives. Actually there is a good possibility they once were available only by prescription. By becoming OTC, they didn't lose their potential for causing side effects or interactions.

References

1. Marion, John Francis. *The Fine Old House*. Philadelphia: SmithKline Corporation, 1980; p. 42.
2. Kahn, E. J., Jr., "All in a Century: The First 100 Years of Eli Lilly and Company."
3. "OTC Review Milestone." *FDA Consumer*, 1984; 18(1):32.
4. Gilbertson, William E. "FDA's Review of OTC Drugs," in *Handbook of Nonprescription Drugs*, 10th ed. Covington, Timothy R., et al., eds. Washington, D.C.: American Pharmaceutical Association, 1993; pp. 28–30.
5. "LYCD-Containing Hemorrhoid Products Have One Year to Reformulate Under Final Rule." *The Tan Sheet* 1993; September 6: 1(28).
6. Kaplan, Jerold Z. "Acceleration of Wound Healing." *Arch. Surg.* 1984; 119:1005–1008.
7. Leary, Warren E. "Report Says FDA Is Lax on Over-the-Counter Drugs." *The New York Times* 1992; February 27:A8.
8. Bob Kniffen, Johnson and Johnson. Personal Communication, January 4, 1993.

9. Merikangas, James R. "Changing Over-the-Counter Drugs While Retaining the Brand Name." *Ann. Int. Med.* 1993; 118(12):988.

10. Weintraub, Michael. "Changing Over-the-Counter Drugs While Retaining the Brand Name." *Ann. Int. Med.* 1993; 118(12):988.

11. Lowenstein, S. R., and T. A. Parrino, "Management of the Common Cold." *Adv. Intern. Med.* 1987; 32:207–234.

12. Taylor, J. G. "The Common Cold," in Krogh, C. M., and Travill L. Caruthers-Czyzewski, eds. *Self-Medications: Reference for Health Professionals.* 4th ed. Ottawa, Ontario: Canadian Pharmaceutical Association 1992; 191–212.

13. Weil, Jonathan. "Antihistamines Are Criticized Before Panel." *The Wall Street Journal* 1992; April 9:B8.

14. Smith, Michael B. H., and William Feldman. "Over-the-Counter Cold Medications: A Critical Review of Clinical Trials Between 1950 and 1991." *JAMA* 1993; 269: 2258–2263.

15. "Which Cold Remedy Is Right for You?" *Consumer Reports on Health* 1994; 6(2):16–19.

16. Ibid.

17. Smith, op. cit.

18. Graham, Neil, et al. "Adverse Effects of Aspirin, Acetaminophen, and Ibuprofen on Immune Function, Viral Shedding, and Clinical Status in Rhinovirus-Infected Volunteers." *J. Inf. Dis.* 1990; 162:1277–1283.

19. "OTC Doxylamine Saccharin-Style 'Hazardous,' Warning Suggested by FDA." *The Pink Sheet* 1991; July 22:T&G 1–2.

20. Ibid.

21. "Doxylamine Officially Placed in Antihistamine Monograph; No Warning Required." *The Tan Sheet* 1994; January 31: 2(5).

22. "P&G Doxylamine-Hepatic Enzyme Induction Clinical Study Results Expected in January." *The Tan Sheet* 1993; July 5: 1(19).

23. "Doxylamine Tumorigenicity Label Warning Rejected by OTC Advisory Cmte." *The Tan Sheet* 1993; July 5: 1(19).

24. Wilcox, C. M., et al. "Striking Prevalence of Over-The-Counter Nonsteroidal Anti-Inflammatory Drug Use in Patients with Upper Gastrointestinal Hemorrhage." *Arch. Intern. Med.* 1994; 154:42–46.

OTC Do's and Don'ts

Making Choices

Selecting the right OTC drug for your symptoms may be a lot harder than you think. Very few people have a clue as to what's in the products they use or how their medicine works. Don't believe us? Here's a short quiz:

How would you use xylometazoline:

Swallowed in a pill?

Smeared on your skin?

Sniffed up your nose?

Inserted as a suppository?

The answer is: sniffed up your nose. Xylometazoline (pronounced zye-low-met-az-oh-leen) is a topical decongestant that shrinks blood vessels to make breathing easier. It is found in **Otrivin Nasal Spray** and **Drops**.

Here's another question for you.

If you have diarrhea, the best medicine is:

phenolphthalein

undecylenic acid

loperamide

triclosan

phenyltoloxamine

First, we admit that trying to pronounce these ingredients is an art in itself, so we're not surprised you are confused. Phenolphthalein (pronounced feen-ole-thay-leen) is a laxative (definitely not the right choice if you have diarrhea). It is found in **Ex-Lax, Correctol,** and **Feen-A-Mint**. Undecylenic acid (pronounced un-da-sigh-len-ick) is an antifungal compound used for jock itch and athlete's foot. It is in **Cruex** and **Desenex**. Triclosan (pronounced try-clo-san) is an antibacterial agent added to soaps such as **Lever 2000** and **Dial**. Phenyltoloxamine (pronounced fen-nel-toe-lox-a-mean) is an antihistamine added to the pain reliever **Percogesic**. If you have diarrhea, the best medicine is loperamide (pronounced low-per-a-mide), the main ingredient in **Imodium A-D, Maalox Anti-Diarrheal,** and **Pepto Diarrhea Control**.

If you knew how to pronounce all these drugs *and* answered the questions correctly, you can shelve this book and apply for an honorary degree in pharmacology. Most people, however, don't know what they are taking. When they go shopping for a product they rely primarily on advertising.

Pushing Your Buttons and Pulling Your Strings

An alien scientist from outer space tuning in on our nightly news would soon conclude that earthlings are plagued and preoccupied with digestive-tract problems—or else we have a love affair with laxatives.

Most people are reluctant to discuss their bad breath, body odor, dandruff, diarrhea, constipation, or gas in polite company, but the characters on the tube seem eager to share their most personal problems with millions of TV viewers. When the authoritative announcer holds up his hands for the umpteenth time to demonstrate how his preparation shrinks swelling of humongous hemorrhoids, aren't you just a little grossed out, or have you become immune to OTC drug ads?

You'd think it would be easy to ignore those silly commercials that warn you of the dangers of dandruff, a dreadful disease likely to turn you into a social outcast unless you use the company's super shampoo. But most of us do worry just a little that we too might offend.

Drug manufacturers are masters at manipulating our insecurities. When they portray some hapless soul with bad breath or, worse yet, body odor, we all cringe in fear that if we're not careful it could happen to us. There but for the grace of **Listerine, Scope, Zest**, and **Ban** go we.

Hogwash! Now we're all for good hygiene. But it's high time we stopped falling for the adman's high-pressure pitch. As we are writing this, Americans spend well over $25 billion on OTC drugs and health and beauty aids each year.[1] Deodorants and antiperspirants alone account for more than $1 billion. Roughly $750 million more gets flushed on laxatives[2]—we're a nation obsessed with regularity.

When it comes to over-the-counter pills and potions, we are our own worst enemies, and we cannot blame anyone else for our foolishness. Sure, the slick ads are tempting, but no one stands in the drugstore with a gun at our heads forcing us to buy **Dexatrim, Excedrin, NyQuil**, or **Slim•Fast**. This is where we all get to play doctor for, by, and on ourselves. It's an interesting game, filled with lots of opportunities both good and bad.

There's the opportunity to save money by skipping a trip to the doctor. Plus you have a crack at relieving the symptoms of something in less time than it takes to get a doctor's appointment. Don't you love it when they tell you it will take three weeks for the specialist to check out your rash, bad back, headache, or whatever? If it's really serious you could be dead in three weeks, and if it's trivial it will probably be long gone. No wonder many people opt for a trip to the drugstore.

Of course there is always the chance that you will completely misdiagnose something that needs medical attention. Or you could select the wrong remedy for what ails you. So if you're going to play this game, the first thing to know is the rules.

Rules of the Road for Choosing OTC Remedies

The first rule is to **Use Common Sense!** Do not attempt to treat anything that seems serious. If symptoms persist or get worse, contact a physician promptly. You are walking a tightrope between trivial complaints on one side and life-threatening disaster on the other. An ulcer may start out feeling like simple indigestion. A brain tumor could initially masquerade as a headache. Treating such conditions with an antacid or painkiller could be deadly. Of course, running to the doctor with every ache or pain is also ridiculous. Strike a sensible balance.

Rule two is **Be Skeptical**. The companies selling OTC remedies are more interested in marketing than in medicine. Ads often promise more than the products can deliver. Most OTC concoctions differ little if at all from those of dozens of competitors, so it's often marketing, not effectiveness, that establishes a winner in the marketplace.

Walk into your local drugstore and start comparing labels. You'll find many products with exactly the same ingredients. One favorite pairing of ingredients is the decongestant pseudoephedrine (30 mg) and the pain reliever acetaminophen (500 mg). This combination can be found in **Bayer Select Maximum Strength Sinus Pain Relief Caplets, Contac Non-Drowsy Formula Sinus Caplets, Dristan Cold Caplets, Maximum Strength Sine-Aid Tablets, Maximum Strength Sudafed Sinus Caplets, Maximum Strength Tylenol Sinus Gelcaps, No Drowsiness Sinarest Tabs,** and **Sinus Excedrin Extra Strength Caplets**.

Ibuprofen is found in **Advil, Aches-N-Pain, Bayer Select Pain Relief Formula, Excedrin IB Caplets, Genpril, Haltran, Ibuprin, Midol 200, Motrin IB, Nuprin, Pamprin IB,** and **Trendar**. There are also more affordable generics. The bulk-forming laxative psyllium is available in **Effer-syllium, Fiberall, Hydrocil, Konsyl, Maalox Daily Fiber Therapy, Metamucil Orange Flavor, Perdiem, Reguloid, Serutan**, and **Syllact**. House-brand psyllium is also available. Bottom line: Shop comparatively for ingredients rather than for brands. You'll save a bundle. If the names seem daunting, enlist the pharmacist in your quest.

Rule three is **Do Your Homework!** This is the most important rule of all. We know people who wouldn't think of swallowing a prescription medicine without first checking on side effects and interactions. Yet these same folks gulp down OTC pills without a moment's hesitation. They don't bother to read the label, check the dosing instructions, follow warnings or precautions, or look up adverse reactions. Part of the problem is that you rarely find side-effect or interaction data on the label. So search it out and when in doubt, ask the pharmacist to fill out the checklist on pages 50–51.

OTC Pain Remedies

W hen the pain reliever **Aleve** (naproxen sodium) showed up on drugstore shelves, Helen was one of the first in line. She has arthritis and had tried aspirin, acetaminophen, and ibuprofen with limited success. The ad "All day strong. All day long" caught her eye. The idea of a new, longer-acting, nonprescription medicine for arthritis really appealed to her.

Like lots of people who hate to waste time reading instructions, Helen threw away the box **Aleve** came in and started popping pills. She took two at a time without bothering to check the label. The print was tiny and there were no obvious dosing instructions. You have to fold the label away from the bottle to find them. Helen had never seen a fold-out label before and it didn't occur to her to check it.

Helen had inadvertently doubled the recommended dose of **Aleve**. She was used to taking two aspirins or two **Tylenol**s, or even two **Nuprin**s, so two **Aleve**s seemed logical to her. She didn't read the warning that adults over age 65 should not take more than one caplet every 12 hours.

Fortunately, Helen didn't end up in the emergency room. When she reported visual disturbances and a terrible bellyache, her son got out the magnifying glass to read the instructions under the flap. Even if she had read the fine print, though, Helen wouldn't have known she was taking a risk. Like most OTC medicines, **Aleve** has no description of side effects on the label so she assumed it was safe.

Aleve is one of the more recent ℞-to-OTC switches. Helen was taking almost as much naproxen as you would find in a prescription dose of **Anaprox** or **Naprosyn**. If she had kept at that level for long she would have been at risk for gastrointestinal bleeding, ulceration, and perforation. Other possible adverse reactions could have included diarrhea, nausea, heartburn, loss of appetite, hepatitis, kidney problems, and dizziness. We worry that millions of people are taking OTC arthritis drugs without realizing the risks.

Baby Boomers Beware: Arthritis Looms

Americans are in pain. Just look at the numbers. The last edition of *The People's Pharmacy* noted that we yearly "fork over $1.6 billion on OTC painkillers."[3] In a decade that figure has jumped to roughly $2.6 billion per year, more than a 60 percent increase.[4] Combined annual sales of **Tylenol** ($698 million) and **Advil** ($328.8 million) surpass $1 billion alone.[5]

As big as this market is now, just wait. Pain-reliever sales are on the verge of exploding, because aging baby boomers are about to discover the joys of arthritis. In 1990 it was calculated that 37.9 million people suffered from joint pain. By the year 2000 that number is expected to be 44 million. The Centers for Disease Control estimates that by 2020 there will be 59.4 million (one in five Americans) complaining of sore knuckles, stiff knees, and painful hips. That is a 57-percent increase.[6]

Please don't get us wrong. We can think of few more important medicines than analgesics. Pain gets your attention. It is like a short in your electrical wiring. Unlike lots of other symptoms, pain cannot be denied or ignored. Fortunately, most pain is temporary and easily treated when we know the cause. Too much stress can bring on a tension headache, easily alleviated by aspirin, acetaminophen, or ibuprofen. A sprain or strain will respond as well.

But sometimes pain is an early warning sign of serious trouble. Treating undiagnosed pain with an analgesic for more than a few days is a little like sticking a penny in your fuse box. You can temporarily override the system, but you would be setting yourself up for a fire. Any pain that persists requires proper medical oversight.

OTC Headache Relief

Let's assume you get garden-variety headaches like millions of other folks. Virtually any OTC pain reliever should be effective. As far as we can determine, none has been shown to be superior to any other. One might argue that a fizzy formulation of aspirin—**Alka-Seltzer,** for example— might go to work a few minutes before an enteric-coated aspirin (such as **Ecotrin**). Whether such a difference is really significant has not been established.

Acetaminophen (**Anacin-3,** APAP, **Panadol, Tylenol,** etc.) is no more effective than aspirin when it comes to headaches, but it will be easier on your stomach. This benefit, however, is relevant only if you have a sensitive tummy, get frequent headaches or rely on a medication more than several times a week. Ibuprofen (**Advil, Bayer Select Pain Relief Formula, Excedrin IB, Motrin IB, Nuprin,** etc.) and naproxen (**Aleve**) should be roughly equal to aspirin and acetaminophen in pain relief, although **Aleve** lasts longer in the body. Most headaches begin to go away within half an hour no matter what you take, so we're not sure the longer action of **Aleve** makes it more desirable. Both ibuprofen and naproxen can be irritating to the digestive tract and can cause ulcers in susceptible people. Again, dose and duration of use are important factors in assessing the risk.

We have always been champions of the less-is-best theory when it comes to medications. That flies in the face of marketing, however, where the motto remains more is better. This is especially true when it comes to pain medications. Consider, for example, the **Anacin** ad that crowed about having "more of the pain reliever doctors recommend most." Their much-touted exotic pain reliever, we're happy to reveal, is plain old unadulterated aspirin, available in plain, unadvertised bottles at any pharmacy for a fraction of the cost of the same ingredient labeled as **Anacin.**

What's true about the **Anacin** claim is that two **Anacin** pills do contain 800 milligrams of aspirin, versus 650 milligrams for two house-brand generic aspirin tablets or competing products such as **Alka-Seltzer, Ascriptin, Bayer, Bufferin,** and **Empirin. Anacin** really has more active ingredient (aspirin, remember?) than these products.

Common sense tells us that more has got to be better. This seems even more obvious when you're sitting there with a splitting headache and would do almost anything for a little relief. If two pills are good, surely four would be twice as strong or would work twice as fast to relieve the pain. We have yet to see any research that proves that to be the case. Take two aspirin . . . any two aspirin . . . and you probably won't have to call anyone in the morning.

The aspirin in **Anacin** won't do you any more good than two generic aspirin tablets. If you really needed more of the painkiller, you could get it by stalking a third aspirin, catching it unaware, and cracking it down the middle with a knife. This will hopefully yield several smaller pieces. Swallowing an additional half a tablet would give you about as much aspirin in your body (800 mg)—and a whole lot more money in your pocket—as one of the highly advertised brands.

Maybe now you are getting the idea how silly these "extra-strength" ads can be. Yet they are effective marketing strategies. As a culture we love bigger, stronger, and more potent. Dose inflation is widespread, and **Anacin** is not the only guilty party. You will also find "extra-strength" **Alka-Seltzer, Ascriptin, Bayer, Excedrin, Tylenol**, etc. Most of these products contain 500 mg per pill. "Maximum strength" brands are also popular these days and we have been predicting "industrial-strength" headache relief for years.

The thing that's aggravating is that the people who create such advertising KNOW better and yet they play on the public's lack of knowledge to turn nonsense into profit. Why the FDA and the Federal Trade Commission (responsible for OTC drug advertising) let them get away with it is beyond us.

We could say one positive thing about **Anacin** for headaches. Scientists have been arguing for years about the benefits of caffeine in relieving headache pain. One standard **Anacin** tablet contains 32 mg of caffeine in addition to 400 mg of aspirin. That means the standard two-pill dose will give you 64 mg of caffeine—about as much as you would get in a weak cup of coffee. A double-blind study (sponsored by the makers of **Anacin**) comparing aspirin and caffeine did prove this combination was slightly superior to plain acetaminophen for relieving tension headaches.[7]

Should you pay more for products (such as **Anacin, BC Tablets** or **Powders, Buffets II, Excedrin Extra-Strength, Vanquish**, etc.) that add caffeine to their formulas? Of course not. If you think caffeine boosts the pain power of generic aspirin or acetaminophen, you could swallow the cheap brand with a caffeine-containing soft drink such as **Coke, Dr Pepper, Pepsi, Mello Yello,** or **Mountain Dew**. A cup of coffee or strong tea would also work.

But be VERY careful not to get into a caffeine cycle. People who regularly drink average amounts of coffee risk caffeine-withdrawal headaches when they quit. A superb study published in the *New England Journal of Medicine* found that people experienced moderate to severe headaches when they abruptly stopped consuming caffeine.[8] The doses were surprisingly low—equal to two and a half cups of coffee or about as much as someone might get from recommended daily doses of caffeine-containing analgesics.

There is a real fear that people who rely on repeated doses of pain relievers containing caffeine might set themselves up for rebound headaches when they stop the medicine. In fact, one of the country's leading headache experts, Dr. Joel Saper, believes that the overuse of almost any nonprescription pain medicine (even without caffeine) might lead to a vicious cycle. He recommends that "analgesics should not be used more than two days per week, and more ideally less often, due to 'rebound phenomenon.'"[9] Someone who has severe, recurrent headaches should be seen by a headache specialist. You might be dealing with migraines, and there are new prescription treatments that are quite effective against this devastating pain.

OTC Products for Menstrual Cramps

No one really knows why some women suffer menstrual pain while others are barely bothered. The prostaglandin theory has taken center stage over the last decade and seems a plausible hypothesis. Prostaglandins have been one of medicine's most fertile research fields. We know that these hormone-like substances are produced by the body and control a wide range of physiological processes, including pain, inflammation, respiration, reproduction, and the contraction of certain types of muscle tissue, like the uterus.

Too much or too little of one or another prostaglandin (there are many different types) may be a factor in pain, arthritis, ulcers, psoriasis, eczema, and menstrual cramps. And we now know that many painkillers, including aspirin and a host of nonsteroidal anti-inflammatory drugs (NSAIDs), work in large measure through their ability to temporarily slow the body's production of prostaglandins.

Painful cramps are believed to be produced in part by uterine contractions caused by prostaglandins. Some women complain of a dull ache that spreads down the lower back and even into the legs. Others say it feels more like a colicky, crampy feeling in the lower abdomen.

No matter how they manifest, menstrual cramps are commonly treated with naproxen (**Anaprox, Naprosyn**) or ibuprofen. Doctors often prescribe **Anaprox** a day or two before the period starts and continue it for one or two days into the cycle. The dose that is recommended in the *PDR* is "550 mg, followed by 275 mg every 6 to 8 hours, as required. The total daily dose should not exceed 1,375 mg."

Now that naproxen is available over the counter as **Aleve**, women have an additional self-treatment option. The OTC dose of **Aleve** is 220 mg (200 mg of naproxen and 20 mg of sodium). Dosing instructions on the label say to "Take 1 caplet every 8 to 12 hours while symptoms persist. With experience, some people may find that an initial dose of 2 caplets followed by 1 caplet 12 hours later, if necessary, will give better relief. Do not exceed 3 caplets in 24 hours unless directed by a doctor."

Ibuprofen is also effective for cramps. In fact, there are a number of companies that have taken advantage of this ingredient to reformulate products that have a reputation for relieving cramps. There is **Cramp Relief Formula Midol IB, Cramp End Tablets, Haltran, Midol 200, Pamprin IB**, and **Trendar**. And of course there are the old favorites, **Advil, Motrin IB**, and **Nuprin**. We suggest the cheapest generic house-brand ibuprofen you can find. The dose usually recommended on the label is "1 tablet every 4 to 6 hours at the onset of menstrual symptoms and while pain persists. If pain does not respond to 1 tablet, 2 tablets may be used but do not exceed 6 tablets in 24 hours, unless directed by a doctor."

Menstrual migraines are seemingly more common than most people realize. These painful headaches can occur around the time of menstruation. Headache specialist Dr. Joel Saper recommends NSAIDs (such as naproxen and ibuprofen) a few days before the anticipated migraine begins. (You will need to keep a regular diary so you can plot your headache in relation to your cycle.) The NSAID is discontinued two to four days after the period begins.[10]

Remember that pain can be a symptom of something serious. A story in the *Wall Street Journal* reveals what can happen when you bypass your internal fuse box: "Other serious disease can also remain undetected for a period with the help of nonprescription drugs. A 32-year-old social worker in Sandy Springs, Georgia, recently discovered that her painful menstrual periods, which ibuprofen pills had alleviated for six years, were actually a sign of endometriosis, a condition of the uterus that is now preventing her from getting pregnant. 'The pills took care of the pain, so I never bothered going to the doctor,' she says. 'I just thought it was normal.' "[11]

OTC Relief for Arthritis and Inflammation

Unlike menstrual cramps or an occasional headache, arthritis lasts. You can have good days and bad days, but generally people with inflamed joints suffer on a long-term basis. There is to date no cure, nor one on the horizon. The best we can hope for is temporary relief. For anyone with chronic pain and inflammation, that means regular use of analgesics, and that is when the trouble starts. Most people can pop a few aspirins, acetaminophens, ibuprofens, or naproxens without getting into major trouble. But daily reliance on pain medication takes a toll.

For one thing there's the stomach. Nonsteroidal anti-inflammatory drugs (NSAIDs) such as aspirin, ibuprofen, and naproxen are notorious for causing indigestion, heartburn, stomach pain, nausea, and loss of appetite. Of far greater concern is the risk of ulcers, which can be extremely serious. Bleeding or perforated ulcers can become life-threatening events, especially for older people.

A review of the epidemiology of NSAIDs shows that people taking these medications have triple the risk of ulcers and GI bleeding.[12] Dr. James Fries, one of the country's leading rheumatologists, has reported that "Conservative calculations, counting only excess deaths, indicate approximately 7,600 deaths yearly attributable to NSAID use in the United States. The Food and Drug Administration suggests figures that are even higher, estimating from 10,000 to 20,000 deaths per year."[13,14] At those levels one must conclude that more people are dying each year from prescribed arthritis medicine than from all illicit drugs (cocaine, marijuana, heroin, etc.) combined.[15]

Most people probably think that the problem lies primarily with prescription NSAIDs such as **Anaprox, Ansaid, Clinoril, Dolobid, Feldene, Indocin, Lodine, Meclomen, Motrin, Nalfon, Naprosyn, Orudis, Relafen, Tolectin,** and **Voltaren.** While such medications can cause serious complications, OTC arthritis drugs can also be a problem. One study found more GI bleeding associated with recent use of over-the-counter arthritis medications than with prescription ones.[16]

How is it that these drugs are so tough on the tummy? Remember that they work by suppressing prostaglandin formation. It is thought that prostaglandins are responsible for inflammation and pain, so if you inhibit these compounds there should be substantial relief. The only trouble is that prostaglandins also serve a protective role in the stomach. When you block their formation you make the stomach far more vulnerable to irritation and ulceration.

Nonprescription NSAIDs are often taken without medical supervision. One woman swallowed 18 ibuprofen tablets (despite the manufacturers warning not to exceed six per day). Even though she experienced considerable digestive-tract distress, and her doctor warned her that she had damaged the lining of her stomach, the experience didn't daunt her. She backed off to nine pills a day and is not worrying because she thinks "the manufacturer's daily recommended dosage of six tablets is probably overcautious." Wrong!

Often there are no early warning signs that damage is occurring. Little ulcers may form and then heal with no symptoms. One day a little sore may turn into a big one that begins to bleed. That is probably what happened to our friend Mike. He's a smart physician at a major medical center. Another aging baby boomer, Mike was experiencing aches and pain for which he self-treated with aspirin (about three or four daily) for quite a few months. One day he woke up feeling really tired, but because it was his daughter's thirteenth birthday he struggled to cope. The next day he could barely drag himself out of bed. Fortunately, his wife dragged him (protesting all the time) to the emergency room where they found a life-threatening bleeding ulcer. After administering several units of blood the staff managed to save Mike's life, but it was a close call.

There are no good ways to tell if this is happening to you but here are a few things to watch out for: persistent heartburn, sudden weight loss, fatigue or lethargy, feeling full before eating your usual amount, or anemia. It would be wise to have a physician monitor your progress if you are taking any OTC pain medicine on a regular basis. Have the physician check your kidney and liver function as well. Ibuprofen and naproxen can both affect these essential organs. Other side effects include skin rash, dizziness, drowsiness, visual disturbances, ringing in the ears, and more. Check the appendix at the end of this book for more detailed information on the adverse reactions and drug interactions associated with **Motrin** and **Naprosyn.**

One way to try and minimize the damage caused by NSAIDs is to take a drug holiday. A few days on and a few days off can give the stomach some time to heal itself. If the pain and inflammation become too intense, acetaminophen may be an alternative during the off days. Although this is heresy, acetaminophen has been found to be helpful against arthritis. For years physicians and pharmacists maintained that acetaminophen was ineffective against inflammation. But a landmark study published in the *New England Journal of Medicine* demonstrated that "in short-term symptomatic treatment of osteoarthritis of the knee, the efficacy of acetaminophen was similar to that of ibuprofen, whether the latter was administered in an analgesic or an anti-inflammatory dose."[17]

In plain English, these doctors found that plain old acetaminophen (**Anacin-3,**

APAP, **Panadol, Tylenol**, etc.) was about as good as the NSAID ibuprofen. They compared 1,200 mg of ibuprofen (the maximum suggested OTC daily dose) against 4,000 mg of acetaminophen—equal to two **Extra Strength Tylenol** (500 mg each)—four times daily. That they were roughly comparable is extraordinary.

So we like an occasional acetaminophen break. But please don't overdose on this drug or take it for granted. We worry about people who consume maximum amounts of acetaminophen. (From our perspective 4,000 mg of acetaminophen is a large dose.) If you do this regularly, or if you like a few beers, a glass or two of wine, or regular cocktails, acetaminophen could be more dangerous than you think.

Too many people assume that **Tylenol** and other acetaminophen products are totally harmless. While it is gentle to the stomach, it can be toxic to the liver and kidneys if taken regularly in large doses. Recent articles point out potential problems with one of America's favorite pain relievers.

Researchers at the University of Pittsburgh discovered that people who weren't eating were at greater risk of acetaminophen toxicity. Writing in the *Journal of the American Medical Association*, they noted that, "Fasting causes several major changes in acetaminophen metabolism and the combined effect of these changes may predispose some individuals to hepatotoxicity [liver toxicity]."[18]

You might not believe that "fasting" would be a problem for many folks, but think about when you have a bad cold or the flu. Feel like eating? Probably not. And yet most cold and flu products on pharmacy shelves contain a healthy dose of acetaminophen. And people in chronic pain may also lose their appetite, especially when the pain is severe. People who are drinkers may also scrimp on food. Since there is a concern that booze may predispose to liver damage, the combined effect of alcohol with lowered caloric intake could lead to a greater risk of liver damage.

There is also serious concern that heavy use of acetaminophen and NSAIDs increases the risk of kidney disease. A study published in the *New England Journal of Medicine* concluded that "This study questions the safety of long-term acetaminophen use (more than 2 pills per day, or more than 1,000 pills overall) and of consumption of large quantities of NSAIDs, but it suggests that aspirin use confers little or no excess risk of renal failure . . . people requiring large quantities of analgesic medicines and those at high risk of renal failure may be best advised to use aspirin for pain control."[19]

Amazing Aspirin

Aspirin remains the gold standard for pain relief and anti-inflammatory activity. All other prescription NSAIDs must be measured against this OTC drug that has been around for almost a hundred years. We are unconvinced that NSAIDs have been found to be substantially safer or more effective. In fact, coated or buffered aspirin may be safer than far pricier prescription arthritis medicines.[20] Unfortunately, familiarity breeds contempt. Like Rodney Dangerfield who "don't get no respect," aspirin is rarely appreciated for the miracle medicine that it is.

There is now overwhelming evidence that aspirin can reduce the likelihood of heart attacks and strokes, especially for those who are highly vulnerable. Results from a major epidemiological study have led researchers to conclude that "If everybody known to be at high risk of vascular disease were to take half an aspirin a day, about 100,000 deaths and 200,000 nonfatal heart attacks and strokes could be avoided worldwide each year."[21] New data suggests that 30 mg may be as effective as higher doses in preventing strokes and there is even some tantalizing evidence that as little as 3 to 10 mg may prevent blood clots.[22,23] At such low levels (one two-hundredth of a normal dose), aspirin is much less likely to irritate the stomach.

More exciting, though, is the growing belief that aspirin may be one of our most effective cancer preventers. The evidence is strong that aspirin lowers the risk of colorectal cancer by up to 50 percent, but there is even data that it may be effective for cancers of the lung, breast, stomach, and esophagus.[24] And researchers are also looking into the possibility that aspirin may reduce the risk of certain kinds of senility such as multi-infarct dementia or perhaps even Alzheimer's disease.[25,26] Of course no one should take aspirin regularly without medical supervision. Even in relatively low doses aspirin can have side effects and some people may never be able to take this drug.

What's Good for Indigestion?

Drug companies have a vested interest in our bellyaches. They love to see us bingeing on billions of burgers, putting away pizza, pickles, and potato chips by the ton, and slurping soft drinks and coffee on the run. Each burp and belch represents another potential **Maalox** moment, or **Alka-Seltzer** fizz. They're also happy to have us gorping down pain relievers such as aspirin, **Advil, Aleve, Anacin, Bayer, Motrin IB**, and **Nuprin,** all of which can add fuel to the fire.

At last count we spend about a billion bucks a year soothing the savage beast in our bellies.[27] Products such as **Tums, Rolaids, Mylanta, Alka-Seltzer, Mylanta II, Mylanta Extra-Strength, Maalox, Pepto-Bismol,** and **Gaviscon** are big sellers. But at the risk of destroying one of America's cherished myths we would like to suggest that treating heartburn with antacids is somewhat illogical.

Acid is essential for proper digestion of food. Think about it for a minute. We put all sorts of weird items into our stomachs—from chips and salsa to peanuts and pastrami. Somehow we must churn all this stuff up, break it down, extract the nutrients, and eliminate the excess. The first step in the process involves enzymes and stomach acid. This is strong stuff. The hydrochloric acid in your stomach is caustic enough to eat through the page you are holding in your hands. So why doesn't it routinely eat a hole in your stomach? The answer is mucus. Your stomach is very good at protecting itself from all those digestive juices. A jellylike coating of mucus normally lines the wall of the stomach and prevents damage. If the tissues become damaged, say by aspirin or another NSAID, the acid may begin to eat away at the vulnerable spot until an ulcer forms.

Trying to neutralize acid in your stomach by popping down antacids is a little like putting your finger in a dike to hold back the ocean. No matter how hard you try, more acid will be made. Even effective antacids can control acid levels for only an hour or two. Some, such as **Rolaids Original,** will provide "relief" (based on a test by Consumers Union's chemists) for just 11 minutes in a simulated stomach.[28]

The point we're trying to make is that attempting to treat heartburn with antacids is actually illogical. To understand why, you have to appreciate what heartburn is . . . and is not. The problem is rarely caused by excess acidity. Remember, the stomach is *supposed* to have acid. The heart of the problem is in the esophagus or food tube that carries food from your mouth to your stomach. At the bottom of this passage is a sphincter—a small ring of muscle—that is supposed to keep food and acid and other gross stomach stuff out. If that sphincter gets weak or lazy, it can allow acid and partially digested food to seep back into the esophagus, which does not have the protective mucus layer that is found in the stomach. This splashback can lead to inflammation and pain—that old familiar burn behind the breastbone.

What few people realize is that lots of things make the esophageal sphincter weak or lazy. Alcohol, chocolate, cigarettes (nicotine), coffee, and peppermint have a negative effect. Many drugs may also weaken this muscle including aminophylline (**Somophyllin**), diazepam (**Valium**), nitroglycerin, progesterone (birth control pills, **Provera**), and theophylline (**Bronkodyl, Slo-Phyllin, Sustaire, Theobid, Theo-Dur, Theolair, Uniphyl**, etc.). Pregnancy, overeating, overweight, stress, and lying down after eating can also contribute to gastroesophageal reflux disease (GERD).

Antacids do not prevent stomach acid, enzymes, or undigested food from seeping back into the esophagus. All they can do is temporarily neutralize the acidity so if the contents splash up into the esophagus they won't be so irritating. This is a little like putting baking soda on your grapefruit so that if it squirts in your eye it won't sting. Wouldn't it be better if you could keep the grapefruit from squirting?

There are ways to keep the sphincter toned up so acid is less likely to end up in the esophagus. First, try to avoid those things that weaken it—alcohol, nicotine, chocolate, coffee, peppermint, cola, and fatty foods. Don't overeat, and don't lie down after eating. Stay away from nighttime snacks. Try to lose weight if you have a spare tire. Raise the head of your bed six to ten inches. Sleep on your left side.

Your body's natural fire extinguisher is saliva. The more spit you make the more saliva will wash down your esophagus and naturally neutralize acidity. It also helps rinse acid back into the stomach where it belongs. Hard candy and chewing gum can stimulate production of saliva. Chamomile tea has also been a time-tested remedy for stomach upset. What was good for Peter Rabbit may be good for you, too. Indian physicians have used banana powder to relieve indigestion. Perhaps a plain banana would be helpful as well.

When discomfort persists, we always encourage medical intervention. Chronic heartburn and indigestion could be a sign of a hiatal hernia, an ulcer, or something worse. If the diagnosis remains heartburn, perhaps **Propulsid** (cisapride) would be appropriate. This prescription drug tones up the esophageal sphincter so that stomach acid can't reflux into your gullet. Only your physician will know if this medication is right for you.

Antacids

If you do decide to try the antacid approach, which products work best? Chemists for Consumers Union tested 29 top brands in a simulated stomach. They were looking for the longest-acting antacids (at least an hour above pH 3—a measure of acid neutralization). Their high-rated brands were "**Mylanta Double Strength** tablets in the Cool Mint Creme flavor and three concentrated liquids: **Mylanta Double Strength** in both Original and Cherry Creme flavors and **Maalox Plus Extra Strength** in the Mint Creme flavor."[29] When these antacids were used in the high-dosage ranges recommended by the manufacturers they provided over 100 minutes of simulated relief.

These antacids and other products such as **Riopan Plus 2, Di-Gel**, and **Gaviscon** contain aluminum and magnesium. These ingredients are often combined because they provide acid neutralization while balancing conflicting side effects. Aluminum can be constipating, while magnesium tends to produce diarrhea. By putting the ingredients together it is hoped you will avoid both consequences. Unfortunately, many people complain that they experience some complications one way or the other.

Aluminum and Alzheimer's Disease

The aluminum and Alzheimer's story is a medical mystery with murky data, FDA inactivity, and lots of money at stake. A decade ago we wrote that "trying to make sense out of the aluminum-Alzheimer's connection is at this moment almost impossible. There are no easy answers." Nothing much has changed in the intervening years.

Our friends at *Consumer Reports* say that there has been "speculation that aluminum may cause Alzheimer's disease, but few researchers now endorse such a link."[30] On that score we would agree. And yet data continues to accumulate suggesting there may be a connection between aluminum and neurotoxicity. But let's begin at the beginning.

It all started when investigators discovered that aluminum had accumulated in the tangled nerve cells of Alzheimer's patients. And when aluminum was administered to animals it produced pathological changes in brain tissue.[31] Certain residents of Guam have appeared at higher risk of ALS (Lou Gehrig's disease) and Parkinson's dementia. In some areas of Guam the water and food are high in aluminum, which may accumulate in the islanders' brains.[32]

In the past, patients who required kidney dialysis sometimes developed "dialysis dementia" because aluminum in the dialysis water accumulated in their brains. (Special aluminum-free water is now employed to prevent this problem.) These patients have also been treated with aluminum-containing antacids to remove excess phosphate from their bodies. New research suggests that the aluminum from antacids may have accumulated in their brains (depending upon the dose and duration of treatment) and contributed to Alzheimer's disease–like changes in brain tissue.[33]

Kidney patients do not present a normal case, however, and so any problems they encounter may not apply to the rest of the population. Nevertheless, some studies have linked higher levels of aluminum in drinking water with Alzheimer's disease, and miners in Canada who breathed aluminum dust (to protect their lungs) had greater brain deterioration over time than miners not so exposed.[34]

So we are still left to wonder whether aluminum is the chicken or the egg. We cannot say whether aluminum contributes to the disease process of senility or whether the secondary accumulation of this metal in brain tissue occurs as a consequence of the illness.

We doubt that there is any risk from cooking with aluminum pots and pans as long as you do not cook anything acidic or salty in them, such as tomato sauce or sauerkraut. For ourselves, we prefer those old-fashioned cast iron or porcelain-covered pans that weigh a ton.

As far as the safety of aluminum antacids is concerned, we don't think the final chapter has been written. We only wish the Food and Drug Administration would take a more active role in trying to resolve this controversy once and for all.

Calcium to the Rescue

There is growing concern that aluminum-containing antacids could be undesirable for another reason. Older women are at a higher risk of osteoporosis, which weakens the bones and makes them more susceptible to fractures. The medical experts at *Consumer Reports* admit that "Long-term use of aluminum antacids can rob the body of calcium, weakening bones."[35]

So while high-potency aluminum antacids such as **Mylanta Double Strength** and **Maalox Plus Extra Strength** are unquestionably the longest-acting products on the market, there are reasons to be cautious about prolonged use. That is why we have turned to a different kind of antacid as our first choice.

Calcium-based antacids work! Products such as **Rolaids–Extra Strength** assorted mints and **Tums E-X Extra Strength** provide low-cost relief. They may not keep going and going, but the high-dose regimen should provide at least one hour of acid-neutralizing capacity.

There is, of course, another reason to choose calcium-containing antacids besides stomach trouble. Most people don't get close to the recommended intake of calcium. Doctors at the National Institutes of Health have reported that half of American adults don't get adequate calcium. Teenagers are probably in even worse shape on this score, especially given the new recommendation that adolescents get 1,200 to 1,500 mg of calcium daily.

Okay, truth time. How's your diet? Really? To reach that level of calcium from food you would need to consume four to five 8-ounce glasses of milk or cartons of yogurt daily. It's even harder to reach the goal if you have to rely on vegetables and other nondairy foods. For example, it would take 8 cups of cooked kale or turnip greens, 21 cups of broccoli, or 30 oranges. Are you even close?

While calcium plays a crucial role in building bones and maintaining their strength, the mineral does much more. It is also important for teeth, nerve transmission, muscle contraction and a host of other physiological functions. Researchers think calcium may help control blood pressure and perhaps even reduce the risk of colorectal cancer.

Osteoporosis, or weakened bones, is the major concern of health experts, however. This killer currently affects 25 million Americans. An elderly person who falls and breaks a hip may be immobilized. Sometimes these patients die from the complications of being bedridden.

Because calcium has been shown to diminish the chance of osteoporosis and because most people do not get adequate amounts in their diets, supplementation is often desirable. Experts now suggest 1,000 mg calcium daily from food or tablets for most adults and at least 1,200 mg for women past menopause, the people at greatest risk of weak bones.

There has been a growing controversy about natural vs. pharmaceutical-grade calcium supplementation. Researchers have found low levels of lead in natural-source calcium carbonate derived from oyster shells or bone meal. Synthetic calcium carbonate found in antacids such as **Tums E-X Extra Strength, Rolaids Calcium Rich**, and **Titralac** liquid offer a cost-effective way of getting this mineral with minimal contamination.

Vitamin D is also an important addition to calcium, because it improves the body's ability to absorb and use calcium effectively. If you get some sunshine on a regular basis, your skin will make the vitamin D you need. Otherwise, 400 units a day is an appropriate supplement.

So if you are going to select an antacid to relieve heartburn and indigestion, why not kill two birds with one stone? Choose one that supplies calcium, a mineral most of us need. But don't overdose. Too much of a good thing is still too much. Limit intake to not more than 2,000 mg of pure calcium a day. Large doses for long periods of time may produce excessive calcium levels and this could get you into metabolic trouble (alkalosis) and be dangerous for people with kidney problems.

Some products list milligrams of calcium carbonate, rather than elemental calcium. Only 40 percent of calcium carbonate is pure calcium, so calculate calcium dose by multiplying the total calcium carbonate mg by 0.4. In the case of

Tums E-X there are 750 mg of calcium carbonate, which equals 300 mg of pure calcium.

Plopping and Fizzing with Alka-Seltzer

We used to badmouth **Alka-Seltzer Effervescent Antacid & Pain Reliever**. It seemed like an irrational combination of ingredients. Why would anyone want to put aspirin together with sodium bicarbonate? If you had an upset stomach, aspirin seemed like the last thing you would want to ingest. **Alka-Seltzer** is also incredibly expensive. Twelve fizzy tablets (six doses) cost us $2.39. For that amount of money you could buy more than 100 aspirin tablets and enough baking soda for hundreds of upset stomachs. And if that wasn't enough discouragement, there was all that sodium. Each tablet contains 567 mg of sodium or 1,134 mg per two-tablet dose. That represents almost half of the daily allowance experts have been recommending.

So why are we now singing the "plop-plop, fizz-fizz" song? First, because sodium bicarbonate is a fast and effective antacid. **Alka-Seltzer** (original formula) provided more than 60 minutes of acid-neutralizing relief in the *Consumer Reports* analysis.[36] **Aquaprin** is a new soluble aspirin with no sodium.

But of far greater value is the soluble aspirin—not for stomach upset or indigestion, but for pain relief and heart protection. We wish there were a plain soluble aspirin product in the U.S. just as there is in Australia. There you can buy aspirin tablets that dissolve in water (**Aspro, Disprin**, etc.). Liquid aspirin is fast-acting and easier on the stomach than pills that have to be swallowed whole.

The fast action of **Alka-Seltzer** would be particularly beneficial if someone suspected he was having a heart attack. A major international study discovered that half an aspirin (160 mg) could reduce the death rate by 25 percent if it were taken by heart attack victims within the first four hours of chest pain.[37] That has led some cardiologists to encourage people to take half an aspirin and call 911 if they think they may be having a heart attack.[38] They believe that if the FDA approved aspirin for heart attack treatment it could save 30,000 lives annually in the U.S. Presumably, the sooner the aspirin starts working the better, and **Alka-Seltzer** produces measurable blood levels within 10 minutes of plopping and fizzing.

As for the high sodium content of **Alka-Seltzer**, we are a little less worried about that issue these days. Sure, some people should always avoid sodium. Those with congestive heart failure or salt-sensitive hypertension should skip the sodium bicarb. They may want to look for **Aquaprin** instead. But for others, a sodium prohibition is probably not necessary.

One word of caution about sodium bicarbonate is in order. Even though a little baking soda in water will alleviate everyday indigestion just about as well as many OTC antacids, you should be aware that it should never be used if you have really overindulged. In other words, if you pigged out, DO NOT reach for the baking soda to relieve the bloated, full feeling. A report from the FDA has warned of an unusual hazard associated with sodium bicarbonate.

A man who had a gigantic Mexican meal took baking soda to relieve his discomfort. Instead of relief, he experienced excruciating pain and passed out. During emergency surgery the doctors discovered that his stomach had a hole in it, apparently caused by the extremely rapid buildup of carbon dioxide gas from the baking soda. Because his stomach had already been stretched to its limits there was no room for the gas to escape. A mini-explosion blew a hole in his stomach.

Fortunately, this fellow's life was saved, but it was a close call. FDA staffers immediately checked the scientific literature for similar events and, sure enough, they did find about half a dozen cases reported since 1845. Apparently five people have died from this bizarre reaction and the others needed emergency surgery.

Clearly, this kind of reaction is a medical rarity, but it reminds us to maintain moderation in all things. If we do overindulge, we should at least be cautious about how we seek relief. Nevertheless, for someone with a rare attack of indigestion without any complicating problems, sodium bicarbonate will do the job without straining the pocketbook.

What Works for Gas?

We aren't supposed to talk about this subject because most folks find it far too embarrassing. We have all sorts of silly terms for it—flatus, wind, toot. But gas is gas, and gross though it may be, it is hard to ignore.

Everyone makes gas. It can be uncomfortable, especially when restrained, noisily embarrassing when you are at a party or in a business meeting, and ultimately smelly. Given that there is a cultural taboo on the topic (except among teenage boys), it's no wonder that a lot of people suffer in smelly silence. Well, we think it is time someone cleared the air and fought the fight for the fart!

We're tired of such euphemisms as "breaking wind" or "passing gas." Whom are we kidding? The correct word is *farting*. Dr. W. C. Watson of Victoria Hospital in London, Ontario, Canada, encouraged his medical colleagues to use the word *fart*. Writing in the *New England Journal of Medicine*, he suggested that once people get used to the word *fart* it would "sound natural and as unremarkable as any other suitable clinical term. I hope that all other clinicians, men of honor and upright standing, will follow this lead. A spark has been struck, a torch has been lit. Let it shine forth and illumine the dark recesses of what has hitherto been that unspeakable thing. I am acknowledging the encouragement of the *Journal*, with fart healt thanks."[39]

Thank you, Dr. Watson, for liberating us. So what causes gassiness in the first place? For a long time physicians told people to stop chewing gum, sipping carbonated beverages, or drinking from fountains. The reason was purportedly swallowed air. But these days the experts in the field (flatologists study the fine art of farting) tell us that gas is created by bacteria that live in our large intestine. These little critters break down undigested carbohydrates. The fermentation process that results produces gas, sort of like the bubbles that emanate from a bottle of champagne, but a whole lot less appealing.

The flatologists say that the normal individual farts about 14 times daily. That equals anywhere from two to eight cups of gas. But some folks pass gas to excess. One poor fellow was urged to keep a fart chart (known medically as a "flatulographic record"). He monitored 141 "events" in a single day. This diary uncovered the culprit, which was milk. Lots of folks have a hard time handling milk and it can lead to gas, cramping, and diarrhea.

Other foods that are notorious for producing farts are apples, beans, bran, broccoli, brussels sprouts, cabbage, cauliflower, dried apricots, onions, prunes, radishes, and raisins. Keep your own fart chart and see which foods are most likely to make you pass gas.

Granola gurus are especially vulnerable. All those fruits, grains, and nuts can do some pretty awful things to your GI tract. But if you aren't willing to give up healthy foods, perhaps it's time for **Beano**. This little gem contains the enzyme alpha-galactosidase, which is supposed to break down the carbohydrates that the bacteria like to feast on. Whether it works or not remains open to debate. Some folks tell us it is fabulous. Others say forget it. For a free sample call (800) 257-8650.

One of our scientific cronies offers a different approach. He says that peppermint tea is just the ticket. Others tell us that activated charcoal (**Charcocaps, Charcoal Plus, Flatulex**) will trap gas in your digestive tract the same way it adsorbs noxious fumes in a gas mask. If milk is the problem, you can buy products, such as **Lactaid,** that contain the lactase enzyme necessary for breaking down milk sugar.

When all else fails, let that gas out. And if you get nasty stares, just use us as an excuse. We found a reference that blames the increasing difficulty with diverticular disease on our passion for polite restraint.[40] No more. Our battle cry is, "Don't fight the fart!"

Devilish Diarrhea

I t can strike at the most inopportune moments—before a speech, on a date, while on vacation. Sometimes it is the body's way of getting rid of nasty stuff you ate. Other times it's a bug, or more likely a virus. Whatever the cause, diarrhea can be embarrassing and uncomfortable. Diarrhea is not a subject for polite conversation and yet it has happened to almost everyone. People can talk about their itches, headaches, sports injuries, and operations without flinching. But diarrhea is off-limits.

The most effective OTC remedy was once available by prescription only. We like loperamide. First, it works. This drug slows down intestinal contractions and helps control fluid loss. It has relatively few side effects and can be safely given to children over six years of age. Loperamide is available in **Imodium A-D, Kaopectate II** caplets, **Maalox Anti-Diarrheal** caplets, and **Pepto Diarrhea Control**.

Side effects are not common with loperamide, but do not drive because you may experience drowsiness, dizziness, or impaired alertness and coordination. Other possible adverse reactions include dry mouth, nausea, vomiting, skin rash, and constipation. Don't use loperamide if you have fever or bloody stools, or if you suspect food poisoning.

We are also big fans of **Pepto-Bismol** (bismuth subsalicylate). It works great against traveler's diarrhea and is rapidly becoming a cornerstone in something called "triple therapy" against stomach ulcers caused by the bacterium *Helicobacter pylori*. It is not entirely clear why **Pepto-Bismol** works so well against diarrhea, but millions of people have been relying on the familiar pink liquid for generations. The "coating action" hypothesis has always seemed a little thin to us, but why mess with success?

The only cautions we can think of are: (1) Never give **Pepto-Bismol** to children who have chicken pox or the flu since the salicylate component may increase the risk of Reye's syndrome. (2) Don't take aspirin at the same time as **Pepto-Bismol**. It would be like doubling your dose. The salicylate ingredient is similar to aspirin and can interact with other drugs in a similar manner. If you are taking any medicines that interact with aspirin, they might also interact with **Pepto**. (3) Don't worry if your mouth, tongue, and stool temporarily turn gray or black. This is a common side effect of bismuth and doesn't seem to be anything to get too concerned about. Obviously, diarrhea that lasts should be diagnosed by a physician.

Saving Your Skin

A ging baby boomers are looking in the mirror and not enjoying the sight. The 40/50-something generations are discovering that they are paying a price for all those years of soaking up the rays. Sun damage is starting to show in the form of lines, red spots, wrinkles, furrows, freckles, and, worst of all, cancer.

Dermatologists tell us that skin cancer has become the most common cancer in the world. Anywhere from 700,000 to 1.2 million cases are diagnosed each year. Fortunately, these basal and squamous cancers are generally curable and do not pose a serious health hazard if caught early enough. They are especially common above the neck, showing up on lips, nose, and ears—places that are vulnerable to ultraviolet radiation from the sun. A bump, a pimple, or any sore that doesn't go away should be examined by a dermatologist. Any spot that appears pearly, thick, or crusted, and bleeds easily also deserves attention.

Melanoma is another kind of skin cancer that is rarer, but it can be a killer.

Over the last decade melanoma has become the fastest-rising cancer in the country. Dermatologists get concerned about any mole that changes in appearance. They look for irregular borders, wedge-shaped notches, and colors of red, white, or blue mixed in with the brown. Any mole that itches or is larger than a pencil eraser could be a problem. See a doctor promptly if you suspect any skin spot.

You would think that with the proliferation of highly effective sunscreens, sun damage and skin cancer would be on the decline. Actually, sunscreens may be part of the problem. The trouble is that they are almost too effective. Before high SPF (skin protection factor) products, most people used to be somewhat sensible about sun exposure. You couldn't spend hours out in the sun without getting a bad burn. People realized that they needed to wear protective clothing, hats, and eyewear. If they were going to spend a lot of time in the sun they needed to develop a tan gradually.

Then the outdoor generation discovered that effective sunscreens allowed hour after hour of fun in the sun with barely a tan, let alone a burn. Our friend Michael Castleman, writing in the magazine *Mother Jones*, presents the paradox quite elegantly: "In the last few decades, millions of people who cherish smoke detectors may have disabled one of nature's equally protective, if annoying, alarms. They've rubbed on sunscreen, never thinking that sunburns, like smoke alarms, might prevent a greater harm. Ironically, sunscreen devotees have turned off their dermatological smoke detectors in the name of preventive medicine."[41]

In other words, sunscreens have allowed us to spend far more time in the sun than we could have gotten away with a few decades ago. Since these products cannot filter all the sun's ultraviolet rays (UVA and UVC may still get through), damage can continue to occur even though we don't see it happening. There is also growing concern that sunscreens won't protect us from the known danger of immune suppression caused by sun exposure.[42]

A highly controversial article published in the *Journal of the National Cancer Institute* reported that sunscreens did not protect mice from melanoma. The researchers went so far as to conclude that "Sunscreen protection against UV radiation–induced inflammation may encourage prolonged exposure to UV radiation and thus may actually increase the risk of melanoma development."[43]

Where does all this sunscreen controversy leave us? You can't undo the damage caused by years of sun exposure. The skin can't forget or forgive all the insults it has experienced. You can prevent further harm, however. Wear a hat and protective clothing, and try to keep sun exposure to a minimum between 10 A.M. and 2 P.M. when the danger is greatest. Use 100-percent UV-filtered sunglasses to protect your eyes. If you do all the above you can slop on a high-SPF sunscreen to at least prevent any further assaults to your tender dermis. We also encourage oral vitamin D (at least 400 units daily) since sunscreens can prevent adequate absorption of this crucial vitamin, which may have anticancer benefits you wouldn't want to lose. Vitamin C and beta-carotene may also be important in protecting the skin and body against ultraviolet damage.[44]

Retin-A to the Rescue

Our favorite acne remedy is **Retin-A** (tretinoin). It has been around for decades, has a proven track record, and offers the added bonus of reversing some of our sun sins. There is now excellent data that **Retin-A** can partially repair sun damage that has accumulated over a lifetime.[45,46] People report **Retin-A** improves the tone and texture of their skin, and causes some of the fine wrinkles to disappear. More impressive, age or liver spots may go away, too. These brown freckles are clearly caused by sun exposure. **Renova** (tretinoin) has been approved by the FDA for wrinkles.

Finally, **Retin-A** may also work against solar (actinic) keratoses. These precancerous skin lesions may start as poorly defined red, scaly spots that sometimes go away, especially if a person regularly uses sunscreen or avoids the sun.[47] Less commonly they can show up as tan, pink or grayish rough bumps. Some people describe them as feeling like having a briar under the skin.

The dean of dermatologists, Dr. Albert KIigman, has used **Retin-A** successfully against these solar keratoses. One approach he has employed is to use **Retin-A** for about a month and then follow it with powerful prescription drugs—**Efudex** or **Fluoroplex** (fluorouracil)—for a couple of weeks. The **Retin-A** apparently helps "blast out" these incipient cancers in two to three weeks instead of the four or five weeks typical with fluorouracil alone—which can make the skin look like a "flaming torch."[48] Obviously, any treatment of solar keratoses requires a skilled dermatologist in charge. The point is that **Retin-A** isn't just for pimples anymore.

Using Retin-A

Please do not take this prescription cream for granted. It can leave your face red, dry, rough, and flaking if you aren't careful. Here are some guidelines. Check with your dermatologist for more detailed instructions.

- Start with a low concentration (0.025% or 0.05%) and work up. You may have to "toughen" up your face gradually over several months. If you have really fair or delicate skin you may have to start even lower with 0.01%.

- Never apply Retin-A after bathing. It should go on dry skin (at least half an hour after washing your face).

- Redness, irritation, flaking or excessive dryness mean you are overdoing it. Either go back to a lower concentration or skip a few days between applications. Always use a moisturizer (such as Purpose) to diminish dryness.

- Keep Retin-A away from eyes, which it can sting. Also avoid applying Retin-A in the folds or cracks near mouth or nose.

- Stay out of the sun or use a high-SPF sunscreen. Retin-A makes the skin far more vulnerable to a bad burn.

- Once you have maxed out on the benefits of Retin-A (usually after a year or so) it may be possible to go to a maintenance program. Two or three applications a week should suffice.

Attacking Acne

We used to think that pimples were the price you paid for passing through puberty. Surely when you reached adulthood zits would be a thing of the past. Sorry to say, a lot of older people are complaining about their complexions. Some women are finding that they break out around their periods, even at age twenty, thirty, or more. And post-pill pimples can be a temporary problems for some women after stopping birth control pills.

Let's destroy some myths. Acne is not caused by dirt. No amount of face washing will clear up pimples. Dermatologists tell us that overzealous washing with medicated soaps and abrasive scrubs can actually make things worse. Gentle washing (with or without soap) no more than two or three times a day is fine. Our preferred soap is **Dove** (either bar or liquid) because it remains one of the most gentle products on the market. *Consumer Reports* ranked **Dove** highly along with **Palmolive Green** and **Pure & Natural** as Best Buys. Alternatives to soap include **Cetaphil** or **Keri Facial Cleanser,** both of which are liquid, nondrying, and effective for removing makeup and keeping your face clean.

Next, forget the special diets. As far as we can tell, neither chocolate nor nuts will make a darn bit of difference. Low-fat foods make sense from a health perspective, but don't worry about a little chocolate now and again.

The Food and Drug Administration has approved three basic ingredients for OTC use against acne—salicylic acid, sulfur, and resorcinol. They are scruffers, that is, they stimulate cell turnover and shedding (otherwise known as keratolytic action). You will find one or more of these compounds in products including **Acnomel, Clearasil Adult Care, Clearasil Clearstick, Noxzema Clear-Ups** pads, **Pernox**, and **Stri-Dex**.

The most popular and aggressively advertised over-the-counter acne remedies contain the ingredient benzoyl peroxide. Despite the commercials, you cannot make acne disappear overnight with one swipe of a cleansing pad.

Benzoyl peroxide is found in a variety of brands including **Acne 5** and **10, Benoxyl 5** and **10, Clear By Design, Clearasil Benzoyl Peroxide, Fostex 10%**

BPO, Loroxide, Neutrogena Acne Mask, Noxzema Clear-Ups Acne Medicated Maximum Strength lotion, **Oxy-10 Daily Face Wash, Pan Oxyl Bar 5** and **10, Vanoxide**, and **Xerac BP5** and **10**.

Although benzoyl peroxide (BP) is widely advertised and sold, there is a cloud over its head. Questions have been raised about the meaning of studies showing tumor promotion in rodents.[49] While we wait for additional test results on carcinogenicity, the FDA has placed BP in bureaucratic limbo—Category III, insufficient data. Particular concern has been raised about whether BP will exaggerate the effect of the sun's rays to cause skin cancer. Until this issue is resolved, we recommend that most cases of acne be treated by a physician. To be truthful, prescription drugs are far more effective and perhaps safer than those available over the counter.

Retin-A has a proven track record against acne, plus the added benefits already discussed (see page 98). Dermatologists sometimes prescribe a topical antibiotic such as clindamycin (**Cleocin T**), erythromycin (**Akne-Mycin, A/T/Solution, Del-Mycin, C-Solve 2, Erycette, Eryderm 2%, Erymax, Erysol, T-Stat 2%,** and **Staticin**), or tetracycline (**Topicycline**) to help control a moderate-to-severe pimple problem. The benefit here is that when such antibiotics are put on the skin, there is far lower risk of systemic (whole body) side effects. Some dermatologists combine a topical antibiotic such as erythromycin with an OTC acne cream containing benzoyl peroxide to improve effectiveness. When all else fails, oral medicine works wonders.

Helping Your Hair

I s there anyone who hasn't had a bad hair day? Maybe the baldy brigade can't complain, but almost everyone else wishes her hair would do something different. People with curly hair envy those with straight. And, naturally, people with straight hair look longingly at those with a mass of curls.

The cosmetics companies have attempted to soothe our insecurities. They have developed shampoos for thin hair, brittle hair, colored hair, limp hair, oily hair, and dry hair. If you've gone shopping for shampoo lately, you might have wondered whether you had wandered into a restaurant by mistake.

If you're in the mood for dessert, you could pick lemon, chocolate, or strawberry mousse. But if you'd rather begin with breakfast, how about eggs, apples, apricots, wheat germ, or honey? If you're a health food purist seeking organic herbs, there's plenty to choose from: aloe vera with keratin, jojoba oil with biotin, henna, yarrow, coconut oil, almond oil, mistletoe, comfrey, rosemary, and ginseng, just for starters.

Shampoo labels also sport a wide range of vitamins, such as vitamin D, vitamin E, or panthenol, not to mention protein enrichers and minerals. Of course, if you're thirsty, you can look for a shampoo with milk, cocamilk, or beer. And if you like vegetables, check out the "**Australian Hair Salad**—an Endoplasmatic Hair Remoisturizer" with extracts of carrot, corn, cucumber, garlic, lettuce, tomato, and pineapple.

Do you get a stomachache just thinking about these shampoos? Your troubles have just begun. Now you need to pick between a "pH-balanced" product and one that's "non-alkaline," and decide whether your shampoo should contain DNA or RNA. And if you really want confusion, just turn over the bottle and look at the list of ingredients. It's hard to imagine anyone except a cosmetics chemist deciphering names like sodium hydroxymethane sulfonate, TEA-lauryl sulfate, FD&C red number 33, triethanolamine dimethicone, and guar hydroxypropyltrimonium chloride.

Confused? Ready to give up and grab the first bottle you find? You're not alone. It turns out that shampoo shoppers are notoriously fickle, ready to switch brands without turning a hair. And no wonder. Many products don't live up to expectations. For one thing, hair is dead. Vitamins, minerals, protein, DNA and RNA, eggs, or beer can't be absorbed into the hair shaft and make it healthier. Most of those fancy additives will be rinsed away with the dirt and the suds anyway.

But if you try to make it simple and just concentrate on whether your hair is dry or oily, you've still got problems. A *Consumer Reports* survey discovered that when people were not told what type of shampoo they were using, people with oily hair usually preferred shampoo formulated for dry hair and vice versa. As one leading hair expert points out, most people have both oily and dry hair on different parts of their scalp. Some shampoos for oily hair strip away too much oil with strong astringents so that after several uses the scalp starts making more oil to compensate. As a result, such shampoos may make the original problem worse.

So what is the answer to the shampoo stalemate? I'm afraid there are no rules that will work for everyone. Trial and error is unfortunately the only true test. For most people who shampoo several times a week, the milder the shampoo, the better. Even baby shampoo may be a good bet. So next time you go searching for a shampoo don't be taken in by long lists of ingredients or hints of gourmet gluttony. Save the vitamins, minerals, wheat germ, and honey for your breakfast cereal and the chocolate mousse or raspberry delight for dessert.

Shampoo should do one important thing—wash oil, dirt, and grime down the drain. Almost all brands do that just fine. *Consumer Reports* tested 50 shampoos and found that they all got hair clean.[50] By the way, so did **Ivory Dishwashing Liquid**.[51] The testers for Consumers Union concluded that searching for the perfect formulation is probably fruitless since people have a hard time telling the difference between shampoos for oily hair versus dry hair. For example, they found that **Fabergé Organics Normal** did the job equally well for both fine and normal hair, allowing for easy combing. And it did the job at a good price. People with fine hair especially liked **White Rain Extra Body** and **Suave Full Body**.

Conditioners Plus

The hottest development in hair care since the last edition of *The People's Pharmacy* has been the evolution of two-in-one products that contain both shampoo and conditioner. As aging baby boomers start covering the gray, they may want something such as **Alberto VO5 for Permed/Color-Treated Hair**. It apparently works quite well for damaged hair. *Consumer Reports* rated highly **Pantene Normal, Pert Plus Normal,** and **Nexxus Ensure** for normal hair and **White Rain Extra Body** and **Suave Full Body** as Best Buys for those with fine hair. If such shampoos leave your hair limp and oily, however, you may want to return to plain shampoo.

Dastardly Dandruff

Dandruff isn't a disease, but you'd never know that if you watch television. Commercials are designed to make you feel as if you'd die of embarrassment if a few white flakes ever showed up on your collar. The message is clear: give up on that promotion you were hoping for and forget your love life. Dandruff will turn you into a social outcast.

Balderdash! No matter how healthy your scalp may be, some scaling and flakiness is to be expected. About a third of the adult population suffers dandruff at one time or another. Dandruff is simply an acceleration of the normal process by which we shed external skin cells. Dandruff occurs when the rate of scalp shedding reaches two or three times normal, and when certain other changes lead to larger-than-normal clumps of cells. That makes what's normally invisible visible.

Dermatologists have been debating the causes of dandruff for decades. They have found that the condition is associated with a rapid turnover of cells on the scalp. Medicated shampoos were thought to slow cell growth. Now researchers believe there may be another explanation to account for severe dandruff. The yeast (fungus) *Pityrosporum ovale* is believed to be an important culprit behind the inflammation, itching, and scaling of seborrheic dermatitis and perhaps even garden-variety dandruff. If you want to impress your dermatologist next time you visit, ask about *Pityrosporum ovale* (Pit-er-oh-spore-umm oh-valley).

If dandruff is caused by a fungus, then anything that beats back this beastie should help control the scruffies. And to some extent most dandruff treatments on the OTC market do help knock down the population of yeast on your scalp. But before you resort to a medicated shampoo, why not try shampooing regularly with plain old ordinary shampoo. This has the virtue of being inexpensive, safe, and, in many cases, remarkably effective. By "regularly" we mean two to three times a week, not twice daily! Some people contribute to their dandruff problem by an active program of scalp abuse. Too much shampoo can dry out the scalp just as too much detergent can dry out your skin.

If regular shampooing doesn't do the trick, how about an inexpensive home remedy? Dr. Robert Gilgor is a smart dermatologist with a lot of good old-fashioned common sense. He recommends the following formula: Mix one part propylene glycol (100 percent) with four parts baby shampoo. The propylene glycol has antifungal properties that seem to keep dandruff under control. You can buy 100-percent propylene glycol from your pharmacist. It is a common ingredient in skin creams and lotions.

If certified dandruff shampoo is what you want, there are lots of good brands on the market. Unfortunately, few people know how to use them effectively. And there's the rub, or rather, the lack of it. We're an impatient bunch at best, used to fast food, instant breakfast, and quick cures. Somewhere on the label of most dandruff shampoos it says to lather up and let the stuff sit there for quite a chunk of time . . . say several minutes or more, at a minimum. But we're not a nation of careful label readers, and besides, five minutes can seem like a l-o-n-g time when you're standing there in the shower with your eyes closed knowing that if any of that stuff drips into an eyeball it's going to hurt.

Now hear this: The effectiveness of dandruff shampoos is closely pegged to the amount of contact time. Anything under the recommended time and you might as well be using pig grease. After spending a lot of money (dandruff shampoos do not come cheap, as you may already have discovered), why wash it down the drain? Learn to sing a five-minute song, get a tape of a five-minute egg cooking, or wear a headband to keep the shampoo out of the eyes and go on with your shower. By the time everything else is squeaky clean, the top will be done, too.

It is also helpful to rotate different types of antidandruff shampoos. If you use **Head & Shoulders, Breck One**, or **Zincon** (which contains zinc pyrithione), you might want to switch to a selenium-based product such as **Selsun Blue** after about six weeks. You could then return or go to a coal-tar brand such as **Neutrogena T/Sal, Ionil T Plus**, or **Zetar**.

Another option would be keratolytic shampoos. These chemical scruffers break down keratin, the hard outer layer of scalp cells, and thus facilitate the removal of this detritus from the head. The two major keratolytic agents are sulfur, in a concentration of 2% to 5%, and salicylic acid in a concentration of 2% to 3%. Among the shampoos containing one or both of these agents in some form are **Cuticura Anti-Dandruff Shampoo, Diasporal, Ionil, Meted, Neutrogena T/Sal, Sebucare, Sebulex Medicated, Sebutone**, and **Sulray.**

If neither the home remedy nor usual dandruff shampoos work well, it's time to consult a dermatologist. One of the most effective treatments for dandruff is a prescription containing the antifungal medicine ketoconazole. Sold as **Nizoral 2%,** this shampoo works extremely well against seborrheic dermatitis and hard-to-treat dandruff. An OTC **Nizoral Shampoo** (1% solution) is one of our favored choices.

If you visit a dermatologist, he or she will be able to determine if the flakes are due to dandruff or to some other cause. Dry skin, which is often aggravated in the winter, occasionally causes scalp flaking. Psoriasis, a condition that causes very rapid cell turnover, might also account for serious snow on the shoulders.

In the Pits with Antiperspirants

We live in a sanitized society. Killing germs and stamping out odors is practically a national pastime. We have deodorant soaps, deodorant tampons, foot deodorants, underarm deodorants, and more recently, genital deodorants. We fork over more than a billion bucks a year to smell sweet.

Now we're as offended by unpleasant smells as the next guy, but enough is enough. Cleanliness may be next to godliness, but this passion for sterilizing our skin and deodorizing body cavities has very little to do with personal hygiene. Seriously, folks, aren't genital deodorants carrying things a bit too far?

Body odor occurs when bacteria normally present on the skin attach to and decompose organic material in perspiration. Since we all sweat to one degree or another, we all smell sometimes. On the average we put out around one-half quart of sweat a day. It is a means of maintaining body temperature and is really an important body process.

Nervous tension and emotional stress can contribute a significant amount of sweat above the normal level. This nervous sweat comes from an entirely different set of pores, and seems to be broken down much more readily by bacteria. There really is a "smell of fear."

Obviously, good hygiene (lots of soap and water) will go a long way toward keeping down both the bacterial level and the accumulation of sweat. This should also help control nasty smells. But you can't shower five times a day, and clearly there are times when you really do need that "all-day protection." Since we cannot keep our underarms clean and dry all the time, an armpit juice is a handy thing to have around. But what to pick?

Some advertisers try to lure you with claims of extra-long-lasting protection while others maintain that their brand goes on dry. Then there's the equivalent of the "**Maalox** moment" strategy—this antiperspirant magically springs into action when you're under heavy-duty pressure.

Since there are relatively few active ingredients in most of the brands on the market, the companies spend incredible sums trying to come up with subtle variations so they can create new and innovative advertising campaigns.

Take a long, careful look at the Personal Care section next time you're at the store. Some armpit products say they're an "antiperspirant" or an "antiperspirant deodorant" while others stick with plain old-fashioned "deodorants."

What's the difference? The key is in the name. It tells you just what the stuff will and won't do. An antiperspirant contains a chemical capable of reducing perspiration by decreasing flow from one of the two types of sweat glands. This is the antiwetness approach. Interestingly, the FDA considers this process a physiological change; ergo antiperspirants are classified as drugs and come under agency review. Deodorants, on the other hand, are intended to mask odor either by adding a perfume or killing germs. They are classified as cosmetics and avoid careful FDA scrutiny. To make matters more confusing—there are gobs of products that claim to be both.

Just how antiperspirants work is still something of a mystery. It was once thought that they reduced wetness because they were astringents—chemicals that caused shrinking and closing of the pores. We now know, however, that many astringents aren't very effective antiperspirants, so scratch that theory. Some researchers think that the chemicals cause sweat ducts to swell. Others offer the hypothesis that the antiperspirants plug up the ducts through which perspiration travels. Suffice it to say, we still don't know exactly what's going on.

One important fact to understand about antiperspirants is that they're not very good at closing off the flow of sweat from the second, "nervous" set of sweat glands. If it's your first date with someone you really like, a speech in front of a big audience, or an important meeting with the boss, all the Industrial-Strength Pit Protection in the world is not going to keep you dry.

In fact, all the antiperspirants can do is reduce—by an average of 20 percent to 40 percent—the flow of moisture. Some are better at the job than that, and some will work better for a given person than another, so when it comes to dampening the flow, a bit of experimentation is in order.

The most popular ingredients in antiperspirants are aluminum salts—aluminum chlorohydrates, aluminum zirconium chlorohydrates, etc. They also have some antibacterial action and therefore diminish odor as well. There are so many brands on the market we wouldn't know where to start. Differences in effectiveness are hard to prove, so trial and error should be your way of selecting a brand.

There is one product that may be more effective—and irritating—than the other antiperspirants. Heavy-duty drippers may want to look for an old-fashioned ingredient called aluminum chloride. It can be found in a prescription product called **Drysol** (20%) or over the counter as **Xerac AC** (6.25%) and **Certan-Dri.**

Here are some tips on getting the most out of an aluminum chloride antiperspirant. Apply it sparingly to DRY skin. These products can be quite irritating, so it is important not to aggravate that by putting them on wet or freshly shaved underarms. The best time to apply any antiperspirant is in the evening before bed. Although most people include antiperspirant in their morning ritual, these products do better if you give them a head start. And don't worry about it washing off. You may find that you need to apply it only two or three times a week.

What about aluminum? One of the questions we are asked most frequently concerns the safety of aluminum, especially in antiperspirants. (See the discussion of aluminum and Alzheimer's disease on page 90.) What we cannot answer is whether there is any danger from such antiperspirants. We have asked world-class dermatologists who study such things for cosmetics companies. About all we get in response is a shoulder shrug. They tell us that there are no good studies or definitive answers. So, at the time of this writing we can say only that we do not know if aluminum is absorbed into the body from an antiperspirant, or, if it were, whether it would pose any danger. Sorry.

So much for wetness. Now there's the problem of odor. Enter the second set of labels—for deodorants plain and simple. A deodorant is something that decreases odor. It can do that by reducing the bacteria, reducing the material they work on, or by simply sloshing on enough perfume to cover up the whole problem.

The antibacterial approach sounds logical, just as it sounds logical that a mouthwash that kills "millions of germs on contact" should be good for something. The problem in this instance is that it's hard to know just which bacteria, in just what quantity, actually cause an odor problem.

So if we don't know what to kill, or how much killing to do, how can the problem be solved? But you should realize by now that lack of information rarely ever stops cosmetics companies. Undaunted, manufacturers put in various "germ killers," such as triclosan, presumably on the assumption that the more bacteria you kill the better off you are. We're not convinced, but antibacterial agents are relatively benign, though some people do develop allergic reactions with continual use.

No matter what antiperspirant/deodorant you select, be aware of the following:

1. These products will be rendered useless if applied to pores that are already sweating. Apply only to a clean, dry underarm.

2. Never apply any of these products immediately after shaving the area, or if there's any kind of a cut or open sore.

3. People differ remarkably in their responses to the various chemicals. If one doesn't work, try another.

4. No antiperspirant will shut off sweat from the "nervous" pores. Don't expect the impossible.

5. Normal antiperspirants reduce somewhat the normal volume of sweat. They will not do the trick if you are an incredibly profuse sweater. In that case you'll need something that contains aluminum chloride.

Antiperspirants form a genre of OTC products in which there is virtually no difference among dozens of competing brands in terms of the active ingredients. The only real differences are in meaningless things such as whether the manufacturer makes it smell like a musk or a meadow, in the packaging, and in the promotion.

As a smart consumer, you'll first decide which of the two or three major ingredients consistently does the job for you and then shop for a product containing that ingredient at the lowest price per application.

Athlete's Foot:
An Itch That's Hard to Scratch

I t's fun to report on categories of OTC remedies in which there have been great strides since the first edition of *The People's Pharmacy*, and this is certainly one of those areas. Athlete's foot is nothing more than a fungus infection. Remember "There's a fungus among us" from grade-school days? Well, athlete's foot is a fungus among the toes, where it takes root and happily grows fully supplied with everything it needs—warmth, moisture, and a friendly surface to live on.

Though we say it's "just a fungus," don't underestimate athlete's-foot infections. They can be downright nasty, especially if you let them run wild before setting up a defense. At first the symptoms may just be a bit of redness between the toes, and a slight itch. Before long, there are deep cracks and fissures; raw, macerated skin; severe itching, burning, and pain.

Anyone who's ever fought the athlete's-foot battle knows that the fungus can be tough to eradicate. One of the reasons for that, scientists have learned, is that the infections are sometimes a mixture of fungus and bacteria, each contributing to the attack on and destruction of the skin between your toes. (When this is the case, an aluminum chloride solution may work wonders.) There is also speculation that our immune systems play an important defensive role. Why is it, for example, that some people can walk barefoot on a wet locker-room floor day after day and never come down with athlete's foot while someone else can pick up the darn stuff after only one exposure?

For a long, long time about the best science could offer over the counter were things such as **Whitfield's Ointment**. These products were generally a mixture of benzoic and salicycic acids, and they didn't exactly cause the fungus to run and hide.

There was also undecylenic acid and zinc undecylenate, which came to you as **Blis-To-Sol, Cruex,** and, **Desenex.** The problem with undecylenic acid was that it could just about achieve a standoff. The fungal infection usually stopped getting worse, but, for many, it never quite went away. Or if the athlete's foot did disappear, it often came back when the medicine was discontinued. Undecylenic acid was better at control than eradication, and it tended to work best on the more superficial infections. People sometimes complained about its odor.

Then along came tolnaftate **(Tinactin).** It was one of the first prescription-to-OTC switches. Eventually the drug became available under lots of brand names including **Absorbine Antifungal Foot Cream** and **Powder, Aftate, Desenex Spray Liquid, Dr. Scholl's Athlete's Foot, Genaspor, NP-27, Podactin, Tinactin, Ting**, and **Tritin (Dr. Scholl's).** This chemical is much more adept at rooting out the stubborn fungal invaders, apparently by disrupting their means of reproduction. It was a major breakthrough in treating athlete's foot—significantly better (and, of course, significantly more expensive) than its predecessors.

Once again there have been advances in nonprescription treatment for athlete's foot. You can now obtain the drug miconazole as **Antifungal Cream–Athlete's Foot** and **Micatin.** This is really a heavy-duty fungal fighter. It's been in use for many years to treat a variety of fungal infections. Many of our female readers might recognize miconazole as **Monistat,** a cream frequently prescribed for vaginal fungal infections and now available over the counter as **Monistat 7.**

Miconazole is a big improvement. So is another formerly prescription-only antifungal—clotrimazole. It is available as **Lotrimin AF Cream** and **Solution** and **Mycelex OTC.** The same compound is found in the vaginal creams **Gyne-Lotrimin** and **Mycelex-7.**

No matter which athlete's-foot remedy you select, it takes a while to get the job done. Fungi are much more tenacious than bacteria, which can often be killed in just hours. So be patient, keep your tootsies nice and dry, and keep using the antifungal goo long after you think you have rid yourself of those beastly yeasties. Eventually you should be able to put your best foot forward . . . without having to scratch it.

Warts, Corns, and Calluses

W hen we were kids we would have given anything for a jar of spunk water. We didn't know what it was, but we knew Huck Finn and Tom Sawyer used it to get rid of warts.

No such luck for us. Our parents dragged us off to doctors, who burned, blistered, froze, or surgically removed the warts. At one time X-rays were actually used to treat recalcitrant plantar warts. Eeeek! No matter what you may have heard, warts don't come from frogs or toads. Warts are caused by a virus that can spread from one part of the body to another, or from one person to another. Although warts have been around for as long as we have records of people, they're still surrounded by much mystery and mystique.

And little wonder. Warts can pop up literally overnight, appearing out of nowhere to stick out their cauliflowery little noses at us in sheer defiance. Like some sort of guerrilla fighter, warts are tough, wily, and seemingly indestructible. Yet left alone, about one-third will disappear of their own free will within a year. Few linger forever.

It's this tendency to disappear as silently and quickly as they came that has through the eons tended to make believers of people who've applied all manner of disgusting material to their warts and then seen them go away. That's what's behind the "success" of spunk water, pennies, potatoes, and dead cats.

That and the power of the mind. Dr. Lewis Thomas was one of this country's foremost medical professors, thinkers, and writers. He was professor of pathology and medicine at Cornell University and president of the Memorial Sloan–Kettering Cancer Center. He described the wart mystery this way: "It is one of the great mystifications of science: Warts can be ordered off the skin by hypnotic suggestion. Not everyone believes this, but the evidence goes back a long way and is persuasive. Generations of internists and dermatologists, and their grandmothers for that matter, have been convinced of the phenomenon."[52]

How the unconscious mind can mobilize the body's immune system, wiping the wart from the body, is one of medicine's mysteries. If it could be solved, we might be on our way to overcoming many of the most vexing problems related to the body's immune capabilities.

Meanwhile, there you are with your warts, and you don't want to wait until your mind makes itself up to will them away, or until they just get up and go. What does the local pharmacy have to offer that might hasten the process?

Before applying anything, make certain you've got a do-it-yourself wart. The only two types safe for home treatment are common warts of the hands or fingers and plantar warts, which occur on the soles of the feet. If you have anything else, or have a simple wart anywhere else, take it to the doctor.

The choice of materials is easy, because in reviewing wart cures the FDA panel on miscellaneous external drug products found only one thing in the "safe and effective" category. That ingredient was salicylic acid in strengths from 5% to 17% in a collodion-like vehicle (such as liquid glue) or 12% to 40% in a plaster vehicle (impregnated into a tape or bandage). The identical ingredient works for corns and calluses.

Some of the brand names are **Clear Away Plantar Wart Remover System, Compound W Wart Remover, Corn Fix, Dr. Scholl's Callus Removers, DuoFilm, DuoPlant Plantar Wart Remover for Feet, Freezone, Occlusal HP, Off Ezy Wart Remover Kit, PediaPath, Wart Fix**, and **Wart-Off.**

A couple of things to know before slathering, slapping, dripping, or pasting on any of these products. First, the preparation is basically skin eater. So don't get it anywhere you don't want skin eaten. Second, salicylic acid works best when it is held in direct contact with the skin and covered with a waterproof material, to hold in moisture. A plaster of salicylic acid fills the bill and can be easily cut, placed over the wart, and changed every few days. Plasters are available in much greater strengths (up to 40%) under names such as **Clear Away Wart Remover System,** and **DuoFilm Patch System Wart Remover.** This greater strength is necessary and acceptable in the plaster.

Third, and most important, do not treat yourself for warts (or any other foot problem) if you have diabetes or circulatory problems. And do be patient. Sometimes it can seem like ages before a wart goes away. Patience is the most valuable aid in successful wart therapy. If nothing OTC seems to work, you may want to give home remedies a whirl (see pages 132–133 in Chapter 6). And when all else fails, see a dermatologist. They can prescribe some powerful drugs that usually work on even the most resistant warts.

For Women Only

For reasons best left to chroniclers of American society, women have been a major target audience for all sorts of "made-up" products. By that we mean products that exist more by virtue of their advertising than anything else. First they were invented, then a "need" was created by intensive promotion.

Drug manufacturers have played on the fears and insecurities of generations of women to create such non-products as vaginal deodorants. Perhaps the most blatant example of a made-up product is "feminine hygiene sprays." At least that's what they were called when first marketed. The FDA finally awakened to the fact that there was nothing hygienic about these sprays, and forced the manufacturers to drop all references to hygiene.

Undaunted, the hype masters convinced goodness knows how many women to pay millions of dollars out of fear that they were suddenly (after having survived many generations without such a product) desperately in need of deodorizing their vaginas.

This is such hogwash that it's unbelievable, but obviously some women bought into the notion. A normal, healthy vagina doesn't need to be dosed and doused with a chemical spray containing perfumes, propellants, and solvents of various sorts. Such compounds could irritate sensitive skin, and there have indeed been reports of adverse reactions to vaginal spray products.

And please don't overdose on douches. The vaginal tract is highly capable of absorbing almost anything that comes into contact with it. Remember, douches contain lots of chemicals that Mother Nature never intended for your genital tract.

While there may occasionally be some medical reason for douching, several studies have reported an increased risk of PID (pelvic inflammatory disease) in women who douche regularly. The force of water may spread bacteria from the vagina into other reproductive organs and lead to infection. This could eventually cause ectopic pregnancies or infertility.[53,54] Ectopic pregnancy can be deadly. We lost Carol, a very dear friend, from complications of an ectopic pregnancy. We would hate for this to happen to anyone else.

The best "feminine deodorant" is still soap and water. If you have an offensive vaginal odor that soap and water can't get rid of, see a doctor. There's a good chance you've got an infection, which should be treated medically, not cosmetically.

Yeastie Beasties

Speaking of infections, one of the most common has to do with fungi, also known as yeast. Other terms for this problem are moniliasis or vaginal thrush. The culprit is usually *Candida albicans*, a fungus that lives on skin and in the digestive tract, and can sometimes be cultured within the vagina when a woman is perfectly healthy and has no symptoms.

For reasons that aren't perfectly clear, this yeast can grab a foothold under a variety of conditions. Broad-spectrum antibiotics can upset the delicate balance of flora and fauna within the genital tract. Cortisone-type drugs, immune-suppressing medicines, obsessive douching, and birth control pills may also increase the risk of infection, as can pregnancy, diabetes, and maybe even pantyhose.

A physician can quickly diagnose yeast by taking a vaginal smear and looking at it under a microscope. And if you have never experienced anything like the discharge and itch, you really need a doctor's diagnosis. There are many infections that can cause vaginal problems, and only yeast will respond well to the antifungal medicines available over the counter.

Remember, too, that sometimes there may be two or three infections coexisting. Some, like *Chlamydia,* are nearly silent and yet can do devastating damage. Untreated, it could result in infertility. So if you have any question at all about whether you have a yeast infection or something else, make an appointment with your doctor. Do the same if your yeast infection doesn't respond to over-the-counter treatment, or if it comes back quickly or repeatedly.

What symptoms should make you suspect a yeast infection? Dr. Marvin C. Rulin suggested the mnemonic COITAL. Here's what it means: the Color of the discharge is white. The Odor is minimal or yeasty. The Itching can be intense. The Texture is thick and lumpy—like cottage cheese. The Amount of discharge is scanty. The Look of the vulva and vaginal tissue is beefy red, maybe swollen.

Your first experience with such symptoms should NOT send you to the drugstore for **Gyne-Lotrimin, Mycelex-7** or **Monistat 7**. Get a doctor's diagnosis first, then pick up your fungus fighters. House-brand generics are widely available. Look for the best price on miconazole or clotrimazole. Any of these products, which come as vaginal tablets, vaginal suppositories, or vaginal creams, can clear up a simple yeast infection if used every night at bedtime for a week. Side effects are uncommon but be alert for burning, itching, or irritation.

More than any other drugs on pharmacy shelves, these vaginal yeast medicines demonstrate the power now available to consumers without a prescription, and the risks we assume when we use it.

Only a few years ago, all these vaginal creams and tablets required a prescription—a doctor's diagnosis. The FDA decided that women who had already suffered through one yeast infection could probably recognize it when it struck again (as they do all too often). But infectious-disease experts worry that some women will self-diagnose incorrectly, use the medicine for too long, and end up with serious pelvic inflammatory disease as a consequence of some other bug going untreated.

We are also concerned about products designed to treat symptoms of yeast overgrowth without curing the underlying infection. We have seen the proliferation of products containing hydrocortisone, diphenhydramine (an antihistamine that can cause an allergic rash), and benzocaine (a local anesthetic that may also trigger contact dermatitis). Please read labels carefully and make sure that the product you buy can deal with the cause of the problem.

If you use good common sense, you can benefit from over-the-counter products. If something doesn't fit the pattern, though, don't waste a lot of time wondering about it. Check in with an expert for guidance. Ask your pharmacist, doctor, or nurse practitioner. You'll end up a wiser and better consumer of over-the-counter drugs.

References

1. Gannon, Kathi. "Tracking OTC/HBC Sales: Drugstores Vs. Food Stores." *Drug Topics* 1993; 137(10): 45–64.
2. Gannon, Kathi. "OTCs: Shelf Busters—Analyzing Nonprescription Drug Trends." *Drug Topics* 1993; 137(2): 34–41.
3. "Best Selling OTCs." *Drug Store News* 1984; May 19:59–67.
4. Elliott, Stuart. "For the Latest in Pain Relief, Try a $100 Million Campaign." *The New York Times* 1994; June 17:D1–D15.
5. Bird, Laura. "P&G's New Analgesic Promises Pain for Over-the-Counter Rivals." *The Wall Street Journal* 1994; June 16:B9.
6. Associated Press. "Boomers' Next Trend: Arthritis." *The Herald-Sun* 1994; June 24:A4.
7. Schactel, B. P., et al. "Headache Pain Model for Assessing and Comparing Efficacy of Over-the-Counter Analgesic Agents." *Clin. Pharmacol. Ther.* 1991; 50:322–329.
8. Silverman, Kenneth, et al. "Withdrawal Syndrome After the Double-Blind Cessation of Caffeine Consumption." *N. Engl. J. Med.* 1992; 327:1109–1114.
9. Saper, Joel R., et al. *Handbook of Headache Management: A Practical Guide to Diagnosis and Treatment of Head, Neck, and Facial Pain.* Baltimore: Williams & Wilkins, 1993, p. 37.
10. Saper, Joel R., et al. *Handbook of Headache Management: A Practical Guide to Diagnosis and Treatment of Head, Neck, and Facial Pain.* Baltimore: Williams & Wilkins, 1993.
11. Cooper, Helene. "Warning: Americans Overuse Over-the-Counter Drugs." *The Wall Street Journal* 1994; January 11:B1.
12. Willett, Laura Rees, et al. "Epidemiology of Gastrointestinal Damage Associated with Nonsteroidal Anti-Inflammatory Drugs." *Drug Safety* 1994; 10(2):170–181.
13. Paulus, H. E. "FDA Arthritis Advisory Committee Meeting: Post-Marketing Surveillance of Non-Steroidal Anti-Inflammatory Drugs." *Arthritis Rheum.* 1985; 28:1168–1169.
14. Fries, James F. "NSAID Gastropathy: Epidemiology." *J. Musculoskeletal Med.* 1991; 8(2): 21–28.
15. Horgan, Constance, et al. "Substance Abuse: The Nation's Number One Health Problem." Prepared by the Institute for Health Policy, Brandeis University for The Robert Wood Johnson Foundation, Princeton, N.J., October 1993, p. 37.
16. Wilcox, C. Mel, et al. "Striking Prevalence of Over-the-Counter Nonsteroidal Anti-Inflammatory Drug Use in Patients with Upper Gastrointestinal Hemorrhage." *Arch. Intern. Med.* 1994; 154:42–46.

17. Bradley, John D., et al. "Comparison of an Anti-inflammatory Dose of Ibuprofen, an Analgesic Dose of Ibuprofen, and Acetaminophen in the Treatment of Patients with Osteoarthritis of the Knee." *N. Engl. J. Med.* 1991: 325:87–91.

18. Whitcomb, David C., and Geoffrey D. Block. "Association of Acetaminophen Hepatotoxicity with Fasting and Ethanol Use." *JAMA* 1994; 272:1845–1850.

19. Perneger, Thomas V., et al. "Risk of Kidney Failure Associated with the Use of Acetaminophen, Aspirin, and Nonsteroidal Antiinflammatory Drugs." *N. Engl. J. Med.* 1994; 331:1675–1679.

20. Fries, J. F., et al. "A Reevaluation of Aspirin Therapy in Rheumatoid Arthritis." *Arch. Intern. Med.* 1993; 153:2465–2471.

21. Aldhous, Peter. "A Hearty Endorsement for Aspirin." *Science* 1994; 263:24.

22. The Dutch TIA Trial Study Group. "A Comparison of Two Doses of Aspirin (30 mg vs. 283 mg a Day) in Patients After a Transient Ischemic Attack or Minor Stroke." *N. Engl. J. Med.* 1991; 325:1261–1266.

23. Lee, Makau, et al. "Dose Effects of Aspirin on Gastric Prostaglandins and Stomach Mucosal Injury." *Ann. Int. Med.* 1994; 120:184–189.

24. Schreinemachers, Dina M., and Richard B. Everson, "Aspirin Use and Lung, Colon, and Breast Cancer Incidence in a Prospective Study." *Epidemiology* 1994; 5:138–146.

25. "Aspirin and Multi-Infarct Dementia." *Physicians' Drug Alert* 1989; August:58.

26. Breitner, J. C. S., et al. "Inverse Association of Anti-Inflammatory Treatments and Alzheimer's Disease: Initial Results of a Co-Twin Control Study." *Neurology* 1994; 44:227–232.

27. Gannon, Kathi. "OTCs: Shelf Busters—Analyzing Nonprescription Drug Trends." *Drug Topics* 1993; 137(2): 34–41.

28. "Antacids: Which Beat Heartburn Best? *Consumer Reports* 1994; 59(7) July:443–447.

29. Ibid.

30. Ibid.

31. Shigematsu, K., and P. L. McGeer, "Accumulation of Amyloid Precursor Protein in Damaged Neuronal Processes and Microglia Following Intracerebral Administration of Aluminum Salts." *Brain Res.* 1992; 593:117–123.

32. Garruto, R. M. "Pacific Paradigms of Environmentally-Induced Neurological Disorders: Clinical, Epidemiological and Molecular Perspectives." *Neurotoxicology* 1991; 12:347–378.

33. Harrington, C. R., et al. "Alzheimer's-Disease-Like Changes in Tau Protein Processing: Association with Aluminum Accumulation in Brains of Renal Dialysis Patients." *Lancet* 1994; 343:993–997.

34. Rifat, S. L. "Aluminum Hypothesis Lives." *Lancet* 1994; 343:3–4.

35. *Consumer Reports*, op. cit.

36. Ibid.

37. ISIS-2 (Second International Study of Infarct Survival) Collaborative Group. "Randomised Trial of Intravenous Streptokinase, Oral Aspirin, Both, or Neither Among 17,187 Cases of Suspected Acute Myocardial Infarction." *Lancet* 1988; ii: 349–360.

38. Horwitz, Nathan. "Wider Scope for Aspirin Urged: Top Cardiologists Say FDA Approval Could Save 30,000 Lives a Year." *Medical Tribune* 1993; 34(9):1

39. Watson, W. C. "Speaking the Unspeakable." *N. Engl. J. Med.* 1978; 299:494.

40. Wynne-Jones, Geoffrey. "Flatus Retention Is the Major Factor in Diverticular Disease." *Lancet* 1975; 2:211–212.

41. Castleman, Michael. "Beach Bummer." *Mother Jones* 1993; May/June:33–37.

42. Mechcatie, Elizabeth. "Sunscreen May Not Protect Against Immunosuppression." *Skin & Allergy News* 1993; March:9.

43. Wolf, Peter, et al. "Effect of Sunscreens on UV Radiation-Induced Enhancement of Melanoma Growth in Mice." *J. Natl. Cancer Inst.* 1994; 86:99–105.

44. "Beta-Carotene Battles Sun Damage." *Men's Confidential* 1993; 11(7):4.

45. "Retin-A Reduced Photodamage in 68% of Subjects Using .05% Concentration." *FDC Reports (The Rose Sheet)* 1990; January 8; 11(2):1–2.

46. Hanahan, John F. "Preliminary Drug Effects Show Continued Success in Photoaging." *Dermatology Times* 1989; October; 10(10):2,4.

47. Thompson, Sandra C., et al. "Reduction of Solar Keratoses by Regular Sunscreen Use." *N. Engl. J. Med* 1993; 329:1147–1151.

48. "Tretinoin Q&A." *Dermatology Times* 1989; March; 10(3):22.

49. "NDMA's Benzoyl Peroxide 13-Week Oncogenicity Studies Expected to Begin by End of Year." *The Tan Sheet* 1993; 1(38).

50. "Shampoos & Conditioners: Heading Off the Hype." *Consumer Reports* 1992; 57(6):395–403.

51. "Shampoos." *Consumer Reports* 1989; 54(2):95–99.

52. Thomas, Lewis. In *The Medusa and the Snail.* New York: Viking, 1979.

53. Washington, A. Eugene, et al. "Preventing Pelvic Inflammatory Disease." *JAMA* 1991; 266:2574–2481.

54. Wolner-Hanssen, Pal, et al. "Association Between Vaginal Douching and Acute Pelvic Inflammatory Disease." *JAMA* 1990; 263:1936–1942.

Sexy Trade Secrets and Home Remedies

Americans have traditionally been self-reliant. The do-it-yourself mentality has long been popular here, perhaps out of necessity. Frontier families taming the wilderness could hardly run to the doctor for every ache or pain. They developed an appreciation for Grandma's homespun wisdom about how to soothe a cough or quiet an itch. In some places, they also came to respect the knowledge of the Indians, whose experience had taught them much about the useful properties of the local plants.

As the country modernized, home remedies fell out of favor. Telephones and automobiles made it possible for most people to get to the doctor and get modern medical treatment. Specialization within the medical profession and increasingly sophisticated drugs and medical technology undermined people's faith in simple remedies.

It was no longer enough to see the doctor; you had to see a specialist. And the specialist would have to do some fancy tests, like an MRI (magnetic resonance imaging) for a backache. By the time you'd spent all that money, a new neurosurgeon or orthopedist, fresh out of medical residency, might be embarrassed to tell you just to go home and rest for a few days, or do some back exercises. Out would come the prescription pad and off you'd go for a heavy-duty prescription pain medicine.

But although medical practice has continued to become more high-tech and specialized than ever, the situation is changing. Americans are disenchanted with a medical system that seems preoccupied with treating disease rather than preventing illness. The public is also starting to revolt against the ever-increasing costs of both medical insurance and physicians' fees. Although by the 1970s the Food and Drug Administration was ready to relegate herbal remedies to history, it is clear that is not happening. People are turning in increasing numbers to alternative or unconventional therapies such as acupuncture or chiropractic. One survey showed one person out of every three had tried at least one alternative therapy within the past year.[1]

This is not simply the desperation strategy of people who can't afford medical care. In a landmark study published in the *New England Journal of Medicine*, researchers found that the people most likely to consult unconventional practitioners were on the whole younger, more educated, and better off than the rest of the people in the study.[2] Study results suggest that "in 1990 Americans made an estimated 425 million visits to providers of unconventional therapy. This number exceeds the number of visits to all U.S. primary care physicians (388 million)."[3] In many cases, such visits are not covered by insurance and must be paid for out of the patient's pocket.

More and more, people are interested in striving for optimal health rather than settling for some doctor-defined "norm." Nutrition and exercise have almost become national obsessions. Self-care and nondrug alternatives are growing in acceptability. The interest in home remedies has grown at the same time.

Doctors don't know quite what to make of home remedies and alternative medicine approaches, and for good reason. In medical school they learn they are supposed to evaluate therapies on the basis of data from well-designed clinical studies. But good double-blind controlled studies of home remedies are mighty scarce, and even mediocre studies aren't easy to find. Still, we're always in favor of good old-fashioned common sense. In this chapter we are celebrating a return to home remedies. We will examine some things you can do without a doctor to relieve a wide range of minor problems. Some of these ideas have been tested and reported in prestigious medical journals; others are just passing notes whose appearance is justified because they simply seem to make sense. And many others come from you, our readers, who have been extraordinarily enthusiastic in sharing the remedies that work for you. Keep sending them in. We love it!

Chicken Soup and the
Case for Self-Treatment

Home remedies are folk medicine, which simply means they are healing methods people use without consulting a doctor. Some home remedies have been passed from generation to generation by word of mouth. Others have come to the attention of medical people who are often skeptical, but who may adopt them if they seem to fit into scientific knowledge of the time. It's always nice to have a medical endorsement for a home remedy, but that still doesn't tell us for sure whether or not it actually works. The home remedies we're about to discuss do have two advantages: they are available without a prescription, and they're easy to use.

Take chicken soup, for example. In fact, taking chicken soup for a cold is just what the Mayo Clinic has suggested in its *Health Letter*.[4] There has actually been some research on the uses of Grandma's favorite "antibiotic," and there's evidence that chicken soup does more to relieve cold symptoms than other hot liquids. By the way, our best source on natural remedies describes chicken soup thus: "Chicken soup is obtained from a hot water infusion of selected parts of the common chicken *Gallus domesticus*."[5]

"Chicken soup," says the Mayo Clinic's distinguished health letter, "is a safe, effective treatment for many 'self-limiting' illnesses (those not requiring professional attention). It is inexpensive and widely available. Side effects are few, with the notable exception of weight gain if it is used excessively. . . ."

"Next time you come down with a head cold," the letter concludes, "try hot homemade chicken soup before heading for the pharmacy. We believe chicken soup can be an excellent treatment for uncomplicated head colds and other viral respiratory infections for which antibiotics ordinarily are not helpful."

So there you have it, straight from one of the most respected institutions in American medicine. A home remedy works. It works well. It works better than anything modern medical science has to offer, and like most home remedies it does the job cheaper than anything you can buy to treat the problem. What's more, the risk of side effects or problems is almost nonexistent, and that's not always true of over-the-counter cold and flu medicines.

There's no doubt about it, home remedies can be great. But that doesn't make *all* home remedies great, useful, or even safe. Like all medication, home remedies have to be used carefully. The most critical factor is deciding when a home remedy is appropriate.

The trick to doctoring yourself lies in knowing when not to do it. Most of the conditions we'll discuss in this chapter are benign ones—those that are uncomfortable, irritating, sometimes even maddening, but not life-threatening. They're the kinds of conditions for which it's unlikely you would be much the worse for wear if another day or two passed without medical attention other than a home remedy. As it turns out, many minor illnesses are "self-limiting." Translation: It will go away by itself in seven days if you take medicine, or in a week if you leave it alone. (That will be $35, please.)

With the national medical tab rapidly running out of control, there's a strong argument to be made for each of us doing what we can to take care of ourselves in situations where such an attempt doesn't run any serious risk of doing damage. It's up to you to use your good judgment and check in with a doctor if your symptoms persist or get worse despite your ministrations. Remember that very young people and very old people often have less resilience, so if you have doubts, check in with their doctors. With that in mind, we present *The People's Pharmacy* guide to doing it yourself. Here are the sexy trade secrets and home remedies that just might help.

Cranberry Juice

For years, women have shared a home remedy that, they claimed, could help prevent cystitis. And for years, doctors scoffed at the possibility that cranberry juice could have any activity against bacteria in the urinary tract. Mostly this was because it didn't seem theoretically defensible. Some enterprising individual came up with the idea that cranberry juice *might* work—by acidifying the urine—and shortly thereafter arguments were raised that making the urine acid would require far too much cranberry juice, and in such concentrated form that it would be virtually undrinkable.

After that, the cranberry juice remedy was relegated to the category of "old wives' tale" by most doctors. But not all. A group of researchers intrigued by laboratory evidence that cranberry juice might keep bacteria from sticking to the lining of the urinary tract decided to find out if the drink could in fact reduce the number of urinary tract infections women suffered.[6] Older women are quite susceptible to urinary tract infections, so they recruited their subjects from the residents of several senior housing complexes and a long-term-care facility. The study was double-blind and placebo-controlled, with the Ocean Spray company developing a look-alike, taste-alike, juice-free drink as the placebo. Urine samples were collected on a monthly basis, along with a history of any symptoms of urinary tract infection.

When the urinalyses were complete and the statistics were calculated, the old wives won. The women drinking cranberry juice had less than half the risk of showing bacteria in the urine. What's more, the women were treated only if the bacteria caused a symptomatic bothersome infection. The cranberry juice drinkers had only about one-fourth the risk of bacteria persisting in the urine month after month.[7]

Women may not always have such good luck with home remedies, but cranberry juice is clearly a keeper. Let us point out, however, that cranberry juice is no substitute for medical treatment of a full-blown symptomatic case of cystitis. In addition to the excruciating pain and disruption it causes, such an infection could have serious complications and needs attention.

Raisins Against Arthritis

N ow that cranberry juice has been vindicated, we're hoping an ambitious rheumatologist will tackle the gin-soaked raisin remedy for arthritis. This one has evidently been making the rounds by word of mouth, fax, and photocopy. Every version we have seen credits the parish newsletter of St. Lucas Lutheran Church in Toledo, Ohio, but we haven't seen the original newsletter, and some details of the story change from one version to the next. The recipe is unchanged, however:

> Empty one box of golden light raisins into a large shallow container. Completely cover the raisins with gin. Let stand, uncovered, until the gin evaporates. Store them in a closed container and eat nine raisins daily.

Apparently Lois (Loehrke? Loebide?) of St. Lucas Lutheran Church got this remedy from a friend of hers in Hyannis, Massachusetts, and found it immensely helpful: "I was able to walk up and down those small steps from the sidewalk to the street outside our Sunday School building without turning sideways to go one step at a time or hanging on to a parked car." A reader in Greensboro, North Carolina, has written to second the endorsement:

> I started the remedy and after about one month I really started noticing a difference in the way I felt. A number of things changed.
>
> 1. I noticed how much easier it was to get out of bed in the mornings. Before, I was so stiff and sore that I had trouble walking. Now I get up without any trouble at all.
>
> 2. I find it much easier to climb stairs. I do volunteer work at one of the local hospitals, and I sometimes have to climb the stairs to get from one floor to another. In the past, I would have to stop halfway between the floors and rest. My knees would be throbbing. Now I can go up 3 or 4 flights without stopping at all.

> **3.** I love to play tennis, but for a while I thought I was going to have to give it up. After the game was over I could hardly move. It was difficult to go on with the rest of my daily activities. Now I play 3 to 4 times a week without a problem. I know that arthritis can come and go, but it has now been about 18 months without severe pain. As long as it keeps working for me I will continue to eat my 9 raisins a day. It sure is cheaper than paying for a lot of high-priced medicine that was beginning to hurt my stomach.

We surely cannot argue with that logic. Once the gin has evaporated, there is very little alcohol left in the raisins to pose a hazard, although alcoholics might need to pass. We doubt there's enough juniper berry extract in those raisins to make any pharmacological difference, either, although one traditional use of juniper is to treat arthritis. We can't imagine why gin-soaked raisins might help, and we can't promise that they will help your aches and pains. Anyone allergic to sulfites will have to forgo this one, because light raisins usually contain these preservatives. To anyone else, all we can say is this remedy probably won't do much harm.

Hiccups

Hiccup home remedies seem to be some physicians' favorite pastime, to judge from the periodic spates of letters describing new cures in prestigious medical journals. First, let's take a stab at understanding hiccups. The diaphragm, a muscle between your chest and abdomen, supplies the power behind every breath. When the phrenic nerve, which stimulates this muscle, becomes irritated, it can produce a spasmodic contraction of the diaphragm. This in turn causes the voice box to close suddenly, which is what makes the distinctive hiccup sound.

Now let's cure it. Get a cotton swab. Have the hiccuping victim open his or her mouth. Place the swab on the roof of the mouth, right where the surface changes from hard (in front) to soft (towards the rear). Rub gently for a minute or so, and kiss those hiccups good-bye. This one was first suggested in a letter to the *New England Journal of Medicine* and republished in the Mayo Clinic's health newsletter, so it's nothing to sneeze—or hiccup—at.[8]

Why does it work? Probably for the same reason many of the traditional hiccup remedies have worked. It irritates the phrenic nerve someplace other than where it's already being irritated, and the two irritations cancel each other out or so overload the system that it just shuts down.

Other remedies reputed to do some good are swallowing hard bread, eating crushed ice, placing sugar at the back of the throat, and pulling the tongue. One of our readers wrote about her husband, who had developed severe hiccups after surgery. Her doctor suggested placing currant jelly under the sufferer's tongue, and that seems to have helped. Each of these actions presumably stimulates the rear of the throat, which may well be the key.

The sugar cure also appeared in the *New England Journal of Medicine*. Dr. Edgar Engelman reported that "one teaspoonful of ordinary white granulated sugar swallowed dry resulted in immediate cessation of hiccups in 19 of 20 patients."[9] Twelve of these poor souls had had their hiccups longer than six hours, and eight of them had endured anywhere from a full day to six weeks of hiccup suffering, so they were surely grateful the sugar worked.

We find brown sugar a bit more palatable, but white may do the job more consistently because of the grainy texture. It has been suggested that for younger patients a few drops of water with the sugar will also help it go down.[10]

In case the Q-Tip or sugar cures don't do the job, here are several other tips from the pages of the *New England Journal of Medicine*. Dr. Jay Howard Herman offered the following suggestion, titled "A Bitter Cure."

Hiccups (singultus) have plagued humanity for ages, often at awkward times. Therapy is tedious, with frequent failures. Granulated sugar taken orally has been previously reported as highly effective; it probably activates a local pharyngeal reflex. Hiccups are commonly associated with ethanol (alcohol) ingestion. We wish to report our success with an alternative remedy that is well known to bartenders, but that we cannot find in the medical literature. All subjects had ethanol-induced hiccups that were unresponsive to traditional treatment. . . . Treatment consisted of oral administration of a lemon wedge of the size served in bars; the wedge was saturated with Angostura bitters and rapidly consumed (except for the rind). Small amounts of granulated sugar were occasionally used to enhance palatability, but they did not increase efficacy. Response was defined as at least a two-hour cessation of hiccups within one minute of treatment. The total response rate was 88 percent (14 of 16 cases), including two cases of initial treatment failure that was overcome after a second treatment within five minutes.[11]

Dr. Herman's hiccup home remedy spurred another note to the *Journal*: "No doubt the remedy of Herman . . . is good, but one does not always have a lemon in the house. I am 81 years old, and I have always found the following to cure hiccups.

"Fill a glass to the top with water, then bend over as far as you can from the waist, and drink all you can from the far side of the glass. You will find that the hiccups disappear."[12]

We told you doctors love hiccup remedies. But here's one we've never seen in any medical journal. A friend swears he has seen a woman cured by having someone hold a $20 bill just above her extended thumb and first finger. The person promises her she can have the bill if she'll just catch it as it slips between her fingers. By talking constantly and releasing the bill at unexpected times, it has invariably fluttered untouched to the ground, and the hiccups have consistently disappeared after just a few rounds. Don't blame us if you lose money trying this.

Any home remedy that works has advantages over the full-fledged medical approach. There are a few reports in the literature of success stopping hiccups in hospitalized patients incapable of swallowing. In one case a patient's rectum was massaged with a (gloved) finger. This approach sounds extremely unorthodox, but it may have fewer side effects than some of the prescription medications that have been tried. The antidepressant amitriptyline, the anti-Parkinson's drug amantadine, the blood pressure medicine nifedipine, the muscle relaxant baclofen, and the heartburn medication metoclopramide have all been used with varying degrees of success, but none is sure-fire.

A final word to the wise: If you know someone suffering from prolonged, incurable hiccups, take note. They could be a sign of something serious, including diseases of the liver, pancreas, esophagus, or bladder. Even some drugs (**Decadron, Hexadol**) can cause hiccups.[13] So if none of our handy-dandy home remedies does the trick and those hiccups persist, it's time to see a doctor for a complete physical examination.

Heartburn—Getting the Right Juices Flowing

A sk most people what you should do for heartburn and they will probably suggest an antacid (see page 90). But if you liked a spoonful of sugar for hiccups, you'll love candy and chewing gum for heartburn.

Okay, we admit that candy and chewing gum sound like the last thing you might want if you suffer from "gastroesophageal reflux," otherwise known as heartburn. But once again, the *New England Journal of Medicine* offers us a simple and elegant home remedy for one of humanity's most common woes.

When stomach acid splashes back up into the esophagus (sometimes referred to as the gullet), it causes irritation and pain. After all, we're talking about hydrochloric acid here—nasty stuff. The body's natural response to this assault is to swallow, which gets most of the acid back into the stomach where it belongs. But that may not be quite enough.

Sucking on a piece of hard candy or chewing a stick of gum can stimulate saliva production, which helps in two ways: it washes the acid down by promoting swallowing, and it serves to neutralize any residual acid left in the esophagus.[14] A soothing cup of chamomile tea or a banana probably wouldn't hurt, either. Both are known for their stomach-settling properties. In short, anything that makes you produce more saliva is going to help you get rid of heartburn.

Doctors once thought that it would take too much saliva to be able to neutralize the acid that sloshes up and causes heartburn. When physicians at the Medical College of Wisconsin published their research showing that sucking on candy can increase saliva production by eight or nine times, it became clear that would be enough to neutralize the acid for most people.

Be aware, though, that the hard candy you choose should not be peppermint. Both chocolate and peppermint, together with tobacco, coffee, alcohol, and several medicines, can make heartburn worse by loosening the junction between the esophagus and stomach. In a sensible home-remedy approach to heartburn, the first step is to eliminate these substances from your life as much as possible. Skipping bedtime snacks, raising the head of your bed, and lying on your left side if heartburn bothers you when you sleep are all things you can do for yourself to manage your heartburn.

Preventing Chinese-Restaurant Syndrome

H ave you ever gone out to eat Chinese food and afterwards suffered from heartburn, flushing, headache, chest tightness, lightheadedness, tingling, or even asthma? For reasons that are still mostly a mystery, some people react strongly to monosodium glutamate (MSG), frequently used in Chinese, Japanese, or Southeast Asian foods.

Until recently, this has meant that sufferers had to forgo these delectable cuisines. Nowadays many restaurants will respond to a request for a dish without MSG. There may also be an antidote.

Researchers have found that vitamin B_6 (pyridoxine) seems to be involved. Students who reacted to MSG took 50 mg of B_6 a day for twelve weeks. When they were again dosed with MSG, they no longer reacted to it.[15] This home remedy may not work for everyone. Especially if you're supersensitive to MSG, we wouldn't recommend that you gobble some vitamin B_6 and then pig out on Chinese food. Try to gradually increase your pyridoxine intake for a couple of months up to—but not beyond—50 mg daily, and perhaps then you could sample the egg rolls or wonton soup. If you have no reaction, the next time out you could be a little more adventuresome.

Hot Relief from Colds

O nce you're not worried about Chinese-restaurant syndrome, a steaming bowl of hot-and-sour soup could help when you have one of those miserable colds where the gunk in your chest is thick and nasty. According to Dr. Irwin Ziment, chief of medicine at Los Angeles County–Olive View Medical Center, spicy foods loosen up respiratory tract secretions, making it easier to cough up that mucky mucus.[16] If going out for Mexican or Szechuan Chinese food is more than you can manage (or if your local eating establishments don't meet the heat standards Dr. Ziment is used to in L.A.), he says you can accomplish the same thing at home with a gargle of about 20 drops of Tabasco sauce in eight ounces of water.

Another ingredient in spicy cooking is garlic, which has long been touted as a cure for the common cold. American physicians prescribed garlic for colds and coughs in the 1800s. More recently, scientists have discovered that garlic has antibacterial and antifungal properties. In fact, garlic extract was used to treat battlefield wounds as recently as World War II.[17] Whether it combats viruses is still unknown.

Does garlic work? A couple of our readers have offered their opinions. One recalls his boyhood:

> I remember a fad of the mid-1930s when syrup of garlic was administered as an antidote for the common cold. It was forced on us by the spoonful at a boarding school in Great Britain by the school nurse, who was something of a sadist. Whether it did any good I don't know. It was indescribably loathsome.

Another relates a more recent experience:

> I was coming down with a nasty cold and decided to try garlic. I put about 20 cloves in a pot of chicken soup. The next day I was fine. Of course, nobody could get near me, but I didn't care because I was feeling so much better.

We can't verify the success of this treatment, but eating that much garlic might help prevent the transmission of colds by keeping people away. There is still no scientific consensus on exactly how people catch or spread colds, but proximity probably plays a role.

Curing the Common Cold

D espite the long-standing traditions of garlic and chicken soup, Americans shell out large sums of money every year on over-the-counter cough and cold remedies.[18] So many of these products contain a sinkload of ingredients—antihistamines, decongestants, cough suppressants, expectorants, pain relievers, not to mention alcohol and caffeine—that sometimes these ingredients work at cross-purposes. For example, the expectorant is designed to loosen mucus and help you cough it up. But when combined with a cough suppressant that keeps you from coughing, there is no way for the expectorant to work. This is not rational. Serious questions have been raised about the effectiveness of antihistamines, and pain relievers/fever reducers could be counterproductive for the immune system's response to the virus. (For more information, see page 72.)

In this light, home remedies for the all-too-common cold make a lot of sense. We have already discussed the benefits of chicken soup and spicy foods such as peppers and garlic. What about vitamin C?

Probably a lot more people are enthusiastic about vitamin C than any other home remedy for colds. We're enthusiastic ourselves, but there is little if any evidence that ascorbic acid can prevent the sniffles. What research seems to show instead is that relatively high doses of vitamin C (about 4,000 mg a day) can shorten the cold and make it milder.[19] Certainly not magic, but nothing to sneeze at, either.

Not surprisingly, there are plenty of skeptics on the value of this vitamin. Just imagine how these guys must have greeted the idea of zinc against colds. Based on very little research, zinc lozenges started popping up in health food stores about a decade ago. For a while they were all the rage, and all because one little girl decided to be stubborn. Scientists at the University of Texas in Austin started the zinc study after they discovered that

a leukemic child refused to swallow a 50-mg zinc gluconate tablet and dissolved it slowly in her mouth instead. When her accompanying cold symptoms disappeared within hours, the investigators looked into the ability of zinc ions to halt replication of diverse viruses. . . .[20]

The Texas researchers took 65 people with fresh cold symptoms and gave half of them zinc gluconate lozenges (2 mg every two hours during the day) for a week. The remainder got placebo lozenges. The results were impressive. More than four-fifths of the people getting zinc got over their colds in less than a week, while more than half of those taking the placebo were still suffering after seven days.[21]

A number of those in the zinc treatment group got rid of their cold symptoms almost immediately: 11 percent reported cold symptoms gone within 12 hours, while 22 percent said their colds disappeared in less than a day.

There were only two drawbacks. Zinc lozenges can be nasty-tasting and irritating to the mouth, and they can cause nausea on an empty stomach. Any follow-up research that may have been done has not gotten much attention. Our anecdotal reports suggests that a lot of children would rather suffer a cold than suck on anything that tastes so awful. So there are still plenty of questions to be answered before we'll recognize zinc as the cure for the common cold.

Before you leave the health food store empty-handed, though, there is one other product you might want to consider. Unfortunately, research is skimpy on this one as well, but tantalizing. Echinacea is an herb that has been used for over a century—well over a century if you consider that American Indians taught the settlers about it. It has a reputation as being helpful in promoting wound-healing and stimulating the immune response.

Word on the grapevine suggests that taking an Echinacea capsule or two as you start coming down with a cold can help ward it off. In fact, in Australia a product that combines Echinacea with vitamins A, C, and E together with zinc and garlic is sold by prescription only in pharmacies. Don't look for such a combo here, though, as it hasn't made it across the Pacific. If you decide to try Echinacea, keep in mind that research findings suggest it may work better for colds if you don't take it all the time. In one study, researchers found that Echinacea boosted cell-mediated immunity after a single dose, but that repeated doses dampened the immune response.[22] You may want to do your own research on this: try it out and see how it works for you.

Will we ever have a truly effective cure for the common cold? It's possible. Research is now proceeding on many fronts and there may one day be an interferon nasal spray that really works without making you sick. Until then, however, you can't beat chicken soup. It is still the safest, tastiest, and cheapest cold treatment we know of.

Mastering Motion Sickness

One of the most embarrassing facts of space flight is motion sickness. NASA astronauts, even experienced fliers who have spent thousands of hours in the air, often lose their lunch on their way into orbit. Almost half the space shuttle pilots have had to cling to airsick bags like nervous passengers on a bumpy flight. This delicate problem has inspired lots of high-level research, and we hope that someday it will trickle down to those who have trouble just moving around on Earth.

Motion sickness can strike sensitive people almost anywhere—in a car, bus, plane, or train. And let's not forget boats. Anyone who has really been seasick knows that death seems like a reasonable alternative.

What causes motion sickness? Why do some poor souls suffer when the car hits a few bumps, while others can ride a roller coaster with glee? The problem seems to arise when the brain receives confusing signals from the inner ear. It is the inner ear, after all, that is responsible for our sense of which end is up in the world. When the messages relayed to the brain from the ear conflict with those from the eyes or with what makes sense, the result can be that sinking feeling in the pit of the stomach.

There are several over-the-counter motion-sickness remedies available, and just about everyone who's ever been seasick has tried at least one of these, such as **Dramamine** (dimenhydrinate), **Bonine** (meclizine), or **Marezine** (cyclizine). The results are usually mixed, with some getting some relief and others left still hanging over the railing. And of those who do get relief, some of them pay for it with side effects such as extreme sedation, which hardly adds to the enjoyment of a day on the water.

If you're prone to motion sickness and are offered an irresistible invitation to go sailing, there's still hope. You just might get relief by bypassing the medicines in favor of a couple capsules of ground ginger.

That's right, ginger. The spice is a remedy that Chinese fishermen have been using for centuries to counteract motion sickness. It's available in pharmacies in Australia, New Zealand, and a number of other countries. We have ourselves tried **Blackmore's Travel Calm Ginger** (400 mg) and wish it were available in the U.S. That's not science, though.

In a test of ginger's ability to control motion sickness, two researchers subjected 36 people who were highly susceptible to motion sickness to a motor-driven revolving chair. This device brings out . . . and up . . . the worst in those prone to motion sickness. About 20 minutes before being blindfolded and entering the torture device, the people were dosed with either **Dramamine**, two capsules (total dose 940 milligrams) of powdered ginger, or an inert placebo. When the chair began to whirl, each person was asked to rate their feelings of stomach upset.

When the results were tallied, the winner in suppressing motion sickness was ginger, which was almost twice as effective as **Dramamine**.[23] None of the people who received a placebo or **Dramamine** was able to stay in the chair for the full six minutes. But surprisingly, over half the subjects who received powdered ginger made it all the way through the experiment.

"We don't recommend that people just take a spoonful of ginger, because it's rather caustic," says one of the researchers on the project. "But a small bit of ginger root ground up and put in a gelatin capsule just might be effective for people who have tried everything else with no effect."

You probably won't be able to find ground-up ginger in your pharmacy, but the local health food store probably has ginger capsules in stock. And if you don't mind filling capsules, the kitchen spice shelf may already hold all you'll need. We have also heard from people who say that slicing up fresh ginger root, pouring boiling water over it and letting it steep makes a tea that's as helpful as any medicine they've tried.

Running Cold on Hot

Most burn injuries happen at home, and this is an instance where a home remedy is not only possible but actually very important. Action taken in the first few seconds can have a strong effect on how serious the burn injury will be.

For many years, medical people couldn't agree about appropriate first aid for burns. There were enthusiastic proponents and equally vociferous detractors for butter, baking soda, and nothing.

But at long last, there's an unequivocal answer about what to do with a burn. Immediate application of cold water or a cold, wet compress is the treatment of choice.[24] This treatment, applied for 20 minutes, "has been shown to reduce the depth of the injury."[25]

One researcher reported a reduction of up to two-thirds in total treatment time and burn severity when immediate cold-water immersion was employed on 150 patients suffering a variety of chemical, heat, and electrical burns, some quite severe.[26] All infections were avoided.

This is an instance where too much of a good thing could be bad, though. Do not rush in with ice. Used directly it's just too cold, and you can wind up causing tissue damage from the cold on top of the tissue damage already present from the burn. A few ice cubes added to a pan of water would be okay.

If a person gets burned, move quickly with that cold water or cold compress. Seconds count, and it doesn't take long to make the difference between a nasty blister and no obvious skin reaction.

For reasons that escape us, there's been a trend toward burn ointments and sprays. This can be dangerous. Most of these preparations contain a local anesthetic (benzocaine is one of the most common ingredients). It can cause a nasty reaction, especially when applied to skin where the first layer or two may already be missing.

Sometimes this skin reaction can actually be worse than the original burn. Where there's a deep burn, you can get in double trouble due to greater absorption of the ointments into the body. Remember, they've been tested and found safe as topical ointments, not as drugs for internal use.

The cold-water treatment is safe and proper first aid for any burn, but anything worse than a first-degree burn confined to a small area should also be seen by a doctor. A first-degree burn involves slight reddening, comparable to sunburn. It's perhaps the most uncomfortable kind of burn, since the tissue is all very much alive and hurting.

Anything beyond a first-degree burn represents a substantial medical threat from infection, lost fluids, and many other complications. Don't play doctor with one of these burns, and don't make later medical help more difficult by gooping up the scene with butter, oil, ointments, or anything else. Get cold water on it first, then get the person to a doctor or an emergency room.

At this point, we can almost hear a chorus of people screaming, "You forgot aloe vera." One reader urged us not to run this "miracle plant down. Hot grease popped into my hand out of the frying pan. I cut a fresh aloe leaf and tied it over my burn. It didn't hurt, didn't blister and healed by the next day."

Fresh aloe vera gel may indeed help relieve pain and speed healing of burns. We think you should try it after the cold water, though. And there are some doubts about how well it may work in promoting healing. Researchers at the University of Southern California found that using a commercial aloe vera preparation on obstetrical incisions actually delayed the healing process. In a study of women who had undergone obstetrical surgery, they found that "Aloe vera had no beneficial effect on wound healing and was associated with a significant delay in healing among patients with a vertical incision."

By the way, there is one kind of burn that isn't helped much by cold water. This is the chemical injury resulting from handling hot jalapeño or red peppers. This type of injury typically strikes people not raised in the Southwest who decide for the first time in their lives to make a "real" Mexican (or Indian) meal.

Unaware of the burning power built into one of these chiles, our intrepid chef washes, seeds, and slices the chiles with bare hands instead of wearing gloves. Within an hour, the poor soul will be uselessly plunging his or her hands into ice water, seeking to put out the fire. A friend of ours spent an entire sleepless night suffering with her fingers in water.

The fire, though, is caused by an oily, alkaline resin called capsaicin. It's insoluble in water, so all the soaking in the world won't help. You have, for all intents and purposes, plunged your hand into a barrel of lye.

If you get Hunan Hand, or Chili Fingers, or whatever you call it, the only things that can help are (a) the passage of time . . . you will live, though this may not seem desirable for a while, (b) mild pain relievers such as aspirin, and (c) a prolonged soak in vinegar. The acid should eventually neutralize the highly alkaline capsaicin. Another soak might be yogurt, which is sometimes suggested as an antidote when you burn your mouth on a potent curry. You might even try holding a slice of raw apple on the burning skin or tongue.

The Sting

Whatʼs the first thing you do after being stung by a bee or wasp? Most people probably scream a little, make futile efforts to remove the stinger, or perhaps make a compress of mud or baking soda. The baking soda might help, but meat tenderizer may be better. A quarter teaspoon added to one or two teaspoonfuls of water (enough to make a paste) should stop pain pronto according to Dr. Harry L. Arnold of the Health Insurance Institute.[27] A little dab will do you.

How does meat tenderizer work? It contains papain, an enzyme extracted from papaya fruit. In addition to breaking down muscle tissue and thus tenderizing meat, papain also does a job on the proteins that make up bee-sting and other insect venom. When it is rubbed into the skin immediately after a sting, the toxic chemicals are broken down before they do damage.

There are fancier ways of finding papain. You can go to your neighborhood pharmacist or health food store and ask for a "digestive aid" containing papain, or buy one from a mail-order vitamin company. Then you'll have a tablet to smash up and make into a paste. There's even a ready-to-use ointment that contains 10-percent papain, but it's available only by prescription—and it's pricey. Still, if you want the enzyme in a ready-to-use form, ask your doctor about a scrip for **Panafil Ointment** (Rystan Company, P.O. Box 214, Little Falls, NJ 07424).

A final tip on using anything containing papain: Do NOT cleanse the wound first with hydrogen peroxide. The hydrogen peroxide inactivates any papain you apply. Just remove the stinger (without squeezing or pushing on it, which will release more venom) and slap on the papain. Meat tenderizer is still cheap, readily available, and relatively easy to use.

One of our readers, who obviously knows his onions, came up with a home remedy for stings that meets all those criteria. He credits his German neighbor with suggesting a cut onion be applied to the sting for at least ten minutes. He reports this works surprisingly well.

When we checked in with the world-renowned onion researcher, Dr. Eric Block of the State University of New York at Albany, he confirmed that a fresh-cut onion might minimize the pain of an insect sting. Onions contain an ingredient that can break down the chemicals responsible for inflammation and discomfort. What we have heard from readers who've tried this remedy suggests, however, that results may vary.

Over the years readers have shared other favorite bee-sting remedies. The most popular usually involve baking soda applied to the affected area. One woman mixes the baking soda together with hand cream to make it stick. Another wrote to tell us that she moistens an **Alka-Seltzer** tablet and, when it starts fizzing, applies it to the sting.

Many folks also turn to vinegar as a sting remedy. Some mix vinegar with baking soda to make a foaming paste. One fellow even combined it with papain:

The lifeguards on Hawaii's beaches told me they use a mixture of Adolph's Meat Tenderizer and vinegar for the stings from the Man of War jellyfish. I mixed it up and used it for wasp and hornet stings. It's fantastic! Just mix enough white vinegar with approximately 2 to 3 teaspoons of meat tenderizer to dissolve it in a jar. Shake well and apply with a cotton ball or clean cloth. I keep a bottle in my fridge all the time and carry it with me on picnics.

After all this talk about what to do once you've been stung, who in their right mind would *want* a bee sting? As strange as it may sound, bee-venom therapy for arthritis was used by the leading doctors in this country between the first and second world wars. Hospital pharmacies stocked an injectable solution of mixed venom.

This therapy fell out of favor for lack of scientific proof. But there is renewed interest in bee stings to treat arthritis or even multiple sclerosis, although research is still scarce. Some people go out and catch bees to sting their sore joints. Others get their doctors to inject bee venom, used for bee-allergy desensitization. Needless to say, no one who is allergic to bee stings should try this treatment, because one sting could trigger a fatal reaction.

If you have any reason to believe that you or anyone who has been stung is in fact allergic to bee or insect stings, then get to an emergency room instantly. People who suffer severe reactions to insect venom can have a life-threatening reaction within minutes, with swelling, wheezing, and shock. Such a situation is a crisis and no time to think about home remedies.

Bites and Itches

Luckily, mosquito and flea bites aren't really dangerous, but the itching can drive you crazy. What happens when a dive-bombing mosquito selects your juicy body as its next meal? What do you do if your dog's fleas decide that they would like some variety in their diet and take a taste of you? How do you respond to the plague of poison ivy?

If you're like most people you swear a little and then smear, spread, or spray some over-the-counter anti-itch gunk on your skin. Some of these products work and some don't, but, fortunately, there's an incredibly simple and effective home remedy. It's available everywhere and is as cheap as anything could ever be. What is this wondrous stuff? Nothing more exotic than water. Hot water, to be precise.

According to some dermatologists, applications of hot water for a brief period of time can provide almost instantaneous relief of itching. And the effects last up to three hours.[28] It sounds crazy, but it really works. The water should be hot enough to be slightly uncomfortable (about 120 to 130 degrees Fahrenheit), but not so hot as to burn. If it's not warm enough, it could make the itching worse.

You can either stick the affected spot under the running water for a second or two, or you can use a washcloth. Several applications should do the trick for a few hours. One reader reported that she was suffering from poison ivy on her hands until she washed her dishes in very hot water. The itching disappeared for several hours, she said.

Obviously, an extensive skin involvement should not be treated in this manner, nor should poison ivy that has blistered. Keep in mind that prolonged heat may be dangerous in certain kinds of skin problems, so make the applications short and sweet. If the skin reaction is severe, it's time to call the dermatologist.

Poison ivy reactions may call for treatment with powerful steroids or antihistamines.

How does this one work its magic? Interestingly enough, it works much as the hiccup cure does—that is, by overloading a nerve network, in this case the fine nerves in the upper layer of your skin. By short-circuiting the itching reflex, your urge to scratch is reduced or eliminated.

Of course the most desirable approach in dealing with an itch is to remove the underlying cause. But when the problem is a mosquito or flea bite, mild poison ivy, or atopic dermatitis (a chronic condition with no known cause or cure), hot water therapy can be a cheap and fast temporary treatment. And it certainly is readily available.

Water for Warts

H ot water may also be a good home remedy for a problem that can otherwise be quite tricky to treat. Dermatologist Samuel L. Moschella has suggested a series of foot baths in hot water for patients with plantar warts—that is, warts on the soles of the feet. Needless to say, surgery on plantar warts usually means a period of staying off the feet while the wound recovers, and some of Dr. Moschella's patients, doctors themselves, have balked at that. They were willing, however, to try an old-fashioned remedy: soak their feet for 30 to 90 minutes weekly in water at 110 to 113 degrees Fahrenheit.[29] After two to three months, two-thirds of them had recovered completely.[30] Dr. Moschella points out that this method, while by no means definitive, has several advantages; it's cheap, it doesn't hurt, it's non-invasive, and it's under the patient's control.[31] That makes it probably worth trying.

Over the years we have learned about a number of other wart remedies from our readers. We have received several testimonials that the application of castor oil two or three times daily has made warts disappear in a month or two. It is inexpensive and safe, though not endorsed by medical opinion.

Other readers favor vinegar. Francis wrote, "Many years ago I had a wart on my finger. When I visited the dentist he suggested I should get rid of it. By then I was ready to try any silly remedy. He told me to soak the finger in vinegar for a half hour morning and evening. After a week the wart disappeared and never returned." More recently we heard from a lab technician who treated a wart the size of a dime by soaking her finger in vinegar and applying a vinegar compress for an hour or two a day. Before she tried this, the dermatologist had unsuccessfully frozen the wart three times. The vinegar worked after about six weeks. She reports, "My husband and coworkers are amazed. They're also glad I don't smell like I'm wearing vinegar perfume anymore."

Gisela suggested an herbal cure: "My six-year-old son had warts on both hands. One Sunday after church an elderly Italian lady told us to use milkweed to get rid of the warts. He applied the milky sap several times a day and before long the warts disappeared. It didn't cost a penny."

Miriam remembered curing a wart at camp. "Furtively taking a raw white potato from the camp kitchen, I waited until after lights out to slice off a thin piece of the spud with my Girl Scout knife. I then rubbed the juice over the surface of the wart. I kept this up for nearly three weeks until the wart shriveled and fell off. Outcome, no wart, no scar, minimum cost (guilty conscience for purloined potato)."

We can't vouch for any of these home remedies, or for hydrogen peroxide (the variety found in drugstores) applied twice a day or vitamin E oil squirted on the wart. None of them is very expensive, though, and it shouldn't hurt to try them. If the person with warts is a child, keep in mind that warts are very susceptible to suggestion. The more persuasive you can make your "cure," the better.

Keeping Bugs Away with Bath Oil

W hen it comes to insect bites, there's no question that prevention is better than cure. But how to keep them from biting? There are about as many home remedies for scaring off biting critters as there are fishermen, hunters, and lumberjacks who've crawled around on the ground. Through the millennia, humans have rubbed themselves with a veritable cornucopia of disgusting things in the hopes that mosquitoes, chiggers, black flies, gnats, and biting fleas, would also be disgusted and thus move on to a more palatable meal.

Rancid bear-grease was a favorite home remedy with American Indians. And according to one authority, when Henry David Thoreau got fed up with the mosquitoes around Walden Pond he "concocted a mess of turpentine, oil of spearmint and camphor that he finally decided was itself more unpleasant than the insect bites."[32] The original **Old Time Woodsman's Liquid Fly** dope contained pine tar, camphor, and citronella, and many lumberjacks in northern New England swore by the stuff. But it's possible friends and lovers also did a lot of swearing when they got close enough to smell anyone so coated.

The one thing that has been proven superior to the competition at keeping skeeters and such away is a chemical called N,N-diethyl-metatoluamide, which for obvious reasons is usually called DEET. DEET has its seal of approval from no less than the U.S. Army. Those folks have tested everything anyone could ever dream up (and a few more besides) for keeping bugs away from our servicemen and -women. After sifting through more than 9,000 preparations, the Army pronounced DEET the chemical of choice.

DEET is available in any number of over-the-counter products. Just read the label and you'll be able to tell which ones have DEET. Those with the highest concentrations are usually more effective, but concern has been raised about the safety of strong formulas, especially for children. There have been reports of rashes, confusion, irritability, insomnia, and seizures. Medical reports have shown that, because DEET can be absorbed into the bloodstream through the skin, the use of DEET can have serious consequences.[33] The use of DEET, therefore, like the use of any medicine, has to be carefully considered against the possible side effects.

If you'd rather avoid DEET, you've got a lot of company that doesn't like serving as mosquito meat, either. Legions are devoted to the bath oil **Skin-So-Soft** from Avon. An investigation in *Consumer Reports*, however, was discouraging for this home remedy. The testers put 500 hungry mosquitoes in a cage. Then the volunteers applied repellents or **Skin-So-Soft** to their arms and stuck them into the cage, and the number of bites were counted. The conclusion was that **Skin-So-Soft** is ineffective against aggressive mosquitoes, although it did deter stable flies a bit.

We have had readers corroborate the magazine's findings, saying that **Skin-So-Soft** is worthless against bugs. But many others disagree vehemently. One woman insisted: *"Consumer Reports* was wrong about Avon **Skin-So-Soft**. I play golf regularly twice a week, and the very few times I've played without **Skin-So-Soft** I've come home with bites and been pestered by bees." Another reader offered the following home remedy: "Here is the best recipe for mosquito repellent—1 tablespoon citronella oil, 2 cups white vinegar, 1 cup water, 1 cup Avon **Skin-So-Soft**. This really works."

How can there be such differences in people's experience? The obvious answer would be the placebo effect. If people believe in something enough, even if it is inactive, they find reasons to see it as effective. It is true that bug bites leave marks and some people may be more "tender and juicy" and appeal more to biting bugs. Others may have body chemistry that combines with **Skin-So-Soft** to discourage bites.

Avon has never marketed **Skin-So-Soft** as an insect repellent. The company finally has taken all the enthusiasts to heart, however, and formulated an insect repellent called **Skin-So-Soft Moisturizing Suncare Mosquito, Flea & Deer Tick Repellent.** It has at least one accepted active ingredient, oil of citronella.[34]

Whether Avon's new product is really better than—or even as good as—its bath oil, you will be able to determine for yourself. This is one of the few areas where you can be your own scientist. Try these remedies, pay attention, and see if they work for you.

Getting Ticked Off

A fter we wrote about **Skin-So-Soft** in our syndicated newspaper column, we heard from a physician in Missouri. According to him, "In writing about Avon **Skin-So-Soft**, you have missed its most important benefit. It keeps ticks off like magic. I hunt in tick-infested areas and the stuff is great."

Ticks are undeniably undesirable critters. There you are, merrily hiking away on a lovely day in the beautiful countryside. Pausing to take in a magnificent view, you glance at your leg and see . . . a tick. Yecch. There goes the fun.

While tick bites are not terribly painful, they can be hazardous. Ticks are vectors—carriers, that is—of several serious diseases, most notably Rocky Mountain spotted fever and Lyme disease. Once one of these little guys leaps aboard, he plants his paired pincers into your skin for a blood sundae. In the course of doing that, all manner of nasty things go from tick to Rick . . . or Sally, or Sam, as the case might be.

Over the years all sorts of ways have been suggested for getting ticks to let go of their hold on people. The first temptation, of course, is to grab the little bugger by the butt and yank him out. After all, there sits the tick, head buried in your arm or leg, tail end waving in the breeze.

The problem with that solution, however, is that violence tends to cause the tick to lose his head, which will remain buried in your skin, where it can get infected and may continue transmitting whatever disease the tick might have had to offer.

The tick trick is to get the thing to back out, on its own accord. You're then welcome to carefully burn it to a crisp or set it free, depending on exactly how much of a nature lover you are.

The old macho approach used to be to light up a cigarette, take a few deep drags to get the tip red-hot, and then touch the cigarette to the tick's hind end. We've also heard that some folks used to pour a little lighter fluid on the tick and light it. That was back when men were men, John Wayne was still around, and most people carried Zippo lighters. It also didn't work very well. Both techniques have been known to produce some rather bad burns.

More modern techniques are available. Some have even appeared in medical journals. If you insist on using a heat technique, you could follow Dr. Joseph Benforado's suggestion as published in the *Journal of the American Medical Association:*

The materials needed are a pocketknife (or similar blade), large nail (eight- to ten-penny size), and matches.
   The procedure is as follows.

1. Warm the tip of the nail in a match flame.

2. Slide the flat of the knife blade under the tick's abdomen.

3. Place the heated nail tip on the tick's dorsal surface [back] so that the beastie is sandwiched between the knife blade and the nail.

4. When the tick's legs begin to wiggle (a response to the heat), turn the knife blade 90 degrees so that the tick, now at right angles to the skin, is "standing on its head."

Keeping the tick sandwiched, raise the blade and the nail slowly away from the skin. The live tick, having released its mouthparts, comes away easily and is then appropriately disposed of. If the legs do not wiggle, the nail is not warm enough and a reattempt is needed. However, the object is to "annoy" the tick rather than to roast it.[35]

As a camp physician, Dr. Benforado apparently had ample opportunity to try out this approach on an almost daily basis. He claims it never failed him.

If, however, the nail-and-knife technique sounds a tad complicated, not to mention a little dangerous, you could try the fingernail-polish trick. This one comes from Dr. Warren Sherman, who generously credits it to the real discoverer—his 15-year-old daughter:

I would like to report a simple and successful method of removing an embedded tick from the skin. This method was suggested to me by my daughter, a 10th-grade student. It was applied successfully on two occasions involving other members of my family, during a recent visit to Cape Cod, Massachusetts. Approximately two drops of clear fingernail polish are allowed to fall from the brush and completely cover the tick. Within seconds the tick will release its bite and back out of the wound. The tick can then be easily wiped from the skin and properly disposed of.[36]

A California physician reports in the *Western Journal of Medicine* that a little petroleum jelly will also do the trick quite nicely:

A simple and safe method of tick removal is to coat the tick with petroleum jelly (such as Vaseline), wait ten minutes and then gently remove the tick with forceps, grasping it very close to the skin of patient or pet. The tick can be removed intact without problems associated with application of strong chemicals or burning. In addition, petroleum jelly–based ointments are readily available in most homes.[37]

One theory to explain the petroleum-jelly tick trick is that the goo so completely covers the tick that it can't breathe. Ticks do breathe, by the way. Faced with suffocation, the tick begins to let go and back out. There is considerable controversy over the effectiveness of all these techniques.

Standard medical advice goes back to grasping the tick with a pair of tweezers and exerting gentle steady pressure until you pull him out. Not too different from first impulse! We have tried petroleum jelly and can vouch for its success, though patience is required. Waiting ten minutes can seem like an eternity when you have one of those beasties imbedded in your skin.

Of course prevention is still the best approach of all. By checking frequently for ticks while hiking, it should be possible to spot them soon after they land, preferably before they've dug in for dinner. If they've already become attached to you, do not panic. Reach for the clear nail polish or the petroleum jelly.

Beautiful Nails from Brittle Ones

When it's nail inspection time, do you feel like hiding? We get a lot of questions about dry, chipped nails. And don't count on gelatin to make things better. The "evidence" to support the use of gelatin to strengthen nails is thin.

If you're a woman, you might get your nails treated with a "nail wrap" consisting of nylon, acrylic, or some other nail-hardening agent. That may give the temporary appearance of improvement, but it could actually make the situation worse, since the treatment tends to make hard, brittle nails even harder and more brittle. We heard just that from one reader:

> I'm writing to share my "secret" for strong nails. Ten years ago I was told to stop wearing nail polish or hardener because it could cause damage. My nails were brittle and always split, which I covered up with polish.
>
> My friend advised me to cut my nails short while they grew out. I followed her advice, and at the end of three short months with no polish they had grown out beautifully. My nails are still long and hard.

Here's another simple solution for you. Dr. Lawrence Norton, an expert on nail disorders, reported to a meeting of medical writers conducted by the American Academy of Dermatology that people with brittle nails should soak their fingers in water 15 minutes a day, three to five times a week. After soaking, the moisture is sealed in with a phospholipid-containing hand cream such as **Complex 15**.

"The fluid content of nails determines to a large extent their pliability and capacity to withstand breakage, reported Dr. Norton. "The relative lack of water in nails is a primary reason for their hardness."[38]

The trick is in getting the nail to absorb some water and then hold on to it. The prolonged soak is needed because the dense tissue of the nail is reluctant to suck up water at first. Once you get it in there, applying a cream or lotion should help keep the moisture in. Dr. Norton advises against overuse of nail polish remover or excess exposure to soap or detergent. These chemicals tend to dry out the nails and make them more brittle.

We have heard that **Epilyt** (Stiefel Labs; 255 Alhambra Circle; Coral Gables; FL 33134; 800-327-3858), sold as an OTC moisturizer, does wonders for rehabilitating nails. Our top-secret source suggested applying it at bedtime and protecting the sheets by wearing plain cotton gloves.

But we also received an interesting note from some folks who run a feed and garden store. Their female customers swear by the hoof moisturizers they keep in stock. They report that 80 percent of the women who buy the products don't use them on horses.

We have no data to back up the claim that such animal "cosmetics" are helpful for people. But ingredients such as lanolin, beeswax, mineral oil, and coconut oil certainly should help brittle, dry nails. If the nearest feed store is in the next state, you may want to check in with the manufacturers yourself. The **Hoofmaker** is from Straight Arrow Products and their number is (800) 827-9815. They also have a product formulated for humans under the brand name **Equenne**.

Fighting Nail Fungus

N ext to chipping and splitting, the nail problem we hear about most is fungus. Fungal infections can make the nail look nasty: munched on, ragged, and yucky. The fungus often thickens and discolors the nail to a sickly yellow-brown hue and may make it hard to trim.

If you've asked a dermatologist about this problem, you may have been told that fungal infections of the nail are notoriously difficult to eradicate, and that the medicine used for treatment is expensive, has potential side effects, and must be taken for close to a year. Even at that, sometimes it's necessary to remove the entire infected nail. Faced with what sounds like medieval torture, many people choose to suffer their fungus quietly, and keep their hands in their pockets or their feet in their socks.

If you're one of those people, we have a pile of home remedies for you. Our readers have done a lot of experimenting on this issue, and we get a lot of letters. Mary told us that her physician suggested squirting vitamin E between the toe and the nail, and that this approach worked. A lot of people wrote to second that one, though very few had discussed this remedy with their doctors.

Jeannine wrote in with an herbal approach, soaking the feet daily in a solution of Pau d'Arco tea. Walter goes one better, suggesting an occasional "booster" soak to keep the fungus at bay. And a listener, Louise, called our radio show to say she'd conquered her toenail fungus by taking Pau d'Arco tea internally. We don't know whether Pau d'Arco tea is safe for long-term consumption.

Margaret sticks with foot baths. A cardiologist, based on his own experience, recommended she soak her feet five minutes a day in a solution of warm, soapy water with a little **Clorox** added—one cup of bleach or less to a quart of water. To this we would add that you should discontinue treatment if any irritation occurs. We've heard from many people that vinegar soaks or foot baths with vinegar added are helpful against toenail fungus. It is our impression that all these home treatments require a fair bit of patience and persistence. Do remember, too, that **Clorox** should not be combined with vinegar or other home cleaning solutions.

We must also warn you that many doctors cringe any time we mention these home remedies. Here is one letter we received:

> As a dermatologist I was disappointed you wrote about home remedies for toenail fungus. These anecdotes are no more credible than the ads we see for quick weight-loss schemes or bust developers.
>
> You should stick with scientifically proven medications and not confuse your readers with dubious treatments that haven't been tested. You do a serious disservice to patients by leading them to waste their money on useless remedies such as vitamin E and herbal teas.

We agree that such remedies are untested and unproven, but they *are* a lot less expensive than conventional treatments. Six months' supply of griseofulvin (prescribed by brand names such as **Grifulvin, Gris-PEG, Grisactin,** and **Fulvicin P/G**) could cost over $500. The new antifungal drug **Sporanox** (itraconazole) probably works better, but it's a lot dearer. One person told us he'd spent $1,800 on the medicine—about $10 a day! He was happy, though, because it worked. For people taking griseofulvin, the usual prescription treatment, there are no guarantees.

If you have a stubborn infection that doesn't respond to home remedies or even prescription medicine, the nail may indeed have to come off. Here's a trade secret that even many dermatologists might not have heard of, so you may have to help your doctor by providing the literature reference.

The secret potion is a mixture of urea, white petroleum jelly, lanolin, and beeswax. The chairman of the Department of Dermatology at Stanford University, Dr. Eugene M. Farber, discovered the urea ointment treatment while traveling in the former USSR. He learned that Russian doctors have apparently been using urea plasters "for many years to remove fungus-diseased nails."[39]

After protecting the skin around the infected nail, the goop is applied and covered with a piece of plastic wrap. Booties or plastic gloves can also be used to keep the nail completely dry. After seven to ten days, you return to the doctor and the nail is removed with no strain or pain.

One of the amazing things about this treatment is that normal nail is not affected. The only thing that comes off is diseased nail. According to Dr. Farber and his collaborator, Dr. David South,

> The procedure has several distinct advantages. It is a nonsurgical method, and therefore intrinsically inexpensive for the patient. Multiple abnormal nails can be treated in one session. The procedure is essentially painless, and apparently without risk of infection or hemorrhage, making it ideal for treating patients with diabetes and others with vascular insufficiency [circulatory problems].[40]

Once the diseased nail is gone, the underlying infection can be treated with a topical antifungal ointment. **Tinactin** (tolnaftate), **Micatin** (miconazole), or **Loprox** (ciclopirox) may be effective. Japanese researchers have reported impressive results using a 2-percent tolnaftate ointment along with a 20-percent urea ointment.[41]

There is one prescription cream containing 40-percent urea paste for nail removal. At one time, this ointment had to be specifically compounded by a pharmacist for each patient according to Dr. Farber's formula.[42] Now it is available by prescription as **Gordon's Urea 40%** (manufacturer: Gordon Laboratories; Upper Darby, PA; 800-356-7870 for physicians or pharmacists).

Moo for Your Favorite Moisturizer

N ow that you've taken care of your nails, what about the rest of the hand? Or the body, for that matter? The body loses moisture that has to be replaced, whether it's on your hands or any other part of you. If you have shopped for a moisturizer lately, your head may be spinning. Shelf after shelf is loaded with an incredible array of products, each claiming to outdo the next.

Needless to say, you can spend a lot of money in your quest for soft, silky skin. **Sudden Change Oriental Pearl Moisture Rich Potion**—$3.59 per ounce—contains "crushed precious oriental pearls." **Nivea Visage Liposome Creme with Vitamin E**—$7.64 an ounce—"visibly improves skin's tone and texture for a smoother, more supple appearance." It is also labeled "Creme Jeunesse aux Liposomes," which means "youth cream with liposomes."

Since moisturizers just help the skin hold in moisture better, you don't need something costly to make your arms and legs feel smoother. Plain old petroleum jelly will do the job, but might make you feel like a greased pig. Perhaps what you need is in another part of the barnyard. Whenever we write about **Bag Balm** and **Udder Cream,** testimonials pour in about their benefits. These products average 50 to 70 cents an ounce.

Carol writes: "A friend of mine who also quilts gave me a sample of **Udder Cream** and I love it! Since I am diabetic, my skin gets really dry and **Udder Cream** helps. I like the texture and the fact that it's nongreasy. I'm getting rid of all my other creams and using just this." Another quilter sews up the case for **Bag Balm:** "Quilters prick their fingers while quilting, and **Bag Balm** is not only antiseptic but also very healing and soothing. **Bag Balm** is the thing to have in your sewing kit!"

Other **Bag Balmers** include a professional harpist who uses it during dry winter weather, combined with white cotton gloves, and a reader who soaks her rough feet and then applies **Bag Balm** to them. Then she'd put on white socks and go to bed. Next morning her feet would be like babies' skin.

Bag Balm and **Udder Cream** are among the cheapest moisturizers on the market and are available from some pharmacies, but you may have better luck locating them at farm or feed stores.

If you can stand it, another good cheap moisturizer is even closer to hand. Our dermatological consultant, Dr. Robert Gilgor, recommends **Vaseline** petroleum jelly after bathing to treat rough and dry skin. For one of our readers who suffered from calluses so rough and dry they ripped her hose, Dr. Gilgor suggested she use petroleum jelly after bathing and then cover it with plastic wrap, keeping it in place with a stocking.

But what about the chef whose hands are red and rough? It isn't very appetizing to know that the person who shaped your meat loaf had just slathered on **Vaseline** or **Udder Cream.** Well, there is a simple, inexpensive—and edible—"hand cream" out there called **Crisco.** Our readers report that cooks, who wash their hands frequently, have long used this product. What's more, we've even heard from women who are convinced that Crisco is better than any cold cream for makeup removal and facial moisturizing.

Homespun Hints

T here are scores of other popular home remedies, many of which don't fit into the categories we've mentioned so far. So let's wrap up this chapter with a little tour of the typical home, concentrating on the kitchen and the bathroom.

Baking Soda

Two things that are stocked in probably every kitchen, and by extension every home medical arsenal, are baking soda and vinegar. Baking soda—sodium bicarbonate—may be kept in the bathroom, too, but we'll just assume you have another box besides the one in the fridge. Besides its utility in cooking, it is a wonderful cleaning agent. Even better than that, it has time-honored medicinal applications.

Probably the foremost medical use for baking soda is as an antacid. It neutralizes stomach acid, liberating carbon dioxide (the baking-soda burp) in the process. And unlike many popular antacids, sodium bicarb contains no aluminum. However, it is high in sodium. So if you are on a salt-restricted diet, take baking soda sparingly, if at all.

Besides burping with it, people brush their teeth with it. Baking soda is less abrasive than some toothpastes and may even be helpful in reducing the risk of gum disease. For denture wearers, baking soda makes a good cleaner.

A combination of cornstarch and baking soda can be dusted on underarms or feet to absorb moisture and deodorize naturally. After all, it works for your refrigerator, doesn't it?

And speaking of smelly feet, one of our readers sent in a baking-soda tip on how to get rid of smelly feet.

> Take a pan big enough for your feet and fill it with water as hot as you can stand. Put two tablespoons of plain old baking soda in the water and soak the feet for thirty minutes for thirty nights.

We don't know if thirty days will do the trick, but it certainly couldn't do any harm and is cheaper than foot deodorants. All of the folks who write to us about smelly feet emphasize the importance of shoes that breathe.

Vinegar

Vinegar is as versatile as baking soda. Used for pickling, marinating, and salad dressings, vinegar is also helpful for any number of common problems.

By its acidic nature, vinegar discourages fungus infections. One ear, nose, and throat specialist recommends a solution made from one part white vinegar to five parts tepid water for the itching caused by fungus in the ear canal. The ear is flushed gently three times a day, and the fungus usually responds. Just make sure the liquid is close to body temperature, because if it is too cool or too warm, it could cause dizziness, discomfort, or even damage.

Another ear specialist prevents swimmer's ear by rinsing children's ears with a combination of half vinegar and half alcohol after they get out of the pool. One woman wrote that her granddaughter's pediatrician prescribed a one-third white vinegar soak, fifteen to twenty minutes daily, for toenail fungus.

Warts, headaches, dry skin? We've received letters suggesting that vinegar will cure those maladies by soaking, drinking, and rubbing, respectively. There's no medical data to back it up, but people do say that it works for them.

One doctor-recommended hint came from a reader who suffered from one vaginal infection after another. Her doctor suggested douching with two table-spoons of white vinegar to a pint of warm water. She said it worked so well, "I haven't been troubled with another infection—and that was three years ago." We encourage women to get a proper diagnosis from a physician. If a vinegar douche is appropriate, common sense would dictate not using a solution that is too strong or too hot.

Vinegar is available in some commercial douche products or could be mixed as the physician suggested, using sterile water. Women should not make douching a regular routine, though, because it has been linked to an increased risk of pelvic infections.

The Rest of the Cupboard

Baking soda and vinegar are the two heavy hitters of the kitchen, but let's see what else is in the cupboard, starting with the spice rack. Alum, once widely used as a crisping agent in canning pickles, can be sprinkled in shoes to control stinkiness, according to one grandfather out there.

Tea is a popular remedy for several complaints. A recent study by the National Cancer Institute found that green tea could possibly reduce the incidence of esophageal cancer.[44]

But our readers lean toward more topical applications. Again for smelly feet: A dermatologist friend says to brew five tea bags in a quart of hot water. Let it cool, then soak your feet for thirty minutes. The main ingredient in tea—tannic acid—is used in many commercial products, including **Ivy Dry, Zilactol,** and **Zilactin,** to control excessive sweating.

Instant tea on a canker sore? According to one reader, it smarts for a few seconds, "but this old family remedy has worked for us. Repeat a few times if necessary." The truth is, tannic acid has been used as an astringent for centuries, and products such as **Zilactin** are even designed for use on canker sores.

Mint tea has long been used as a folk remedy in many different countries for generations. Of all the remedies for indigestion, mint tea is probably one of the least expensive and innocuous, not to mention the tastiest.

And don't forget about coffee, which has a wide variety of actions on the entire body. It can affect heart rate, raise blood pressure, stimulate the nervous system, and increase digestive-tract motility. That's why one reader wondered if it was just his imagination or was his morning cup of joe acting like a laxative? It probably wasn't his imagination.

A couple on their honeymoon didn't foresee the bride's asthma attack. With her medication left far behind, she almost panicked when the wheezing started. "I remembered reading in your book that coffee can act as an emergency treatment for asthma. Three cups controlled my attack and I didn't have any more trouble. The rest of the honeymoon was great."

When you're finished with your coffee you can dye your hair with the grounds. The editors of *Sassy* magazine asked hair expert Richard Stein for a natural hair-color agent, and he offered the following: mix a quarter cup blackstrap molasses with one tablespoon used coffee grounds, a tablespoon of dried rosemary, and a tablespoon of your favorite conditioner. Put this stuff on clean, damp hair and wash it out after twenty minutes.

If coffee and tea aren't for you, how about tonic? A reader suffering from leg cramps was told by her doctor to drink a glass of tonic water every afternoon. She says it worked for her. A pharmacist told one of his customers to try drinking buttermilk in order to get rid of his long, painful siege of cold sores. "I tried it," he wrote. "It's easy and cheap and it has really cut down on the number of fever blisters I have suffered."

The Bathroom Cabinet

Canker sores and cold sores find relief in the bathroom medicine cabinet, but not from prescription drugs. One woman made this suggestion:

> I suffered frequently from canker sores and tried everything but nothing worked. Finally, a wise lady told me about baking soda. Now when I feel a sore coming on I brush my teeth and rinse my mouth with baking soda, and haven't had a canker sore since.

Another reader suggested putting **Pepto-Bismol** on a canker sore several times daily, while someone else would send you back to the kitchen to daub yogurt on it.

If you have athlete's foot instead of canker sores, take that hair dryer, set it to high heat, and point it at your toes. After three days of drying the toes for a full minute, one reader got rid of his athlete's foot for good. Drying out the toes can create an inhospitable environment for fungus, but dermatologists sometimes recommend antiperspirants with aluminum to accomplish the same thing.

Baby shampoo is not only good for the hair, but "removes every bit of eye makeup, including mascara (even so-called waterproof mascara) and does not irritate the eyes. Nor does it dry the delicate skin surrounding the eyes," according to one reader. Another reader said her ophthalmologist suggested the same thing. And it's a lot cheaper than most cosmetic cleansers. Of course, common sense dictates that you rinse well after cleaning.

Much Ado About Toilet Seats

A nd while we're in the bathroom, what about toilet seats? We're not suggesting you can catch anything from them, but a lot of people worry about this aspect of sanitation. They are particularly concerned about using them away from their own homes.

It all started innocently enough when we received a letter from a reader who wanted to know how to sterilize the seat in public restrooms. Back pain made it difficult for her to crouch over grungy seats in theaters, gas stations, and fast-food restaurants.

While a search through the medical literature turned up no cases of horrible diseases from sitting on the toilet, this is still a frightening prospect for many. Hovering over the toilet seat can cause urinary difficulties, including reduced flow and an increased susceptibility to bladder infection.[44] This news, however, does not make women feel better about sitting down on a seat of questionable cleanliness. Sterilizing a public restroom toilet seat is virtually impossible. According to microbiologist Chuck Gerba, the only way to sterilize a toilet is to douse it with alcohol and set it aflame.[45] This is not practical! Do not try this at home, or anyplace else, for that matter.

Although some readers use alcohol wipes to clean the seat or a dilute bleach to disinfect it, most prefer disposable paper seat covers. We don't know how well they work against microbes, but they are inexpensive and provide a certain psychological comfort.

One disquieting fact did turn up in the medical literature. Public restroom surfaces are commonly contaminated with invisible intestinal bacteria. Microbiologists found these not only on toilet seats but also on flush and tap handles and doorknobs, which bothers us a lot more.[46] Undoubtedly some of these bacteria get there from people's hands; bacteriologists also worry about aerosolization, which is what happens when you flush. Teeny water droplets, some complete with microbial passengers, are flung into the air in an almost undetectable mist. When it settles, those bugs are left on the surfaces where they landed. That's why one expert recommends that even in your own frequently cleaned home you should keep the toothbrushes as far away from the toilet as possible. [47]

Should you use alcohol wipes on the tap handles? Should you open the door with a paper towel after washing your hands? Should you disinfect your home toilet bowl every day? Sadly enough, we have no answers to these questions, and don't even know if we have anything to worry about. One last tip, though: If you have a choice of stalls in a public bathroom, use the first one. Gerba says, "Everyone avoids that one because they think everyone else uses it."[48]

Danger: Home Remedies

T here you have it: our bag of helpful home hints, most of which have some evidence to support their safety and efficacy. We do need to remind you, though, that home remedies can have a dark side.

Many home remedies don't do anything. There's probably little danger in that except for prolonging your discomfort a bit. There are certain cures, however, that can be far, far worse than the problems they're supposed to treat. And the danger may not be obvious.

Take, for example, the seemingly innocuous practice of putting baking soda on an infant's diaper rash. This remedy is based on the logic that (1) the problem is a highly acidic environment caused by the ammonia in the urine, which should be offset by the alkaline baking soda, and (2) baking-soda soaks are often recommended as first aid for adult rashes, bites, and other skin irritations.

The problem, according to an article in the medical journal *Pediatrics*, is that when applied to an infant's rash, baking soda may be absorbed much more than it would be in an adult. The infant, with immature kidney function, has a limited capacity for clearing the bicarbonate, and the result can be a serious disruption in the acid-base balance of the body.[49] When it comes to babies, extra caution is in order before you smear anything on their skins. They absorb chemicals more readily and are less able to handle them. That's why many of the unpleasant reactions to the insect repellent DEET were reported in infants or young children, and why you're not supposed to use sunscreen on a baby less than six months old.

Herbal Hazards

When it comes to home remedies, none are held in higher esteem than herbs. We tend to think of herbs as gentle things with almost magical powers to heal when rubbed, swallowed, or otherwise applied to the body. This positive attitude is reflected in a large number of books on herbs published in the last several years, and an incredible expansion of the herbal section in your local health food store. Many otherwise sensible and cautious people who wouldn't dream of taking medicine without checking its side effects throw caution aside when they encounter those attractively packaged herbal medicines.

There are indeed roots and herbs with marvelous curative powers. After all, many of our modern medicines are derivatives of herbs. The important heart drug digitalis (**Lanoxin** or digoxin) is from the foxglove plant, the anticancer medicines vincristine and vinblastine are derived from the Madagascar periwinkle, and **Taxol** for ovarian cancer was developed from the Pacific yew.[50]

So what's the problem? Well, there are several. First of all, herbs can be strong medicine, both good and bad. Socrates died drinking an herbal tea, as you may recall.

Herbal products are widely used in certain other countries. In Germany, a standardized extract of ginkgo is one of the most commonly prescribed medications.[51] Where they are accepted as orthodox medical agents, they get the same sort of oversight as pharmaceuticals and there is greater recognition that they may have adverse effects.

But because herbs are hardly regulated at all by the FDA, the potency of herbal remedies varies enormously. This is magnified by the many methods of preparing them. Since systematic clinical testing is rarely done, we know little about the indications and effectiveness of herbal medicines. Worse yet, we may not have good information on adverse reactions, and so we're forced to rely on anecdotes that show that herbs can sometimes cause harm.

One story concerns the 80-year-old relative of a physician who had suffered diarrhea for two months, and had lost considerable weight. The old woman was, needless to say, greatly depleted and the doctors were about to put her through a grueling series of tests when her relative found a bottle of "dark brown liquid" on the kitchen table.

"She told me," reports the doctor, "that this was an alcoholic extract of herbs, which she had prepared herself according to a recipe she had read in a popular phytotherapeutic magazine. . . . [T]he [old Swedish] recipe included laxative herbs such as aloe, senna, rhubarb, and jalap and diuretic herbs such as juniper berry and radix ononidis (restharrow root) in high doses."[52] Placed on a diet of fruits and vegetables, the woman promptly overcame her diarrhea and regained her former vigor.

Four patients taking Chinese herbal medicines for arthritis or back pain suffered even more serious consequences when they came down with the blood disease agranulocytosis and accompanying life-threatening infections. One of the four died.[53]

The herbal concoctions they had been taking turned out to contain both aminopyrine and phenylbutazone as undeclared ingredients. Aminopyrine was once available as an over-the-counter product, but was removed from sale in 1938 because of its known propensity for causing agranulocytosis. Phenylbutazone is used by physicians to treat inflammation, but is used with great care because it too is known to cause blood abnormalities. Yet the herbal remedy was available without a prescription.

This incident and another in which a woman developed severe lead poisoning from another Chinese herbal cure illustrate the problem: It is impossible to know everything that's in an herbal tea or preparation, since the material isn't subject to consistent quality control or testing. Chinese herbal mixtures may contain unlisted medications, sometimes powerful prescription drugs with potentially serious side effects.

Even if the product is strictly herbal material, it's almost impossible to know what the dose limits might be, since rarely, if ever, are there any clinical studies that would help establish the boundary between rational and dangerous use of herbal medicines. Herbal medicines, like any other medicine, should be kept safely locked away from children. Toddlers have had to be treated for poisoning when they ingested a number of tablets of a traditional Chinese product called Jin Bu Huan.[54]

Some home remedies now known to be dangerous ought to be avoided. One is the notion that you should rub snow on frostbitten tissue. It makes things worse by further chilling the skin and constricting blood vessels. Much better is gradual warming in tepid water.

Camphor (camphorated oil—a mixture of camphor and linseed oil) is extremely toxic when taken orally and has accounted for far too many poisonings in the past, especially when parents confused it for castor oil. Children are also susceptible to lead poisoning when they are given certain remedies that may have been passed down from their grandparents. Azarcon and greta, traditional treatments for constipation in families of Mexican descent, have been implicated in a number of incidents. Other cases have been linked to the use of paylooah or surma, which are Asian traditional medicines.[55]

Even something as simple as licorice root or sassafras could be dangerous. Licorice can deplete the body of potassium and cause fluid retention, serious consequences for anyone with high blood pressure. Sassafras-root bark contains sassafras oil, which has been shown to be a cancer-causing chemical in animals. Comfrey may be carcinogenic and toxic to the liver; it should not be taken orally, although it's possible poultices may help wound healing.[56]

Those are traditional herbs that can be dangerous. But home remedies—with possible hazards—are being invented all the time. We first heard about people using **WD-40** on stiff joints from the owner of our local hardware store. He was surprised at how many older folks relied on this remedy for rheumatism.

Our can of **WD-40** claims that it "stops squeaks, protects metal, loosens rusted parts and frees sticky mechanisms." There is no mention anywhere on the label about arthritis. When we combed the medical literature, we could find no studies to support its usefulness for arthritis. *Dr. Dean Edell's Health Letter* suggests that massaging sore joints with almost anything, even **WD-40,** may make them feel better, especially if you believe in it.

Obviously, this is not an FDA-sanctioned remedy and there may be risks. For one thing, you may absorb some of the petroleum ingredients through your skin. And NEVER breathe the spray. There is a report in the medical journal *Chest* that describes a case of chemically induced pneumonia in an elderly woman who overused **WD-40** for her sore back and shoulders.

Many home remedies are helpful and inexpensive. But we need to be careful to keep familiarity from breeding contempt or carelessness. Like any medications, home remedies need to be used with caution, moderation, and common sense. Don't forget, symptoms that persist deserve medical attention.

If you've got a home remedy you've found helpful, we'd love to hear about it. We might even write it up in our newspaper column or the next edition of *The People's Pharmacy*. Please send your reports to:

Graedons People's Pharmacy: Dept. HR
P.O. Box 52027
Durham, NC 27717-2027

References

1. Eisenberg, David M., et al. "Unconventional Medicine in the United States: Prevalence, Costs, and Patterns of Use." *N. Engl. J. Med.* 1993; 328:246–252.
2. Ibid.
3. Ibid.
4. "Chicken Soup and the Common Cold." Mayo Clinic Health Letter, October 1984, p. 5.
5. "Chicken Soup." *Lawrence Review of Natural Products*. St. Louis: Facts & Comparisons, 1987.
6. Avorn, Jerry, et al. "Reduction of Bacteriuria and Pyuria After Ingestion of Cranberry Juice." *JAMA* 1994; 271:751–754.
7. Ibid.
8. "Why Hiccups Start and How You Can Stop Them." Mayo Clinic Health Letter, September 1984, p. 3.
9. Engelman Edgar G., et. al. "Granulated Sugar as Treatment for Hiccups in Conscious Patients." *N. Engl. J. Med.* 1971; 285:1489.
10. Margolis, George. "Hiccup Remedies." *N. Engl. J. Med.* 1972; 286:323.
11. Herman, Jay Howard, and David S. Nolan, "A Bitter Cure." *N. Engl. J. Med.* 1981; 305:1054.
12. Brenn, Ethel. "Sequel on Singultus." *N. Engl. J. Med.* 1982; 306:1115.
13. LeWitt, P., et al. "Hiccup with Dexamethasone Therapy." *Ann. Neurol.* 1982; 12:405–406.
14. Helm, James F., et al. "Effect of Esophageal Emptying and Saliva on Clearance of Acid From the Esophagus. *N. Engl. J. Med.* 1984; 310:284–288.
15. "Chinese-Restaurant Syndrome." *Nutrition and the M.D.* 1982; 8(12):1.
16. "Cold Medicines." *Glamour,* May 1984, p. 345.
17. "Garlic." *Lawrence Review of Natural Products*, Olin, Bernie R., ed. St. Louis: Facts & Comparisons, April 1994.

18. "Consumer Expenditure Study." *Product Marketing* 1984; 13(8):22.

19. Long, Patricia. "The Power of Vitamin C." *Health* 1992; October 6:66.

20. "Sniffles and Sneezes 'Take Two Zincs . . .'" *Medical World News,* February 13, 1984, pp. 41.

21. News Front. "Zinc Speeding Recovery from the Common Cold." *Modern Medicine,* July 1984, p. 43.

22. "Echinacea." *Lawrence Review of Natural Products.* St. Louis: Facts & Comparisons, 1990.

23. Mowrey, Daniel B., and Dennis E. Clayson. "Motion Sickness, Ginger and Psychophysics." *Lancet* 1982; 1:655–657.

24. "Heat and Cold as Analgesics." *Medical Letter* 1970; 12:3–4.

25. Chatten, Milton J. "Disorders Due to Physical Agents," in *Current Medical Diagnosis and Treatment,* Krup, Marcus and Milton Chatton, 1983. Los Altos, CA: Lange Medical Publications, 1983, p. 963.

26. Shulman, A. G. "Ice Water as Primary Treatment of Burns." *JAMA,* 1960; 173:1916–1919.

27. Arnold, Harry L. "Immediate Treatment of Insect Stings." *JAMA,* 1972; 220:585.

28. Sulzberger, M. B., et al. *Dermatology Diagnosis and Treatment.* Chicago: Yearbook, 1961, p. 94.

29. LoCriccho, J., Jr., and J. R. Haserick. "Hot Water Treatment for Warts." *Cleveland Clinic Quarterly* 1962; 29:156–161.

30. "Hot Water Soaks Said to Be Effective for Plantar Warts." *Skin & Allergy News* 1989.

31. Dr. Samuel Moschella, Lahey Clinic Medical Center, personal communication, June 29, 1994.

32. Bulkeley, William M. "'Deet, by Any Name, Doesn't Smell Sweet to a Pesky Mosquito." *Wall Street Journal,* May 26, 1983, p. 1.

33. "DEET's Downside." *Consumer Reports.* July 1993, pp. 455–458.

34. "S.C. Johnson's Off! Ads 'Sabotage' Avon's Skin-So-Soft." *FDC Reports—The Tan Sheet* 1994; 2(23):16.

35. Benforado, Joseph M. "Removal of Ticks." *JAMA* 1984; 252:3368.

36. Sherman, Warren T. "Polishing Off Ticks."*N. Engl. J. Med.* 1983; 309:992.

37. Shakman, Robert. "Tick Removal." *Western J. Med.* 1984; 140(1):99.

38. "New Formula Offers Hope for Chronically Brittle Nails." American Academy of Dermatology, news release, March 22, 1984.

39. "Diseased Nails Are Easily Shed with Urea Treatment." *Medical World News*, February 5, 1979, p. 88.

40. Farber, Eugene, and David South. "Urea Ointment in the Nonsurgical Avulsion of Nail Dystrophies." *Cutis* 1978; 22:689–692.

41. Ishii, Masamitsu, et al. "Treatment of Onychomycosis by OD Therapy with 20 Urea Ointment and 2 Tolnaftate Ointment." *Dermatologica* 1983; 167:273–279.

42. South, David A. and Eugene M. Farber. "Urea Ointment in the Nonsurgical Avulsion of Nail Dystrophies—A Reappraisal." *Cutis* 1980; 25:609–612.

43. "Green Tea: More Than Just a Soothing Brew," *The New York Times,* June 15, 1994, p. C1.

44. Moore, K. H., et al. "Crouching Over the Toilet Seat: Prevalence among British Gynae-cological Outpatients and Its Effect on Micturition." *Brit. J. Obstet. and Gyn.* 1991; 98:569–572.

45. Roach, Mary. "How to Win at Germ Warfare." *Health* 1994; 8(4):77–80.

46. Scott, Elizabeth, and Sally F. Bloomfield. "A Bacteriological Investigation of the Effec-tiveness of Cleaning and Disinfection Procedures for Toilet Hygiene." *J. Applied Bac-teriology* 1985; 59:291–297.

47. Roach, op. cit.

48. Ibid.

49. Gonzalez, M. D., and R. J. Hogg. "Metabolic Alkalosis Secondary to Baking Soda Treat-ment of a Diaper Rash." *Pediatrics* 1981; 67:820–822.

50. "Pharmaceuticals Plants: Great Potential, Few Funds." *Lancet* 1994; 343:1513–1515.

51. Ibid., 1514.

52. Eichler, Ingeborg. "Cryptic Illness from Self-Medication with Herbal Remedy." *Lancet* 1983; 6(12):356.

53. Ries, Curt A., and Mervyn A. Sahud. "Agranulocytosis Caused by Chinese Herbal Medi-cines. *JAMA* 1975; 231:352–355.

54. "Jin Bu Huan Toxicity in Children—Colorado, 1993." *MMWR* 1993; 42:633–636.

55. "Lead Poisoning Associated with Use of Traditional Ethnic Remedies—California, 1991–1992." *MMWR* 1993; 42:521–524.

56. "Comfrey." *Lawrence Review of Natural Products*. St. Louis: Facts & Comparisons, 1990.

Part III

Prescription Drugs

7

Drug Interactions:
When 1 + 1 May Equal 3

"The time has come," the Walrus said,
"To talk of many things:
Of shoes—and ships—and sealing-wax—
Of cabbages—and kings—
And why the sea is boiling hot—
And whether pigs have wings."

—Lewis Carroll
Through the Looking-Glass

D rug interactions are the Achilles' heel of the medical profession. The laws of nature no longer hold true. This is a crazy world where one plus one equals three, where down may very well be up, and surely pigs have wings. In fact, mixing medicines is very much like playing Russian roulette. You never know when a particular combination will produce a lethal outcome."

When we wrote those words two decades ago in the first edition of this book, we had no idea how prophetic it would be and how many people would be interested in this issue. Drug interactions seemed like a pretty esoteric topic, one that only a pharmacologist could get excited about. We were amazed when thousands of letters started pouring in about the various combinations of drugs people were being given.

All of a sudden, what had been of only theoretical concern became all too real. Readers related horror stories that sent chills up and down our spines. One woman from Orlando, Florida, wrote about her sister:

> **M**y sister was taking Valium, Lanoxin, Enduron and Emfaseen every day. When her ankles swelled her doctor prescribed Lasix and Inderal.
>
> I was with her when she asked the doctor what medication she should stop while she took these new prescriptions. He told her just to add them to the others.
>
> She became extremely weak and lost ten pounds of fluid very suddenly, so she went back to the doctor. He just told her to keep taking all the medicine. When she complained that all the drugs were making her feel weak and tired, he answered, "If playing bridge and going to the hairdresser means more to you than getting well, then do whatever you like."
>
> Naturally she did what her doctor told her to. She died a month later, a senile old lady, though she had been an active, outgoing person before. The death certificate just read "cardiac arrest." That only means her heart stopped beating, but I think all those medications killed her.

Of course there is no way to prove whether this woman did indeed die from drug interactions, but the medications she was taking could easily have been responsible for her symptoms of fatigue, disorientation, and confusion. The diuretics **Lasix** (furosemide) and **Enduron** (methyclothiazide) almost definitely depleted her body of potassium, a life-threatening situation for anyone taking the heart medicine **Lanoxin** (digoxin). Low potassium levels predispose people taking digitalis to potentially fatal irregular heart rhythms. As if that weren't enough, **Inderal** (propranolol) may have removed what little reserve was left in a heart already failing.

This is only one case, but we have received many, many other heart-wrenching letters. We'll never forget the story of the young mother who was put on **Reglan** (metoclopramide) for her heartburn, **Asendin** (amoxapine) for depression, **Halcion** (triazolam) for insomnia, and **Valium** (diazepam) for anxiety.

This combination turned her into a zombie, barely able to walk or talk. One of her drugs (**Reglan**) could have brought on insomnia, anxiety, and depression by itself, and also produced drowsiness and dizziness. The other medications prescribed to treat the insomnia, depression, and anxiety only added to the problem by increasing her sedation, disorientation, fatigue, and faintness. When a new doctor advised her to stop all medications abruptly she went through hell and even weeks later was having a terrible time sleeping.

Who's in Charge?

Trying to avoid drug interactions is a little like trekking blindfolded through a treacherous swamp full of ravenous reptiles. Your guide may not realize there is a man-eating alligator behind you, but even if he warns you about that hazard, he might miss the quicksand ahead, or the poisonous snake about to drop out of a tree right on top of you.

Obviously no one in his right mind would venture into such a situation without being prepared. Yet every time you mix medicines you could be risking dangers that are equally unexpected and life-threatening. Perhaps even scarier, your trusted guide, the doctor, may be as blind as you are to the dangers ahead.

There is no good way to predict in advance which drugs will be incompatible. The Food and Drug Administration has not required pharmaceutical manufacturers to test new compounds for interaction potential. And the feds have no organized, systematic, scientific method for collecting information on interaction problems. As a result physicians have to play a deadly game of blindman's buff whenever they prescribe more than one medication.

Only after severe adverse reactions occur or the bodies start stacking up do reports show up in the medical literature. But physicians and pharmacists have to be incredibly vigilant to detect this information because there is no central clearinghouse or efficient way to alert health professionals to interaction hazards.

Even when such interactions appear in reference books and computer databases (often years late), many overworked physicians may be unaware of the dangers of mixing certain compounds. How does this sort of thing happen? Why do people end up receiving prescriptions for numerous medications that should never be taken together?

Several factors are responsible. First, of course, is the fact that an enormous number of medications are available by prescription with more being introduced constantly. Add to that the hundreds of thousands of over-the-counter remedies, all of which also have the potential to interact with each other and with prescription medications, and you begin to grasp the immensity of the situation.

Another part of the problem may be arrogance. Too many doctors either assume they know all the essential information about the drugs they prescribe or wish to appear knowledgeable in front of their patients. Just how would it look, they think, to have to flip through a "crib sheet" like the *PDR* (*Physicians' Desk Reference*) or a drug interaction handbook while a patient watches?

But that's just plain foolishness and false pride. It is absolutely impossible for any human being to remember all the relevant side effects and cautions associated with the thousands of prescription drugs on the market, let alone know how all of them interact with each other. It would take a computer to keep track of all the possible permutations and combinations. Most people would be delighted if their doctor took a few extra minutes to look up drug interaction precautions.

The risk of experiencing an adverse reaction increases astronomically as the number of drugs a person takes goes up. Take aspirin, for example. Americans down 80 million aspirins a day—more than 29 billion pills a year. That's enough for every man, woman, and child to swallow 117 tablets annually. So many people are gorping down an aspirin a day to ward off a heart attack or a stroke that they almost take this drug for granted.

But aspirin interacts with dozens of other drugs to produce unexpected and occasionally serious problems. Even when an interaction is reported, physicians may not realize its significance. For example, an article appeared in the *Journal of the American College of Cardiology* in December 1992 titled "Counteraction of the Vasodilator Effects of Enalapril [**Vasotec**] by Aspirin in Severe Heart Failure."

Vasotec is one of the most prescribed drugs in the world. It is extremely helpful for patients with heart failure and high blood pressure. But this article suggested that as little as one aspirin could reduce the effectiveness of Vasotec: "In patients with severe heart failure, concomitant use of aspirin could compromise the beneficial actions of angiotensin-converting enzyme inhibitors [such as **Vasotec** and **Capoten**], particularly on symptoms and survival. . . ."[1]

The results of this study were astounding and have implications for hundreds of thousands of heart patients. We were so concerned about this research that we contacted the manufacturer of **Vasotec** (Merck) not once, but several times to get a reaction or at least some guidelines for physicians and patients.[2,3] After all, with millions taking aspirin and millions taking **Vasotec** it is quite likely there would be a lot of overlap.

What we got back was classic company CYA (Cover Your A**) gobbledygook. Dr. Charles M. Alexander, Director of Professional Services for Merck, acknowledged that the authors of the research "concluded that in patients with severe heart failure, aspirin decreased the effectiveness of enalapril. . . ." He continued, "[L]ong-term studies are needed to confirm these results."[4]

No one we talked to at Merck would commit to instituting such studies and the company fell back on a tired chestnut: "Merck does not recommend the use of its products in any manner other than as described in the prescribing information." Of course there is no mention of such an interaction in the prescribing information, so you and your doctor are on your own.

We have belabored this point to demonstrate how difficult it can be to get answers to these extremely thorny questions. If aspirin diminishes the benefits of **Vasotec**, doctors and patients need to be told so they can take appropriate countermeasures. Unfortunately, at the time of this writing we are no closer to an answer than we were when the research was published in 1992. And Merck is the Cadillac of drug companies. If it can't do better than CIA (Cover Its A**), then you can imagine what some of the less reputable drug manufacturers do.

Whether aspirin affects blood pressure control with drugs such as **Vasotec** or **Capoten** is also unresolved. We received a letter describing the following episode: "A friend told me that you recently had an article regarding the side effects of aspirin and **Vasotec**. In December I took four 325 mg pills of **Ecotrin** [coated aspirin] for back pain and was on either 5 or 10 mg of **Vasotec** twice a day when my blood pressure went up to 210/90 and my nose bled profusely."

No one can say that aspirin was responsible for this hypertensive crisis. There is no way to track such interactions. Merck says it has logged only three aspirin-and-**Vasotec** interactions since the drug was marketed. That could mean either that it's not a problem or that no one has bothered to report such interactions to the manufacturer.

We asked a question at the beginning of this chapter—Who's in charge? By now you should realize that the answer is no one. No one is flying this plane—not the drug company, not the FDA, and not your doctor. We're up there on our own and we'd better be as informed as possible if we want to avoid a crash. By the way, never stop taking aspirin or **Vasotec** without medical supervision! These drugs are life savers; aspirin prevents blood clots, heart attacks, and strokes, and **Vasotec** protects the body from the ravages of hypertension, heart failure, and diabetes! (See page 192 for more on the benefits of aspirin.)

Killer Combinations

Most drug interactions are merely annoying—increased drowsiness or dizziness; perhaps some nausea and diarrhea. A little known factoid, for example, is that iron supplements can reduce absorption of thyroid hormones such as **Synthroid** and may lead to symptoms of hypothyroidism (fatigue, dry skin, weakness, constipation, cold intolerance, brittle fingernails, etc.). This may make people feel uncomfortable, but shouldn't pose a substantial health threat.

But every once in a while someone stumbles across a life-threatening drug interaction. These tragedies rarely show up in premarket testing. It may take months or even years before someone discovers that a particular combination is deadly.

Take the example of **Seldane** (terfenadine). This antihistamine took the market by storm when it was launched in 1985. At last there was an allergy treatment that didn't put you to sleep. Tens of millions of prescriptions were written for **Seldane** and it quickly became the most successful allergy treatment in the pharmacy. But then the darker side of **Seldane** began to surface.

Dave Flockhart and Raymond Woosley are clinical pharmacologists at Georgetown University. They are extraordinary human beings—heroes—asking crucial questions and coming up with important answers. Stephen Fried, an investigative journalist, interviewed them in *The Washington Post Magazine* about the flaws in drug testing:

We can tell you a story," Flockhart began, and they proceeded to tag-team through their research into the antihistamine Seldane and its occasional association with heart arrhythmias [irregular rhythms]. . . .

"Seldane was the 10th most prescribed drug in the country," Woosley cut in, "and it was just about to go over-the-counter," meaning that the drug was about to become available without prescription. "Buried in the experiments were some arrhythmias, patients blacking out. . . . So, there was a case at Bethesda Naval Hospital where a woman was on ketoconazole [**Nizoral**] for a fungal infection and took a friend's Seldane and started blacking out. They called in clin pharm, looked into it as a drug interaction, and ended up presenting it to Carl Peck [who was then director of the FDA's Center for Drug Evaluation and Research]. It was an arrhythmia. It turns out the company had a bunch of these cases and called them overdoses.

"The company stand is, 'We thought it was an overdose. The parent compound [in the drug] was found in high levels.' What happens, we now know, is, when you take it with this other drug, the parent compound builds up—and that's what causes trouble. . . . Carl Peck was telling me that the company wanted to come up and talk to him about going OTC. Carl said, 'Why don't you come up, but the question is going to be if it stays on the market at all.' . . . It didn't go over-the-counter, and Seldane now carries this big boxed warning [about possible interactions with ketoconazole as well as erythromycin]. So you can see why there is a disincentive to the drug company to find out what was wrong with this drug."

Flockhart jumped in. "This is representative of the kind of research that never gets done. . . ."[5]

Adverse drug reactions and interactions are slow to trickle in to the FDA, but by 1992 the agency had 64 cases of serious irregular heart rhythms, 16 heart attacks, and 4 deaths associated with **Seldane**.[6] Seven years after its introduction the feds woke up to the danger and forced the manufacturer to send out strong letters to doctors warning about a potentially life-threatening **Seldane** interaction with the antifungal drug ketoconazole (**Nizoral**) and the antibiotic erythromycin (**E.E.S., E-Mycin, ERYC, EryPed, Ery-Tab, Ilosone, PCE,** etc.).

Even after 600,000 "Dear Doctor" mailgrams were sent to physicians, pharmacists, and nurse practitioners, the lethal combination continued to be prescribed. A 29-year-old woman died from cardiac arrest after **Nizoral** and **Seldane** were taken together. An article in *Journal of the American Medical Association* noted that "Recent case reports involving this combination suggest that a satisfactory awareness of this potentially fatal drug-drug interaction in the prescribing community has not been achieved."[7] In a classic understatement, these physicians went on to note that "The efficacy of the 'Dear Doctor' warning mechanism in relation to altering physician prescribing habits is not known. This terfenadine-ketoconazole example may indicate a suboptimal impact on physician practice."[8]

In diplomatic doctorspeak these researchers have just said that the system doesn't work. So there you have it. Uncovering dangerous or deadly interactions is slow business. We suspect that a lot of interactions *never* get discovered. The bodies have to stack up pretty high before they get anyone's attention. Years can go by before the FDA requires an announcement. And, worst of all, even when "Dear

Doctor" letters get sent out with great fanfare, prescribing patterns may not change.

The number of drugs that interact in dangerous, if not lethal, ways is staggering. For starters, anyone taking popular prescription drugs such as **Calan** (verapamil), **Capoten** (captopril), **Coumadin** (warfarin), **Dilantin** (phenytoin), **Dyazide** (HCTZ, triamterene), **Hismanal** (astemizole), **Inderal** (propranolol), **Lanoxin** (digoxin), **Lopid** (gemfibrozil), **Maxzide** (HCTZ, triamterene), **Mevacor** (lovastatin), **Paxil** (paroxetine), **Pravachol** (pravastatin), **Procardia** (nifedipine), **Prozac** (fluoxetine), **Tagamet** (cimetidine), **Theo-Dur** (theophylline), **Vasotec** (enalapril), **Zocor** (simvastatin), and **Zoloft** (sertraline) had best make sure their physicians and pharmacists are doing their homework and can warn about any serious interactions.

How to Protect Yourself from Drug Misadventures

C ertainly not all drugs interact dangerously, but whenever you take more than one medicine at a time, the potential exists for a drug-drug interaction.

There are several other reasons why this problem has become so severe in recent years. When we were growing up we had a family doctor—the good old GP, or "general practitioner." He took care of every member of the family for just about everything that ailed us. He even made house calls. Since he prescribed all our medicines he could keep track of everything we were taking. And when we got the prescriptions filled we always took them to the neighborhood pharmacy where old "Doc" Sidon filled them and took a few minutes to chat and discuss family health matters.

Today we're in the era of specialty medicine. It sometimes seems there's a specialist for each body part, external and internal. If we have a stomachache we are referred to the gastroenterologist. If our head hurts, it's off to the neurologist. Trouble peeing?—see a urologist. It's not at all unusual for a person to be seeing three or more physicians, and that's where the worst drug-interaction dangers often lurk.

You'd be amazed how hard it is for the right hand to talk to the left hand even in the same hospital. We have been amazed how often charts never make it where they are supposed to go. One office forgets to forward something to another. Unless Doctor B has reason to get your medical records from Doctor A, *and* Doctor C, he or she will have only one way of knowing what medications you're taking. That's right—the patient.

Of course, a careful doctor will always ask, but if you count on that to protect you it's likely you'll eventually get hurt. Some doctors are very aware of drug interaction problems; others don't give it a lot of thought. Some doctors might never think you'd even consider seeing anyone else. If your doctor does not ask what other medications you may be taking before he prescribes, tell him anyway. Of course, this means that you have to be aware of all the drugs you take. Knowing that you take "a little white heart pill" or a "blue water pill" isn't enough.

Make sure you know the names and strengths of all the drugs you take and how often you take them. Make a list if necessary and keep it in your wallet or purse at all times. And don't forget to include vitamins, OTC medications, herbal remedies, wine, and cigarettes. People who smoke metabolize drugs differently, and alcohol may also affect prescribed medication. Pin down your doctor about the chances of a drug interaction. If he doesn't know it automatically, he may be prompted to look it up.

This may prevent not only dangerous interactions but also duplications. We are constantly amazed at the number of times a reader will send us a list of the drugs he is taking and on that list will be the same medicine twice. For example, someone might have received **Lanoxin** from one doctor and digoxin from another. Different names, but the same identical drug (one is the brand name, the other its generic equivalent). Such duplication can lead to dangerous overdoses and toxic reactions. Perhaps it's time to look for a neighborhood pharmacy again. There are so many drugstores these days, many of them chains with the druggist squirreled away in back behind a partition, that it is hard to form a personal relationship with a pharmacist. But today's pharmacists are better trained than ever before and in many cases know even more about drug interactions than the doctor. In fact, many pharmacies now have computers that immediately red-flag potentially hazardous drug combinations.

If you can find a pharmacist who cares and is willing to communicate valuable health information, it could be worth your while to buy all medicines from that person. And that includes over-the-counter remedies. Cold remedies, pain relievers such as ibuprofen (**Advil, Bayer Select Ibuprofen, Haltran, Midol 200, Motrin IB, Nuprin,** etc.) and naproxen (**Aleve**), antacids, and even vitamins can interact with prescription drugs.

And don't forget alcohol. It can interact with dozens of other drugs or chemicals. By the way, alcohol is often an ingredient in many nonprescription medications such as **NyQuil Nighttime Cold/Flu Medicine Liquid** (50 proof), **Pertussin PM Liquid** (50 proof), **Comtrex Liquid** (40 proof), **Vicks Formula 44M Cough and Cold Liquid** (40 proof), **Medi-Flu Liquid** (38 proof), **Contac Severe Cold & Flu Nighttime Liquid** (37 proof), and **Tylenol Cough with Decongestant Liquid** (20 proof).

If the pharmacist keeps a patient profile that lists all the prescriptions, over-the-counter medications, herbal remedies, vitamins, and minerals you are taking, he can prevent duplication and drug-drug interactions. Of course, a good rule of thumb is to try and limit all drug consumption to as few things as possible. In the event you must take more than one medicine at a time, check with your doctor and your pharmacist about complications.

Hospitals Can Be Hazardous to Your Health

T hat is an inflammatory statement if ever there was one—something you might expect from the Graedons. But hold on to your hat . . . this comes from the respectable and conservative Board of Trustees of the American Medical Association. In June 1994 this prestigious group of physicians offered their colleagues some extraordinary observations and recommendations.[9] Here are some of the highlights of the AMA report:[10]

- "Roughly one out of 25 patients experienced an adverse reaction while in the hospital."[11]

- "Medication errors were the most common cause of nonoperative adverse events, occurring in 19.4% of the 1,133 affected patients."

- "Fortunately, a large majority of the adverse events did not result in serious disability. . . . However, 2.6% of the affected patients suffered permanent disabling injuries and 13.6% died."

- "Medication error is a common ground for malpractice litigation. In 90,000 malpractice claims over a period of 7 years, medication error is the second most prevalent and second most expensive."[12]

- "Physicians are mostly responsible for prescribing errors. . . . Errors are often introduced by illegible handwriting, misspelling and the use of inappropriate abbreviations in written orders. . . ."

- "When a patient is attended to by more than one physician, errors may result if an individual physician prescribes medication without consulting with other colleagues."

- "Physicians should evaluate the patient's total status and review all existing drug therapy before prescribing new or additional medications (e.g., to ascertain possible antagonistic drug interactions)."

- "Written drug or prescription orders (including signatures) should be legible. Physicians with poor handwriting should print or type medication orders. . . . Medication orders should be clear and unambiguous."

Do you believe that? For 20 years we have been preaching this message till we were blue in the face. We have been assailed, denounced, and otherwise criticized for bashing doctors. Then comes the most conservative group of doctors you can find—the Board of Trustees of the AMA—and they say (1) Medication errors are common and could be prevented; (2) Physicians often make mistakes—wrong drug, wrong dose, wrong combination; (3) Drug errors are often caused by illegible handwriting and Latin abbreviations; (4) Drug interactions are a real problem and need to be reduced.

Studies show that the average hospital patient will gulp an astounding nine drugs in the course of his or her visit.[13] Many will get the dubious benefits of more than 20 pills and potions while hospitalized. Nothing brings this home better than a personal example. Let us tell you about William. At 70 he was one of the most active, capable people that we knew. He worked eight-hour days, cut his own lawn (with a push mower), and had a mind that was sharp as a tack. Normally William was a cautious person who would think twice and ask plenty of good questions before taking any medicine.

William's doctor wanted him to go into the hospital for some tests. It was not supposed to be a big deal—some X-rays and blood work—but in the hospital William almost died because of a series of mistakes leading to drug complications. Almost from the moment he walked in the door, hospital policy undermined his confidence.

Wanting to be a good patient, William did not complain though he suspected all was not right. The nurses not only insisted that he take sleeping medicine he did not need, but also kept making him swallow all sorts of other pills without telling him what they were or why he had to take them. If he had been less reluctant to protest, he might not have received the wrong medications and suffered a life-threatening drug reaction. It took him months to recover, and he never did regain his full former vigor.

What happened to William is not an isolated event. An analysis of medication errors at 40 hospitals uncovered a startling 3,427 mistakes in a year.[14] The wrong medicine was given in the wrong way for the wrong reasons. Sometimes the right drug was administered too often, while other times the right drug wasn't given at all.

Even when the medicine is given correctly—that is, according to the doctor's instructions—there can be problems. Dr. Marion Friedman, writing in the journal *Postgraduate Medicine,* relates the following:

> In the past several years I have seen several cases in my own practice which I feel involved iatrogenic problems [problems induced by the physician or by the care prescribed]. One was a sudden death which I attributed to interaction of digoxin and quinidine. Another involved a patient with daily fever spiking to 104°F, evidence of newly acquired liver damage, severe leukopenia, and marked lymphadenopathy, all produced by tetracycline. The patient rapidly recovered after discontinuing tetracycline use.[15]

Dr. Friedman also found that increasing confusion and eventual coma in one elderly man was at first attributed to a stroke but actually resulted from the ulcer drug **Tagamet.** When this drug was stopped the patient "regained complete alertness within 24 hours."[16]

Adverse psychological or behavioral reactions to drugs are far more common than most physicians realize. Estrogen and progesterone can cause depression in some women. Men may find they are fatigued or down in the dumps while on heart and blood pressure medicines such as **Blocadren** (timolol), **Inderal** (propranolol), or **Lopressor** (metoprolol). Even something as seemingly innocuous as **Reglan** (metoclopramide), a remedy for heartburn, can bring on the blues.

Patients who complain about feeling down in the dumps may then be given antidepressants such as **Elavil** (amitriptyline) or **Prozac** (fluoxetine) to counteract the side effects of their blood pressure medications. If the choice is **Elavil** they may become confused and disoriented from the drug combinations. In the case of **Prozac** they may experience anxiety and insomnia, for which an antianxiety agent such as **Xanax** (alprazolam) may be prescribed. This is sometimes referred to as the vicious-cycle syndrome—one drug causing side effects for which another is prescribed, and another, and another until the patient is a walking drugstore.

An article in the *Journal of the American Medical Association (JAMA)* has provided some startling statistics. When 34 people diagnosed as having delirium from "unknown causes" were reexamined, 38 percent of them were found to be having a toxic reaction to prescribed drugs. Add to that group the 17 percent of the diagnosed "major depression" cases, and the nearly one-third of the "adjustment disorder" patients who also were having delirium due to drug reactions and you get a pretty significant percentage of patients whose problem was their "cure."[17]

A lot of people were just sick of their drugs, and a lot of doctors didn't realize the cause of the problem. Dr. Friedman admits quite candidly that one patient he witnessed "almost died from the effects of tetracycline and the other from those of procainamide, even when each had been seen by a number of physicians and was under hospital supervision."[18]

How to Protect Yourself While in the Hospital

There are ways you can help protect yourself against drug errors and interactions when in the hospital:

- *Number one*—Never swallow any tablet, capsule, or liquid, or accept any shot or suppository without knowing exactly what you are being given and why. This is especially important if you've been moved to a new room, or if the nursing shift has just changed. If you've been put in Mrs. Smith's bed, someone could be giving you Mrs. Smith's medication.

- *Number two*—Make sure you know what the risks and benefits of the medication are and never forget that you have the right to refuse any medicine. Just because they have taken your clothes away in the hospital doesn't mean you have given up your rights, too. If you feel intimidated by the nurse or doctor, get a family member to stand up for you. When in doubt say no. Make someone explain precisely why they want you to take drug X. We know of one man who almost died because the nurse insisted he take a penicillin-type antibiotic although he told her he was allergic to penicillin.

- **Number three**—Always tell the doctor, nurse, medical student, pharmacist, or any other health worker you see what medications you're taking. Do not assume the information is in your chart or that it has necessarily been seen and remembered.

- **Number four**—Most important, report any side effects so it can be determined whether or not what's supposed to be making you better isn't in fact making you sick. Don't leave home without a healthy dose of skepticism to swallow with the medications you will almost inevitably be offered while in a hospital.

What Is a Drug Interaction?

What is a drug interaction anyway? A drug-drug interaction is simply a situation where two or more compounds, finding themselves together in your body, produce unwanted, unpredictable, or unfortunate complications.

When two drugs are taken simultaneously, they may go about their pharmacologic business without affecting each other in the least. That would be the best of all possible worlds, but don't count on it working that way because you are literally betting your life on the outcome.

A more likely possibility is that one medication will give an extra kick to either the therapeutic or toxic effects of the other. This is where 1 + 1 starts to add up to trouble very quickly. For example, someone who's taking tranquilizers can court death by drinking too much. The two drugs together (remember, alcohol is a drug) sedate more heavily than either alone. Some pretty famous actors and musicians have ended up stone cold because of this kind of combination.

That's an example you have read about over and over ad nauseam. Here is one we'll bet you—and probably your doctor—have never heard of.

Grapefruit juice is a wonderful beverage. We love it—tart, high in vitamin C, not as sweet as orange juice. All in all a great way to start the morning. BUT . . . grapefruit juice contains flavonoids—naringenin, quercetin, kaempferol—that can alter liver enzymes and affect drug metabolism. The result is that grapefruit juice can boost the blood levels of certain drugs and increase the risk of side effects. Heart and blood pressure medicines such as felodipine (**Plendil**) and nifedipine (**Adalat, Procardia**) are affected.[19,20,21]

We have also received personal communication from clinical pharmacologist David Flockhart of Georgetown University that **Seldane** (terfenadine) may be altered by grapefruit juice.[22] As we have already pointed out, increased blood levels of **Seldane** can be extremely hazardous, if not lethal. The powerful immune-suppressing drug **Sandimmune** (cyclosporine) may also be modified by grapefruit juice. Bottom line—even something as simple as your morning glass of grapefruit juice could interact with certain medications.

Okay, you now have an idea how one drug can increase toxicity of another. How about $1 + 1 = 0$? This happens when the antibiotic tetracycline is taken with milk or milk products (yogurt, cream in your coffee, cottage cheese, ice cream, etc.). Antacids and multivitamins with minerals can also wipe out virtually all benefit from tetracycline. Imagine a situation where a woman has the sexually transmitted infection *Chlamydia*. This organism can cause infertility if left untreated. The drug of choice is tetracycline. Yet if a woman were to swallow this medicine in the morning and take a calcium supplement or have a little yogurt or cereal with milk, she would not get any antibiotic effect.

Someone with Lyme disease might also be prescribed tetracycline. Something as simple as a vitamin-and-mineral supplement could reduce effectiveness and make a cure more difficult.

Less common but no less significant is the interaction between barbiturates (pentobarbital, phenobarbital, secobarbital, etc.) and oral contraceptives. Imagine a woman who suffers from tension headaches. She could easily receive a prescription for **Fiorinal,** which contains the barbiturate butalbital along with aspirin and caffeine. Do you think the doctor will warn her that this headache remedy could possibly interact with her contraceptive to reduce its effectiveness? In our experience, not likely.

But butalbital, as well as other barbiturates, may increase the metabolism of oral contraceptives and reduce their effectiveness. This could lead to spotting and breakthrough bleeding, not to mention an unwanted pregnancy.[23] A number of penicillin-type or tetracycline-type antibiotics may also reduce effectiveness of the Pill. We know of several unplanned pregnancies that resulted when a woman taking oral contraceptives also got a prescription for an antibiotic with no caution from her doctor.

Sometimes interactions can be predicted based on knowledge of the drug's expected behavior in the body. Other times the interactions come as quite a surprise. New drugs are often the biggest problem because it may take several years and hundreds of thousands of human "guinea pigs" before physicians realize through trial and error that certain combinations are dangerous.

Even something as simple as a laxative can indirectly interfere with another drug. The speeding up of gastric motion can hinder normal absorption. That means less of what you need winds up getting into the blood so it can go to work.

Most times a drug interaction is unwanted and harmful, but on occasion it can be exploited to a patient's advantage. Giving an antidote for a particular poison is a beneficial drug interaction. When a person overdoses on a narcotic such as heroin or morphine the first thing the emergency-room physician does is administer **Narcan** (naloxone), a narcotic "antagonist." Within seconds a patient who is comatose and on the verge of dying from respiratory depression will wake up and start breathing normally.

We know that all this must seem confusing. How about an example to help straighten out this mess? Meet Mr. Deagan. Except for a little high blood pressure he had the blessing of good health his whole life. But at age 64 Mr. Deagan developed a painful case of thrombophlebitis as a result of several blood clots forming in the veins of his legs. His doctor prescribed an anticoagulant called **Coumadin** (warfarin) to thin his blood and prevent more clots from developing.

Mr. Deagan did just fine on the **Coumadin.** Periodically he went in for a blood test to make sure the drug was working. Everyone was happy. But then Mr. Deagan started complaining of indigestion and stomach pain. He had been under a lot of stress at work and, having had an ulcer once before, he figured he should visit his ulcer doctor, pronto. Sure enough, an ulcer it was and out came a prescription for **Tagamet** (cimetidine). Mr. Deagan didn't think to mention he was also taking **Coumadin,** and the gastroenterologist didn't ask if he was taking any other medicine.

Mr. Deagan was delighted to find that his stomach pain disappeared almost as soon as he started taking the **Tagamet,** but within several days he noticed that his gums were beginning to bleed after brushing his teeth. That was disturbing, but not scary. Then his stools turned black and tarry. Now Mr. Deagan was worried.

He immediately went to the doctor's office and while there had a routine blood check-up. The doctor was amazed. Mr. Deagan's blood wasn't clotting as expected because it was far too "thin." He had been hemorrhaging into his digestive tract (showing up as black, tarry stools) because the anticoagulant **Coumadin** had reached a dangerously toxic level in his blood. What could have gone wrong?

What happened was **Tagamet.** This ulcer medicine can affect liver enzymes and slow metabolism of other drugs. Mr. Deagan was no longer able to eliminate **Coumadin** as fast as he had before and so the drug began building up in his body. If he hadn't gotten to the doctor and had his dosage reduced he might have died from abdominal hemorrhaging or bleeding into the brain.

Mr. Deagan's case is purely hypothetical, but it could have happened just this way. There are reports in the medical literature of people who did in fact hemorrhage because they were taking **Tagamet** and **Coumadin** simultaneously.

Avoiding Dangerous Drug Interactions

How can you or your doctor predict the potential for an adverse drug combination before getting caught with your chemical defenses down? There are no ironclad guarantees, but there are a lot of steps to take, each of which greatly reduces the risk of suffering needlessly.

- **Make sure the doctor knows everything you are taking.** The first thing to do before you even leave the house to see your doctor is to write down every single pill you take, including all nonprescription drugs, herbs, and vitamins. We cannot stress this enough. The list may be longer than you think. If that seems like too daunting a task, pack all the bottles and vials in a brown paper bag and take it with you for evaluation.

- **Whenever you get a new prescription ask about interactions.** Ask the doctor if the drug interacts with alcohol, any foods, OTC drugs, etc. And after you've asked the doctor, ask the pharmacist. This is an excellent means of double-checking information, and in many cases you will find the pharmacist a much more current and aware source of interaction information than the harried doctor. After all, drugs are the pharmacist's sole concern. Make no apologies for double-checking. It's you who will suffer from any mistakes.

- **Become your own best expert.** In Part V of this book you will find 100 of the most commonly prescribed medicines. We have attempted to list some of the more important drugs that interact with these "best-sellers." If you see a potential incompatibility, please contact your physician and pharmacist for more details.

- **Reduce or eliminate alcoholic beverages while taking prescription drugs.** Booze can interact with an incredible number of drugs or chemicals in a potentially harmful way. A good rule of thumb is to try to limit all drug consumption to one thing at a time, and if you must take more than one medicine, check with your doctor or pharmacist about complications.

- **Watch out for food and drug interactions.** The classic example of this is the inactivation of tetracycline by milk or dairy products. But brussels sprouts can diminish the anticlotting effects of the blood thinner **Coumadin**. Licorice may make the diuretic **Lasix** (furosemide) more hazardous because it speeds elimination of potassium. And oatmeal and bran could diminish the absorption and effectiveness of the heart medicine **Lanoxin** (digoxin).

If you find this whole issue of drug interactions fascinating and perhaps a little alarming, you will want to obtain our book *The People's Guide to Deadly Drug Interactions* (St. Martin's Press). It goes into far greater detail on the most dangerous drug interactions to watch out for. You will also learn about foods, herbs, and vitamins that can interact with a wide range of medications. Remember, information is your best protection!

The People's Pharmacy®

References

1. Hall, Donald, et al. "Counteraction of the Vasodilator Effects of Enalapril by Aspirin in Severe Heart Failure." *J. Am. Coll. Cardiol.* 1992; 20:1549–1555.
2. Greenberg, Bram, Director, Professional Information, Merck Sharp Dohme, April 23, 1992.
3. Walker, R. W., Manager, Scientific Information, Merck and Company, April 24, 1992.
4. Alexander, Charles, M., Director, Professional Information, Merck Human Health Division, December 29, 1993.
5. Fried, Stephen. "Prescription for Disaster." *The Washington Post Magazine* 1994; April 3:12,30.
6. AP. "Warning Is Being Issued for the Drug Seldane." *New York Times* 1992; July 8:A20.
7. Honig, Peter K., et al. "Terfenadine-Ketoconazole Interaction: Pharmacokinetic and Electrodarciographic Consequences." *JAMA* 1993; 269:1513–1518.
8. Ibid.
9. AP. "AMA: Doctors' Sloppy Writing Spells Danger for Patients." *The Herald Sun* 1994; June 14:A10.
10. Board of Trustees, American Medical Association. "Medication (Drug) Errors in Hospitals." (Resolution 512, I-93) Introduced by the House of Delegates at the 1993 Interim Meeting.
11. Leape, L. L., et al. "The Nature of Adverse Events in Hospitalized Patients." *N. Engl. J. Med.* 1991; 324:377–384.
12. Physician Insurers Association of America. "The Medication Error Study, 1993."
13. Jick, Hershel. "Drugs—Remarkably Nontoxic." *N. Engl. J. Med.* 1974; 291(16):824–828.
14. Long, Glenda. "The Effect of Medication Distribution Systems on Medication Errors." *Nursing Research* 1982; 31(3):182–191.
15. Friedman, Marion. "Iatrogenic Disease: Addressing a Growing Epidemic." *Postgraduate Medicine* 1982; 71(6):123–129.
16. Ibid.
17. Hoffman, Robert, S. "Diagnostic Errors in the Evaluation of Behavioral Disorders." *JAMA* 1982; 248:964–967.
18. Friedman, op. cit.
19. Bailey, D. F., et al. "Interaction of Citrus Juices with Felodipine and Nifedipine." *Lancet* 1991; 337:268–269.
20. Edgar, B., et al. "Acute Effects of Drinking Grapefruit Juice on the Pharmacokinetics and Dynamics of Felodipine—and Its Potential Clinical Relevance." *Eur. J. Clin. Pharmac.* 1992; 42:313–317.
21. Fuhr, Uwe, et al. "Inhibitory Effect of Grapefruit Juice and Its Bitter Principal, Naringenin, on CYP1A2 Dependent Metabolism of Caffeine in Man." *Brit. J. Clin. Pharmac.* 1993; 35:431–436.
22. Flockhart, David, Personal Communication, November 16, 1993.
23. Tatro, David S., Ed. "Drug Interaction Facts." St. Louis: Wolters Kluwer, 1994.

8

Preventing Heart Attacks: With and Without Drugs

In the movie *Sleeper,* Woody Allen portrays a character who goes into the hospital for an ulcer operation. Through a mishap he ends up in a deep coma and is placed in a life-support capsule. Two hundred years later he is awakened by scientists and finds an incredible new world.

In this future society, things that used to be good for you—wheat germ and organic rice—are now bad; cigars, hot fudge, and steaks are now good.

Well, we haven't been asleep for 200 years, but we still feel a little like Rip Van Winkle. Over the last two decades there have been so many flip-flops in the world of heart research that it's hard to know what to believe anymore.

- **Margarine and vegetable shortenings were once thought to be good for you, while butter, avocados, and olive oil were bad news.** Now that's all reversed—the Mediterranean diet is hot!

- **Salt was a sin. Even healthy people were supposed to stay away from salt.** Now a huge international study says salt's not that big a deal if you don't have hypertension.

- **Eggs were evil—full of cholesterol, said the experts.** Shrimp was off limits for the same reason. False alarm. New research shows eggs are okay and shrimp was never a problem.

- **Nuts are loaded with fat. The experts told us to cut back.** Now they say that walnuts lower cholesterol and the risk of heart attack.

- **Diabetics (late-onset) were told to eat high-carbo diets and lay off fat.** Recent research says that's baloney. More monounsaturated fats improve diabetic control.

- **Alcohol was trouble: it increased blood pressure and put a strain on the heart.** New wisdom: alcohol in moderation is fine. It protects the heart.

- **High cholesterol was the enemy. Low cholesterol was the goal.** Now controversy reigns. Can cholesterol go too low?

- **Type A personality was deadly.** Hard-driving, impatient executives were supposed to be at risk of a heart attack. Researchers now say high-powered, hurry-up types are safe. It's the cynical, hostile, angry responses that harm the heart.

- **The bottom-line advice: Eat less fat and exercise more.** But how do we explain the French paradox? In France, where they aren't fanatical about exercise and eat heavy cream, Brie, nuts, red meat, and foie gras, the death rate from heart disease is one of the lowest in the industrialized world. Go figure.

Is Butter Better?

For the last 20 years if you asked the average person what he was supposed to spread on his bread, the answer would likely have been margarine. It was made from vegetable oils and had no cholesterol, which, as everyone knew, was supposed to clog up your arteries.

The trouble with such simplistic advice is that it's rarely based on real research. It seemed logical, therefore it must be true. But the trouble was that no one bothered to ask the critical question—Does it work?

The data is finally in and margarine isn't marginal. Scientists at Harvard followed 85,095 registered nurses for eight years. They didn't actually follow them around, but the researchers did give these women questionnaires every two years and then compared diet to disease.

What they found was incredible and heretical. The women who consumed more margarine were at substantially increased risk of coronary heart disease (CHD). Even more amazing was the finding that "consumption of cookies and white bread was significantly associated with higher risk of CHD. Intake of butter, not an important source of *trans* isomers, was not significantly associated with risk of CHD. . . . Consumption of beef, pork, or lamb as a main dish was not significantly related to risk."[1]

Bizarre! The world was turned upside down. All of a sudden margarine was worse than butter or red meat. In fact, while butter and red meat were not associated with an increase in heart disease, cookies, biscuits, cakes, and white bread were, presumably because they were baked with hydrogenated vegetable fats. These Harvard researchers concluded that instead of reducing the risk of heart disease, such oils may actually have "contributed to the occurrence of CHD."[2] Greek researchers have come to much the same conclusion based on similar data.[3]

Margarine is made by chemically treating vegetable oils. This hydrogenation process takes liquid oil and turns it into solid fat, giving it texture and shelf life. This allows margarine to look and taste more like butter. But this chemical conversion creates terrible *trans* fatty acids (TFAs). By the way, other vegetable shortenings are also hydrogenated. Mother Nature never made anything like TFAs.

Several years ago, many fast-food chains bowed to pressure and switched from beef tallow to partially hydrogenated vegetable oils. This change was supposedly made in the interest of improving health. It turns out that these oils contain about 30 percent *trans* fatty acids whereas beef tallow contains only 3 to 5 percent.[4] Tropical oils such as coconut and palm oil have also been traded for these chemically modified vegetable oils. Could it be that in their haste to help, the "experts" have actually done harm?

There is growing concern that the *trans* fatty acids, which are formed when vegetable oils are hydrogenated, increase levels of bad LDL cholesterol in the body.[5,6] They also lower good HDL cholesterol, and may promote blood-clot formation and atherosclerosis.[7] Dutch researchers found that *trans* fatty acids actually produced changes in lipid ratios (good HDL cholesterol to total cholesterol) that were worse than saturated fats, which have gotten so much bad press over the years.[8]

Dr. Walter Willett is chairman of the nutrition department of Harvard's School of Public Health. He is America's leading nutritional epidemiologist, overseeing two major studies of nurses (totaling 237,000 individuals) and other health professionals (52,000). As one writer described him, "Willett is no wiggy twig-muncher. He's spent his life learning the lessons of science."[9]

In a recent issue of the *American Journal of Public Health*, Dr. Willett made some amazing comments:

Although the percentage of coronary heart disease deaths in the United States attributable to intake of *trans* fatty acids is uncertain, even the lower estimates from the effects on blood lipids would suggest that more than 30,000 deaths per year may be due to consumption of partially hydrogenated vegetable fat. Furthermore, the number of attributable cases of non-fatal coronary heart disease will be even larger. . . .

The occasional use of butter or lard will not have any important effect on health, and the fatty acid composition of lard and beef tallow, which contain mainly unsaturated fats, may not be as unhealthy as generally believed.[10]

Did you read that? He's talking nutritional heresy. Butter better than margarine? If this were the Middle Ages we don't doubt that Dr. Willett would be stoned or burned at the stake. But remember, he is no granola guru. With his M.D. and Dr.PH degrees, and his chairmanship at Harvard, this man is a heavy hitter. So whom do you trust: Walter, or a food industry promoting hydrogenated vegetable oils that are cheaper to make and have a longer shelf life? We're betting on Walter.

The Incredible Edible Egg

A lot of people don't think of eggs as edible anymore. They've been told for decades that eggs have cholesterol and they are not part of a heart-healthy diet. Balderdash!

Sure, eggs have some cholesterol in the yolk. But dietary cholesterol is not the big problem everyone made it out to be. Danish investigators decided to measure the impact of egg consumption on lipid levels. Now you would think that this kind of research would have been carried out decades ago, given such stringent prohibitions against eating eggs. But until this study we haven't seen any decent effort to answer the basic question of what eggs do to cholesterol levels.

The results are earth-shattering. They gave 12 men and 12 women two boiled eggs every day for six weeks (on top of their usual diet). They measured blood fats before the study, after four weeks, after six weeks, and then four and six weeks after ending the egg experiment.

And the envelope please: total cholesterol did go up "8% after four weeks, and 4% after six weeks of extra egg consumption." But that increase was accounted for by an increase of 10% in good HDL cholesterol. And it is HDL cholesterol that is thought to be important in protecting the heart from atherosclerosis. So this was great news. More important, the critical total cholesterol/HDL cholesterol ratio "was unchanged." Triglycerides actually went down 15% after four weeks and bad LDL cholesterol was unchanged at six weeks.[11] The researchers concluded that

"A moderate egg intake should not be rigorously restricted in healthy individuals."[12]

Okay, we have shaken your belief system. Are you ready for a wonderful story? Dr. Fred Kern, Jr., is in the Department of Medicine, Division of Gastroenterology, University of Colorado School of Medicine. He specializes in cholesterol metabolism. He presented the following case report in the pages of *The New England Journal of Medicine*:

An 88-year-old man who lived in a retirement community complained only of loneliness since his wife's death. He was an articulate, well-educated elderly man, healthy except for an extremely poor memory without other specific neurologic deficits. . . . His general health had been excellent, without notable symptoms. . . . He had no history (according to the patient and his personal physician of 15 years) of heart disease. . . .

The patient's poor memory impaired the accuracy of the dietary history, but his consumption of 20 to 30 eggs a day was verified. Although he could not remember the duration of this eating pattern, his physician attested to its presence for 15 years; a friend, for even longer. He always soft-boiled the eggs and ate them throughout the day. He kept a careful record, egg by egg, of the number ingested each day. The nurse at the retirement home confirmed the daily delivery to him of approximately two dozen eggs. . . . Efforts to modify the behavior had been unsuccessful. The patient stated, "Eating these eggs ruins my life, but I can't help it."[13]

The amazing thing about this story is that the patient's lipid levels were incredibly normal. Total cholesterol was 200. His LDL cholesterol was 142 (130 to 159 is fine) and HDL cholesterol was 45.[14] His all-important ratio of total cholesterol to HDL cholesterol was below the target of 4.5.

It seems this fellow's body had adapted to his humongous egg consumption. He had no signs of heart disease and was in fact amazingly healthy. What's the take-home message? Well, please don't start overdosing on eggs. But if you get an urge for a boiled or poached egg now and again, go for it. Eggs are a nutritious, low-fat source of protein and current research suggests that they may not be as dangerous as we have been warned. But who knows what next year will hold.

Cholesterol Controversy

By now we suspect that your faith has been somewhat undermined. The pillars of a healthy lifestyle are starting to crumble. Are you ready for another temblor?

The loudest shouters in the medical mafia have been decrying dastardly cho-lesterol for decades. This demon was responsible for all our cardiovascular ills. If only we poor slobs would stop eating eggs, butter, and red meat we could get our cholesterol levels down below 200 and we would all be saved from heart disease. And if we were too lazy or gluttonous to accomplish this goal there were some marvelous drugs that could do it for us.

Would it were that simple. The cholesterol controversy has been bubbling for years. Not only have important questions been raised about the connection be-tween diet and cholesterol, but also the value of drug therapy has been called into question.

That sounds like heresy. On December 13, 1984, a consensus panel report from the National Institutes of Health had just reiterated the conventional wis-dom: "lowering cholesterol can reduce the incidence of coronary artery disease and save lives." All Americans were encouraged to follow the American Heart As-sociation's "prudent" diet, "which emphasizes fruit and vegetables, restricts egg yolks to no more than two a week, and specifies lean meat, skim milk, and low-fat cheeses."[15]

Just two weeks later, on January 4, 1985, an article in *Science* summarized the problem:

> But despite what the panel said there is no irrefutable evidence from clinical trials that cho-lesterol-lowering saves lives. And it is not as though no one has tried to get evidence. Over the past 20 years there have been nearly two dozen clinical trials of cholesterol-lowering. These trials involved at least 50,000 people at high risk for heart disease selected so that they would be most likely to benefit from lowered blood cholesterol if it helps at all. But these trials failed to show that cholesterol-lowering prevents deaths from heart disease.[16]

Now fast-forward to the 1990s. The cholesterol controversy heated up. A Finnish study looked at the effect of cholesterol treatment on the only thing that really matters—mortality. In 1974 1,222 Finnish executives with risk factors for heart disease were recruited into a study. They were told about diet, exercise, and smoking. If high blood pressure or cholesterol were a problem, the executives were treated with drugs—defined as "intervention." The results, published in 1991, rocked the cardiology community.[17]

An editorial in the *British Medical Journal* by Dr. Michael Oliver, of Britain's National Heart and Lung Institute, summarized the Finnish results and their im-plications:

I t found that over the 10 years after the trial ended cardiac deaths and total mortality pro-
gressively increased in the intervention group compared with the controls [untreated]. This
finding, together with reports of an increase in non-cardiac deaths related to drug treatment
for hypercholesterolemia should make many doctors, health educationalists, managers, and
politicians reconsider the value of current policies for the primary prevention of coronary heart
disease. . . .

Although this is the first report of increased mortality from coronary heart disease after
multifactorial interventions, previous reports have suggested that mortality from coronary
heart disease does not necessarily fall with intervention to reduce multiple risk factors. . . . We
are now learning to live with the fact that lowering cholesterol concentrations in men at high
risk does not reduce total mortality and may actually increase non-cardiac mortality.[18]

Dr. Oliver has also pointed out the disturbing fact that 30 to 40 percent of people who suffer heart attacks don't have high cholesterol levels.[19] Obviously this
story is a lot more complicated than most physicians would like to admit.

In three of the largest and best-designed studies to date,[20,21,22] scientists found
that lowering risk factors like cholesterol and high blood pressure did not reduce
the risk of death from heart disease, and appeared in some cases to increase the
risk of dying from other causes. Even when the results of six prevention trials were
pooled (meta-analysis) it was found that treatment with drugs appeared to increase
the risk of death from accidents and violence.[23] Two prominent epidemiologists
concluded:

I t is difficult to justify the general use of cholesterol-lowering drugs when the data available
from clinical trials fail to show reductions (and may show increases) in mortality . . . With the
current uncertainty surrounding the benefits and risks of cholesterol-lowering drugs in primary
prevention we suggest that their general use, other than in patients with severe familial hyper-
lipidemias, should await the result of these trials.[24]

To make matters even more confusing, there have never been any studies
showing that older women benefit from cholesterol reduction. In fact, one study
found that elderly women (over 70) had better survival stats if their cholesterol levels were higher rather than lower. According to the researchers, "At the present
time, there is no definitive basis for recommending lipid-lowering treatment in elderly men and women [above 65 to 70 years of age]."[25]

If the data on cholesterol are such a mess, why haven't physicians become more cautious? Once again, the loudest shouters rule the roost. Several of the editorials we have cited above were published in journals that aren't widely read. A Swedish researcher believes that investigator bias may also play a role:

> **L**owering serum cholesterol concentrations does not reduce mortality and is unlikely to prevent coronary heart disease. Claims of the opposite are based on preferential citations of supportive trials. . . . Authors of papers on preventing coronary heart disease by lowering blood cholesterol values tend to cite only trials with positive results. The impression of success presented to doctors is false because the numbers of controlled cholesterol-lowering trials in which total mortality and coronary mortality were reduced equal the numbers in which they were increased.[26]

In other words, when scientists commit a lot of energy and resources to a project, they like to feel that they are doing something important, with a potential for improving lives. Writing a grant proposal to get to do research that can cost tens of millions of dollars means they have to be big league, highly regarded by their colleagues. The most persuasive people get their research funded and then are able to convince other doctors that whatever they're doing—lowering cholesterol, for example—is a good idea. If the results don't confirm expectations, they tend to be ignored, excused, or explained away.

Take angioplasty for example. In this procedure a "balloon" is inserted into a clogged coronary artery, inflated and the plaque is squished so the blood can flow more readily again. This technique can work well for many, but quite often the arteries block up again. To try and prevent this "reocclusion" or "restenosis," physicians conducted a large multicenter study with the drug **Mevacor** (lovastatin), hoping that the medication would keep arteries open. More than 200 patients were treated with **Mevacor** starting about a week before angioplasty and continuing for six months afterwards.

Bad LDL cholesterol dropped on average 42 percent. This probably made the doctors feel very good. The placebo group (angioplasty without **Mevacor**) did not have such a beneficial effect. But when the cardiologists actually looked at the state of the coronary arteries with angiography (dye tests), they were mighty disappointed. There was no difference between placebo and **Mevacor**. Both groups had about 45 percent reclogging of the arteries.[27]

Such a finding could have shaken the confidence physicians have in lipid-lowering drugs in general. But the chief investigator of the study, Dr. William Weintraub, insisted that the disappointing results shouldn't discourage doctors from prescribing such drugs to prevent heart disease: "This finding has interesting implications, because people have thought that atherosclerosis and restenosis are similar. Now we have fairly good evidence that in fact they [do not involve] the same process. One is clearly related to lipids; the other is not."[28] By insisting that "restenosis is different," physicians can feel secure that lowering cholesterol with drugs like **Mevacor** is worthwhile. We hope they are right.

Too Low Cholesterol?

A cardiologist friend of ours has a favorite expression—"you can't have too low a golf score or cholesterol reading." He may be wrong. There is a surprising amount of data that doctors have tried hard to disregard. Japanese investigators discovered that when men had total cholesterol below 178 and women below 190 they were at greater risk of cerebral hemorrhage (bleeding strokes).[29] The Honolulu Heart Project found that when Japanese-American men had cholesterol levels lower than 150 they were four times more likely to die from a bleeding stroke than if their levels were higher than 190.[30] And an American study uncovered the scary observation that if men had diastolic blood pressure above 90 *and* low cholesterol (under 160) they experienced a sixfold increased risk of death from cerebral hemorrhage.[31]

Perhaps the most impressive and anxiety-producing results were "based on a meta-analysis of deaths of 524,000 men and 125,000 women . . . [that] concluded that serum cholesterol concentrations below 4mmol/l [154 mg] are associated with an increased risk of death from cancer, respiratory disease, trauma, and digestive diseases."[32,33] Interestingly, the excess deaths don't appear in studies that involve diet and exercise, but do show up in drug intervention trials.[34]

The dawning realization that there may be dangers from too low as well as too high cholesterol is a hard pill to swallow, especially for drug companies. Millions of men and women are taking cholesterol-lowering medications in the hope that they will reduce the risk of heart disease and prolong life.

There is evidence that drugs like **Lopid** (gemfibrozil), **Mevacor** (lovastatin), **Pravachol** (pravastatin), and **Questran** (cholestyramine) can lower the chance of heart attack. But will they actually help people live longer?

Lowering cholesterol with drugs may be a little like driving with your foot on the brake as well as the gas—you may not make as much progress as you would like. Although deaths from heart attacks drop, people may be more likely to die from accidents, cancers, and other causes.

Dr. Stephen Hulley and his colleagues at the University of California in San Francisco shook the cardiology establishment with an editorial in the journal *Circulation*. They concluded that "There is no association between high blood cholesterol and cardiovascular deaths in women." The relatively few studies of women suggest that the risks of heart attack from high blood cholesterol are offset by the possibility of a stroke when cholesterol drops.

It is shocking that large numbers of people take these medications although doctors don't know for sure what the long-term consequences may be. This is especially true for women and older people.

In the editorial, Dr. Hulley questioned the wisdom of widespread prescribing of cholesterol-lowering drugs. "The overriding ethical obligation is to do no harm. Particularly when considering the long-term use of drugs for people who are in good health, the burden of proof falls on the proponents of intervention."[35]

Drug companies have convinced doctors that their expensive medications are worthwhile because they lower cholesterol numbers. Until recently no one questioned whether those lower numbers translated into better health. Unless they do, it is hard to justify both the cost and the possibility of side effects.

But before you even begin to contemplate giving up on cholesterol-lowering drugs, talk it over with your doctor. There are clear circumstances where such medications save lives, especially when cholesterol levels are very high because of genetic factors. Any decision to stop any medicine needs to be made jointly with a physician.

The French Paradox

There is one other piece of evidence that ought to make all of us a little leery of draconian measures to get our cholesterol levels down. That is the experience of the French. For the past several years, researchers have been trying to explain the "French paradox": French people have long ignored current dietary restrictions and have continued to eat butter, cheese, and foie gras despite their reputation for raising cholesterol. To the consternation of cardiologists, heart attack rates in France are the lowest in Europe and half those in the U.S.[36]

Obviously, heart disease is far more complicated than researchers once thought. Some hypothesize that French wine consumption may be the protecting factor.[37] Others suggest that French mineral waters, high in magnesium, may also be beneficial. Or perhaps the French lifestyle is less stressful.

What's a Body to Do?

By now we suspect you are feeling frustrated with all the contradictions, controversy, and confusion. There might be a temptation to say the hell with it. We too are getting mighty tired of reading about *trans* fatty acids, low-density lipoprotein cholesterol, triglycerides, hydrogenated vegetable oils, saturated fats, apolipoproteins, and goodness knows what else. It seems as if the coronary crazies constantly keep coming up with some new risk—the fat factor of the month. As our favorite cartoon character, Opus of *Outland,* once said: "FAT FAT FAT FAT!! I'M SICK OF WORRYING ABOUT FATS!"[38]

Please don't interpret our cautiousness as cynicism. We sincerely believe that people can do lots of things to protect their hearts and reduce the risk of heart attacks with and without drugs. As we said early in this chapter, we are big fans of Dr. Walter Willett, chairman of the nutrition department at Harvard. Walter is big on the Mediterranean diet and so are we. After all, heart attack rates in Greece and Crete have classically been 90 percent lower than those in the U.S. even though these folks take in as much as 40 percent of their calories from fat. . . . mostly olive oil.[39] According to Dr. Willett, "The message to eat less fat is likely off-target. What seems important to health is the type of fat. People need to realize that some kinds are beneficial."[40]

Instead of spreading your bread with margarine, why not dip it in a little olive oil flavored with garlic? We can't imagine why anyone would ever use any other kind of oil unless it were avocado oil. Like olives, avocados contain mostly mono-unsaturated fat (64 percent vs. 72 percent for olive oil). One Australian study discovered that a diet high in avocado oil actually improved lipid ratios far more than a low-fat diet.[41] Next on our list of favorite fats comes canola oil at 62 percent mononounsaturates.

Garlic

When it comes to food, we are very big on garlic and onions slathered on, in, and around as many foods as possible. The garlic research has become quite elegant of late. Over the last 20 years there have been dozens of studies demonstrating garlic is beneficial for the heart.

The *Annals of Internal Medicine* is only the most recent journal to publish positive results on this topic. The October 1, 1993, issue of the respected publication contained an overview of garlic research. Dr. Stephen Warshafsky and his colleagues at New York Medical College concluded, "The best available evidence suggests that garlic, in an amount approximating one-half to one clove per day, decreased total serum cholesterol levels by about 9% in the groups of patients studied."

One double-blind placebo-controlled study published in *American Journal of Medicine* (June 1993) confirmed that dried garlic-powder tablets (brand name **Kwai**) also lowered cholesterol.[42] Not only does garlic lower cholesterol, but also it seems to prevent or dissolve blood clots. And new data suggests that **Kwai** garlic pills may also prevent oxidation of bad LDL cholesterol, a process that is thought to be crucial in the development of heart disease.[43]

We like our garlic au naturel, though. One of our all-time preferred meals would be broiled salmon (well brushed with olive oil, thank you very much). We might add some rice and definitely veggies—like broccoli. And then a salad. Mama

Graedon's best and simplest salad dressing calls for ⅓ olive oil to ⅔ cider vinegar. Squeeze in two to three fresh cloves of garlic. Salt and pepper to taste. She adds feta cheese and onions to give it some pizzazz. It's simple and tasty and great for your heart.

By the way, remember all that hoopla about the dangers of salt? The Intersalt Cooperative Research Group signed up more than 10,000 subjects from 32 countries. They found that salt had a minimal effect on blood pressure.[44] One expert concluded that "The Intersalt project showed there is no relationship between sodium intake and blood pressure."[45] In China, for example, where they consume almost twice as much salt as people in Hawaii, blood pressure was lower.

This doesn't mean you should overdose on pretzels and sauerkraut. Some people are salt-sensitive and retain fluid if they take in too much salt. And people with high blood pressure or heart failure should definitely be cautious. But for healthy folks who are sensible, salt is not a sin.

Magnesium

Speaking of minerals, we are very big on magnesium. Researchers have known that hard water (water that is high in magnesium and calcium) seems to protect against heart disease. Not only does magnesium appear to lower blood pressure, but also it may be good for irregular heart rhythms, heart failure, and angina. It is often the missing mineral in our diet and many blood pressure pills deplete the body of this crucial element. Of course, too much magnesium will have you running to the bathroom—after all, it is the primary ingredient in MOM (milk of magnesia). Keep intake under 400 mg. Anyone with kidney problems or atrioventricular heart block should avoid magnesium, however, unless directed by a cardiologist.

Potassium is also important! A recent editorial in the *New England Journal of Medicine* suggests that one reason so many large blood pressure studies have not demonstrated desirable outcomes is because the diuretics that were used deplete the body of potassium and magnesium.[46] This can lead to the ultimate in adverse reactions—cardiac arrest. A study in the *Annals of Internal Medicine* (October 1, 1995) revealed that people taking potassium-depleting diuretics were about twice as likely to die from sudden cardiac arrest as those taking diuretics that preserved potassium. For a list of high-potassium foods turn to page 197.

Cutting Back on Meat

According to our hero, Walter Willett, "If you step back and look at the data, the optimum amount of red meat you should eat is zero."[47] That may be a little too extreme for some folks, but we agree with Walter that most people eat too much meat—but for a reason that the average consumer, or even his physician, has never heard of.

Many years ago we stumbled across a fascinating book called *Beyond Cholesterol: Vitamin B₆, Arteriosclerosis, and Your Heart,* by Edward R. Gruberg and Stephen A. Raymond (New York: St. Martin's Press, 1981). They had done an amazing amount of research and discovered that when meat is broken down in the body the protein is eventually converted to a byproduct called homocysteine (pronounced homo-sis-tay-een).

We now know that too much homocysteine is a major risk factor for atherosclerosis or clogged coronary arteries. Too much of this nasty stuff also contributes to clogged arteries in the brain. This is proven research, not even up for debate. What is new and exciting is the discovery that older people appear to have much higher levels of homocysteine than previously appreciated, and this may substantially increase their risk for heart attacks.[48]

What is fascinating is that two vitamins—folate (folic acid) and vitamin B_6—can dramatically reduce elevated homocysteine levels. Vegetarians, by avoiding meat and eating fruits and vegetables high in these nutrients, may be saving their hearts by keeping homocysteine levels down rather than because of the low-fat nature of their diet.

Dr. Willett and his colleague Dr. Meir Stampfer wrote an editorial in *JAMA* about this research. They concluded that "an elevated homocysteine concentration may contribute to a substantial fraction of myocardial infarctions (and perhaps other cardiovascular outcomes) in the United States." They note that "five servings of fruits and vegetables as part of a good diet would bring the folate and vitamin B_6 intakes of most persons to levels adequate to prevent high homocysteine levels."[49]

If you can't manage that kind of diet, then a little vitamin insurance might be good heart protection. We aren't recommending anyone else follow our lead, mind you, but we do consume 25 to 50 milligrams of vitamin B_6 and 400 to 800 micrograms of folic acid daily. We also dig into the veggies.

When Gruberg and Raymond wrote their book *Beyond Cholesterol* in 1981, no one paid much attention. Too bad. They were ahead of their time in recommending B vitamins. They might have been right. Walter Willett seems to think so. Now you know the secret, too.

If your doctor has never heard of the homocysteine theory of heart disease, have him or her check it out in the *Journal of the American Medical Association* (December 8, 1993, and October 4, 1995). And make sure your doctor reads the editorial by Willett and Stampfer!

Vitamin E and Thee

We love vitamin E. This is one of the most fascinating vitamins you will find and perhaps one of the most valuable. The antioxidant properties of this nutrient may make it an excellent heart protector.

The most important question cardiologists have yet to answer is how plaque forms in coronary arteries. Oxidation may be the clue to the mystery. This chemical reaction is often destructive. In nature, oxidized iron is rust. In our bodies, oxidized bad cholesterol (LDL) may be picked up by macrophages (scavenger blood cells) and incorporated into the walls of arteries. There it seems to damage the lining of these blood vessels, attracting more cells that eventually form plaque.

If this theory is correct, perhaps we should pay more attention to ways of preventing oxidation. Vitamin E is an antioxidant. Preliminary research suggests that it may help reduce the risk of heart disease.

A study reported at the American Heart Association annual meeting suggests that taking a supplement of 100 IU of vitamin E daily for two years or more can reduce women's risk of heart disease by 46 percent. Men also benefit, but perhaps less dramatically. A different study reported at the same meeting showed a 26 percent drop in heart disease among men taking vitamin E.

Hostility and Your Heart

Another sacred cow of cardiology was slain in the 1990s when the Type A personality bit the dust. Remember how we were told that people who were highly competitive, constantly striving for achievement, hard driving, and impatient were at high risk of a heart attack? We were warned that if we had a difficult time waiting in line at a restaurant or a checkout counter we were in big trouble.

Well, it turns out that impatience and competitiveness are probably not a problem after all. Once the scientists examined what it was about the so-called Type A personality that was truly hazardous, they came up with hostility as the key factor. Drs. Redford and Virginia Williams, authors of the fabulous book *Anger Kills*, (New York: Random House, 1993), have determined that it is cynicism and aggression rather than ambition that is so hard on the heart.

People who mistrust others, become upset or irritated easily, are quick to find fault, and harbor angry feelings are at increased risk of heart attacks.[50] There is good evidence that hostility revs up the nervous system. Adrenaline and cortisol flood the body, affecting a wide range of physiological processes. Blood pressure goes up, the heart beats more rapidly, blood flow increases, fat is released into the bloodstream, cholesterol is created, blood platelets become stickier, the immune system is activated, and coronary artery disease becomes more likely.[51,52]

What can you do if you are easily annoyed or provoked by other people's rude or thoughtless behavior? First, buy a copy of Redford and Virginia Williams' book, *Anger Kills*. It provides a wonderful set of strategies to control cynicism, anger, or aggression and stop hostile thoughts, feelings, and urges.

Some hints include: (1) Placing yourself in the other person's shoes. (2) Forcing yourself to listen without interrupting. (3) Shouting to yourself internally to "Stop it" when you have hostile feelings. (4) Distracting yourself when feeling riled. (5) Learning how to laugh at yourself. (6) Trying to trust other people and stop punishing their trivial errors. (7) Substituting firmness for aggressiveness. (8) Finding time to meditate. (9) Practicing understanding and forgiveness. (10) Imagining that this is your last day on earth.

We especially like the way Redford and Virginia conclude their book:

No matter how you live, eventually you will die. By controlling your aggression, anger, and cynicism, by other good health habits, by luck and good genes, you may delay your end. This may or may not be a destiny you can steer.

You have some control over the kind of life you will look back on in your final hours. Each day of your life, don't let your initial angry or cynical reactions prevent you from moving on to a more positive focus. If you choose to work at it, you can enjoy a life with less hostility and more heartfelt happiness.[53]

A Drink to Your Health

First a disclaimer. Alcohol causes an incredible amount of suffering in the world. Millions of people cannot drink in moderation and their alcoholism causes misery for themselves and their loved ones. Too much alcohol damages the entire body, especially the brain, the heart, and the liver. So, anyone who cannot handle alcohol, please skip this section.

For those who can manage a little wine, one or two cocktails, or a few beers and not get into trouble, we have some great news for you. Drinkers have significantly less heart disease than teetotalers. That is now established beyond a shadow of a doubt. It is not entirely clear how alcohol protects coronary arteries, but new data shows that it raises good HDL cholesterol.[54]

There is also some fabulous data that suggests red wine may prevent the oxidation of bad LDL cholesterol,[55] perhaps in a way similar to that of vitamin E and garlic. Alcohol may also be helpful by preventing blood clots that lead to heart attacks and by reducing the risk of gallstones.[56] We were pleased to discover that the benefits of alcohol were more pronounced for people who exercise.[57]

Exercise, Exercise, in the Morning When You Rise!

All right. You are eating all the right foods, but those love handles don't seem to want to disappear, even though you're careful about calories. And stress is part of your lifestyle, no matter how hard you wish it would go away. For hundreds of years people have had a simple solution to these two problems and it didn't cost a dime. Our forefathers had a great way of coping with anger and frustration. They'd go out and chop wood, or engage in some other vigorous work and they often felt better afterwards. They didn't need a thousand-dollar, all-in-one stair-stepper/rowing machine to get the job done.

Exercise is great for a sense of well-being and it is one of the most effective ways to maintain body weight at a desirable level. Losing the old spare tire is one of the best methods for controlling high blood pressure. Exercise can relieve stress, aggressive feelings, and just plain make you feel good.

One of the most comprehensive investigations into the question of physical activity and coronary heart mortality was carried out among longshoremen in the San Francisco Bay area from 1951 to 1972. A total of 6,351 workers were studied in order to determine whether the type of work a man did could influence the health of his heart. It was discovered that those longshoremen whose jobs required vigorous physical exercise had a lower rate of heart attacks than other longshoremen who were less active (light or sedentary type of work). The authors concluded that heavy energy-expending work can serve as a protective mechanism against the development of coronary artery disease.[58]

Not everyone has the "luxury" of a physically demanding job. Since most of us have occupations that do not require the kind of protective exertion that longshoremen get, does that mean we are condemned to die from a heart attacks? Absolutely not. Recreational physical exercise may not be as regular or sustained as on-the-job activity, but it can serve a protective function and make us feel better about ourselves.

New research from Finland suggests that the more leisure-time physical activity people engage in, the better their fitness and the lower their risk of heart attack.[59] Based on this and previous studies it is apparent that substantial benefit can be obtained by exercising for 30 to 60 minutes three to four times a week.

Now don't rush out to start jogging five miles every day or stair-stepping your way to heaven. The quickest way to a heart attack is unaccustomed, unsupervised, and overdone physical activity. One recent study found that people who are out of shape "face 100 times their usual risk of a heart attack if they suddenly rouse themselves to split wood, lug furniture or otherwise work up an unaccustomed sweat."[60] That research found that intense exercise in the unfit could be responsible for 4 percent of all heart attacks and represent as many as 60,000 each year.

Research published in the *New England Journal of Medicine* made it crystal clear: "Heavy physical exertion can trigger the onset of acute myocardial infarction [heart attack], particularly in people who are habitually sedentary."[61] So if you find yourself at the airport trying to make a tight connection, please DO NOT run to catch that flight unless you are in excellent shape. And don't shovel snow if you are unaccustomed to strenuous activity. Far too many people die from such exercise if they aren't used to it.

So watch out! Couch potatoes must be cautious if they decide to start burning extra calories. Medical supervision is a must. Your doctor should be more than willing to recommend a safe program of exercise after he or she has done a complete medical checkup in order to determine your capabilities. The best exercise program is one that schedules regular activity. The consensus seems to be that at least three sessions should be planned each week. Thirty minutes to one hour should be sufficient to provide adequate conditioning. After a brief period of warm-up calisthenics, get into total-body exercise such as bicycling, vigorous walking, jogging (moderate), or swimming.

Don't be a dummy and start exercising in hot weather or after a meal. That is a quick way to end up flat on your back. It is also wise to avoid a superhot shower right after your workout since that can put a strain on the cardiovascular system. Just cool down slowly for ten or fifteen minutes and then take a moderately warm shower.

Who's at Risk?

B efore you turn to the next section ("Doing It with Drugs," page 190) it's time to be honest with yourself. Doctors like to think in terms of risk factors. It is a useful exercise. There's one issue that none of us can do anything about and it may be the most important of all—our heredity. Genes are a very important factor in heart disease. If Dad died of a heart attack before age 60 and Mom has angina, then we are also likely to be highly vulnerable. We can't yet change our genes, but we can modify other risks.

High blood pressure, overweight, cigarette smoking, psychological stress, physical inactivity, improper diet, high cholesterol, sluggish thyroid gland, soft water, excess coffee-consumption, and even pollution have all been implicated in one way or another as contributing factors to heart disease. Probably no one thing causes a heart attack; rather, a combination of many of the foregoing elements can increase your chances significantly.

How can you tell if you are eligible for coronary artery disease? There is no simple test that reveals susceptibility. Obviously high blood pressure is important. If you carry around a spare tire, if you sit in a chair all day and rarely exercise, if you smoke, if you are under a lot of tension, and if you feel hostile and mad at the world much of the time, your life-insurance salesperson is not going to be very happy.

Physicians like to run expensive electrocardiogram tests to measure the state of the heart. Unfortunately a single office exam is a poor predictor of heart capability. It is impossible to tell from this whether an individual is eligible for a heart attack. An exercise electrocardiogram or stress test is, however, a valuable tool in the diagnosis of heart disease. By recording heart activity during exercise, often on a treadmill, it is possible for a trained clinician to detect many coronary abnormalities well ahead of time.

According to an article sponsored by the American Heart Association and published in *JAMA*, "Exercise testing should be performed routinely in all men who reach thirty-five years of age, especially in those with coronary risk factors, in order to maximize the benefits of early preventive and therapeutic interventions. The exercise test should be repeated at least every five years in those over 35 and yearly in those who demonstrate an ischemic response (reduced blood flow)."[62] Such a stress test should always be done before someone embarks on an ambitious physical fitness program.

There are also newer and more sophisticated tests available. Ultrasound or echo cardiograms can tell you a lot about blood flow through the heart. Angiograms can tell you the state of your coronary arteries. PET scans will be able to reveal blockage without injecting dye directly into the arteries, but such tests are extremely expensive.

The Bathroom Mirror

Another test that is much simpler and won't cost you a dime is only as far away as your nearest mirror. Just look at your face. Over two decades ago doctors from the Division of Cardiology at the Mount Sinai School of Medicine in New York discovered that patients with coronary artery disease frequently showed up with "diagonal earlobe crease."[63] What was that again? You read right. Earlobe crease. For reasons that are not entirely clear (genetic? physiological? hormonal?) people with clogged arteries seem to have greater chance of having a diagonal fold, crease or wrinkle in one or both of their earlobes.

What is so amazing is that the association has held up surprisingly well for more than 20 years in study after study.[64,65] A report in the *New England Journal of Medicine* confirmed that earlobe creases and perhaps even ear canal hair may be markers for heart disease:

> The earlobe crease has been demonstrated to be significantly associated with coronary-artery disease in specific populations. Patterns of hair growth have previously been suspected as possible risk factors for coronary-artery disease. We investigated both the earlobe crease and ear-canal hair. . . .
>
> The earlobe crease was found to be significantly associated with coronary-artery disease and significant difference was seen between men with and without coronary-artery disease in the presence of ear-canal hair. . . . The combined presence of ear-canal hair and the earlobe

crease was found to be significantly associated with coronary-artery disease. Moreover, combining the earlobe crease and ear-canal hair yielded the greatest sensitivity (90 percent) and the lowest false negative rate (10 percent).[66]

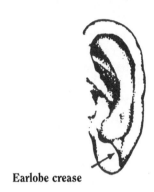

Earlobe crease

Baldies, Beware

It seems unfair that hairy ears and earlobe creases might be markers for heart disease but there's an even crueler factor. Take a peek at your scalp. How's the hairline? An editorial in *JAMA* titled "Is Baldness Bad for the Heart?" reviewed data "suggesting that male pattern baldness in men under 55 years of age is associated with an increased risk of myocardial infarction (MI) [heart attack]."[67]

Epidemiologists at Boston University compared 665 men having first heart attacks to 772 admitted to the same hospitals for non-heart-related conditions. They found that a little receding hairline was not a problem. But men under age 55 who had mild to moderate loss on top of their head had roughly a 30-percent increased risk of heart attack. For those with "extreme baldness" the risk went up over 300 percent.[68] Such an observation is not new. For more than 25 years investigators have been accumulating data to suggest that baldness may be a predictor of heart disease.

There is even an hypothesis to explain the data. Male pattern baldness is thought to be related to a metabolic byproduct of testosterone known as DHT (dihydrotestosterone). This chemical is also known to contribute to enlarged prostate glands. Whether it is bad for the heart remains to be discovered. But the high hostility and heart attack connection might also have something to do with excessive amounts of DHT.

It is worth noting that men who lack the enzyme (5α-reductase) that converts testosterone to DHT don't get bald. There is now a drug (**Proscar**—generic finasteride) that chemically blocks the enzyme and helps shrink the prostate gland. Preliminary data suggests that it may be helpful against male pattern baldness as well. Whether it will help the heart or not is still undetermined.

So what should we make of this bathroom-mirror testing procedure? Not everyone with hairy ears, an earlobe crease, or a bald pate is a candidate for a coronary. But these markers just might serve as early warning signs of coronary artery disease. Please don't panic, but such signals could have valuable consequences. Why not schedule a talk with your physician or a cardiologist just to be on the safe side? But don't let him scedule you for triple bypass surgery just on the basis of the mirror test. That's not the point of this esoteric information.

The bottom line is that people at higher risk (and that includes abdominal adiposity or bulging-belly syndrome) should use any and all risk factors as motivation to get their act together. The body doesn't always give off early signals that something is going wrong. When it does, we should listen.

Doing It with Drugs

You've eliminated all those nasty saturated and *trans* fatty acids from your diet. You've substituted monounsaturated oils, and you're eating all the right foods—lots of fruits and veggies, pasta, some fish now and again, and perhaps some chicken. Your salad has onions and garlic and you're sipping some wine and munching nuts. (Research has shown that nuts reduce the risk of heart attacks and deaths from heart disease.[69] And a lovely little study of California Seventh-Day Adventists found that one to three ounces of walnuts daily could have a surprisingly beneficial impact on cholesterol ratios.[70])

But no matter how hard you try, your cholesterol level makes your doctor frown, and the all-important total cholesterol to HDL cholesterol ratio is over 4.5. What do you do now? First, do not feel guilty. There has been a tendency to blame the victim. Millions have cut back on fat, eliminated eggs, stopped eating red meat, and still have not seen cholesterol levels substantially change. In his heretical article, "Cholesterol Myth," Thomas J. Moore pointed out that for many people, dieting has hardly any effect on cholesterol levels.[71]

Some individuals really do see tremendous progress when they reduce their fat consumption. But a surprising number just don't get dramatic results. For them, drugs may be appropriate. Although questions remain about the benefits of cholesterol-lowering medications (see previous discussion), there is a time and a place for everything. This is especially true if there is a strong family history of heart disease and hyperlipidemia (elevated blood fats).

Fiber Free-for-All

Psyllium can be one of the cheapest and easiest first steps in lowering total cholesterol. Studies have shown that this soluble fiber can reduce cholesterol levels from 5 to 15 percent.[72,73] There are lots of psyllium products on the market, including **Correctol Powder, Fiberall, Hydrocil Instant, Konsyl-D, Metamucil,** and **Modane Bulk**. You can also buy generic house brands of psyllium hydrophilic mucilloid for a lot less money.

Now, let's be perfectly honest about this stuff. It is a bulk-forming laxative, which means it swells in intestinal juices. Psyllium is not irritating to the digestive tract, won't make you run to the bathroom like some cathartics do, and will not create a laxative habit. The soluble fiber (milled from blond psyllium seeds or ispaghula) grabs on to cholesterol and bile acids in the digestive tract and helps escort them out of the body with the stool. More expensive prescription drugs like **Questran** (cholestyramine) and **Colestid** (colestipol) work on a similar principle. These compounds used to be prescribed quite frequently. Research showed that they could lower coronary heart disease, but side effects such as constipation, indigestion, nausea, stomach pain, bloating, gas, and a gritty aftertaste have made them less popular these days.

Niacin

One of the cheapest and most effective drugs to lower bad LDL cholesterol (15- to 40-percent reduction), reduce troublesome triglycerides (35 to 55 percent), and raise good HDL cholesterol (increase of 10 to 35 percent) is a vitamin. Niacin (also known as nicotinic acid) is vitamin B_3. Unlike lots of other cholesterol-lowering treatments, niacin has actually been shown to reduce heart attacks and improve total mortality statistics. And this protection seems to persist for years after niacin has been discontinued.[74]

Besides being inexpensive, another nice thing about niacin is that we have had a lot of experience with this compound. Doctors have *prescribed* it for decades to reduce the risk of heart disease. We emphasize the word *prescribed* because in the doses that are used, niacin can not be considered a simple do-it-yourself vitamin. An editorial in the *Journal of the American Medical Association* states the issue succinctly: "Taking large does of niacin is not dietary supplementation, but rather the taking of a drug."[75]

Niacin has lots of unpleasant side effects and a few serious ones. When taken in doses over 1,000 mg, people often complain of flushing, tingling, itching, fatigue, nausea, heartburn, diarrhea, blurred vision, and headache. Niacin can also do damage to the liver and raise enzyme levels. It can activate stomach ulcers, make blood sugar hard to control for diabetics, and bring on an attack of gout. People with a history of glaucoma, diabetes, gout, liver disease, or ulcers should not take niacin.

Because of the flushing, tingling, and itching, a lot of people have opted for slow- or sustained-release formulations instead of immediate-release crystalline niacin. Such products may be easier to tolerate, but when prescribed in doses of 2,000 to 3,000 mg they are more likely to cause liver damage. One study uncovered a hepatotoxic effect in 52 percent of patients taking sustained-release niacin versus 0 percent in immediate-release niacin.[76]

If niacin is considered as an option, it requires careful supervision and monitoring by a physician. Frequent liver-enzyme tests are essential. Treatment should start with very low doses (100 to 200 mg) and gradually be increased to the desired level. Newer research suggests that total daily doses in the 1,000- to 1,500-mg range may be beneficial even though they are one-half to one-third as much as is usually prescribed.[77] Some doctors recommend one aspirin tablet about 30 minutes before taking niacin with food to reduce the flushing.

Astounding Aspirin

Speaking of aspirin, this could be one of the most miraculous drugs ever invented. Besides the obvious benefits against pain, fever, and inflammation, aspirin is one of the few drugs that has proven itself capable of preventing heart attacks and strokes *and* prolonging life. That is something few other drugs can brag about.

A meta-analysis or overview of 300 aspirin studies involving 140,000 people led to the observation that aspirin is one of the most cost-effective drug interventions available to doctors. The conclusion: "If everybody known to be at high risk of vascular disease were to take half an aspirin a day, about 100,000 deaths and 200,000 nonfatal heart attacks and strokes could be avoided worldwide each year."[78] Not bad for the cheapest drug in the pharmacy.

Aspirin may also be valuable first aid for heart attacks. English heart specialists writing in the *British Medical Journal* suggest that "in emergencies—for example, acute myocardial infarction [heart attack]—a daily dose of at least 160 mg to ensure rapid onset of action seems sensible."[79] One large study showed that if half an aspirin was given within the first four hours of onset of chest pain, it could reduce mortality from heart attacks by 25 percent.[80,81] Of course anyone who suspects he is having a heart attack should also call 911 (in some cases, 999) and get to an emergency room immediately.

What is still unclear is the optimal dose of aspirin to reduce the risk of blood clots that can lead to strokes and heart attacks in the first place. A recent review in the *New England Journal of Medicine* suggested "a daily dose of 75 to 100 mg is based on findings that this dose is as clinically efficacious as higher doses and is safer than higher doses."[82] Some experts have even suggested that half (40 mg) of a baby aspirin may be optimal.

Of course, even small doses of aspirin can produce problems for some people. That is why anyone who takes this drug for more than a routine headache or muscle sprain needs to be supervised by a physician. And some people (those with an aspirin allergy, history of ulcers, asthma, severe uncontrolled hypertension, or other bleeding disorder) should never take aspirin unless a physician has weighed all the consequences and is totally in control.

For a complete understanding of the benefits and risks of aspirin, and lots of practical news you can use, you may want to obtain a copy of our book *The Aspirin Handbook: A User's Guide to the Breakthrough Drug of the '90s* (New York: Bantam, 1993). It will also tell you which other medications could be dangerous in combination with aspirin.

Cholesterol-lowering Powerhouses

The drugs doctors love to prescribe these days are the enzyme inhibitors **Mevacor** (lovastatin), **Pravachol** (pravastatin), and **Zocor** (simvastatin). These are pharmaceutical best-sellers, especially **Mevacor**. What makes them so popular is their ability to block the body's cholesterol-making machinery at an important step. They lower bad LDL cholesterol and total cholesterol with fewer side effects than traditional drugs.

Some people do experience adverse reactions, though, including digestive-tract upset, headache, and rash. Liver enzyme elevation occurs in 1 to 2 percent of patients and therefore needs to be monitored. Muscular pain, fatigue, or weakness are symptoms that require immediate medical attention. For a more detailed overview please check **Mevacor, Pravachol,** and **Zocor** in Part V at the end of this book.

Lopid (gemfibrozil) is another popular prescription item. It not only lowers cholesterol and triglycerides, but also is one of the few medications that can raise levels of good HDL cholesterol. It can increase the risk of gallstones, though, and can occasionally cause digestive-tract problems. See a more complete discussion of **Lopid** in Part V.

Hypertension Treatment

There is no debate that high blood pressure increases the risk of coronary heart disease, stroke, congestive heart failure, and kidney disease. There is, however, some controversy about how to measure blood pressure, when to treat it, and the benefits of drug therapy.

The very first thing that you have to learn is how to take your own blood pressure. The detection of hypertension is too important to be left up to your doctor, and that goes for its presence as well as its absence. For all kinds of reasons, a blood pressure determination in a doctor's office may not reflect the true state of your cardiovascular system. The very act of entering a doctor's office can raise your pressure over the "normal" limits. And when the doctor walks into the room, wowee-zowee!

Doctors in Milan, Italy, decided to measure the effect the doctor can have on patients' blood pressure. Researchers call this white-coat hypertension. What they found was incredible! Within two minutes of walking into a room, the doctor caused an elevation of approximately 27 points in systolic pressure and 15 points in diastolic pressure. Heart rate also jumped up.[83] What's so fascinating about this research is that it included both hypertensive as well as normal patients.

There are other problems as well. This will shock you, but the cuff that is wrapped around your arm could easily be the wrong size. A recent review of blood pressure measurement noted that "96% of primary care physicians habitually use a cuff size that is too small rather than too large, and that only 25% even have a large cuff available."[84,85] The reason this is so crucial is that an undersized cuff will tend to overestimate your blood pressure by as much as 10 to 30 points. So people who have big arms, either because they have been working out and have nice muscles, or because they have been overeating and putting on the pounds, could be misdiagnosed hypertensive if measured with a standard cuff.

Lots of studies have demonstrated that home determinations are usually lower than "official" office measurements and they can be even more reliable in determining the effectiveness of treatment. What you must understand is that there is no such thing as a constant, stable blood pressure reading. Our blood pressure varies minute by minute and hour by hour throughout the day. We have watched as someone's reading went up more than 20 points in a matter of seconds. Anxiety, fear, exercise, food, sex, sleep, and talking can all have a significant impact on your blood pressure. That's right, even talking can increase your reading.[86] So when the nurse or doctor tries to "relax" you by chatting during blood pressure measurement, there is a good chance your numbers will be elevated.

In a brilliant overview of blood pressure detection, Dr. Thomas Pickering of the Hypertension Center at New York Hospital–Cornell Medical Center offered the following insight:

To paraphrase Talleyrand's statement that "war is much too serious a thing to be left to military men," the measurement of blood pressure is much too serious to be left to physicians. Surveys of physicians' measurement techniques have shown them to be frequently inadequate, with large discrepancies between what is recommended and what is done in practice.[87]

Measuring Blood Pressure at Home

There is an easy way for you to determine whether or not you have high blood pressure—learn how to take it yourself. For one thing, you can do it in the peace and quiet of your own house, an atmosphere more reflective of your regular blood pressure anyway. Second, and even more important, you will be able to record your pressure frequently over a long period of time in order to chart fluctuation. You may also spend a good part of the day at work so you should also take periodic readings there.

Since it is not the occasional increase in pressure but rather the sustained elevation that is of concern, who but you is best equipped to measure blood pressure frequently? Keep a diary of readings you can show your physician. A blood pressure monitoring device should be as much a part of everyone's home as a thermometer. Just as a diabetic needs to keep track of blood sugar, someone with hypertension needs to keep tabs on his blood pressure.

It used to be that the only way you could measure your blood pressure properly was with a stethoscope and a sphygmomanometer—the inflatable arm cuff and pressure gauge used at the doctor's office. But using a stethoscope can be tricky. It requires perfect placement over the brachial artery, which is right around the elbow where the fold is formed when the arm is bent. Then you have to listen carefully for subtle sounds of blood whooshing through that artery as air is slowly let out of the cuff. This isn't always easy, and even doctors and nurses can make mistakes.

Fortunately, times have changed. Over the last decade we have seen a revolution in electronic wizardry. Calculators that used to cost a bundle can now be purchased for a few dollars. The price of fancy digital blood-pressure monitoring devices that were sold to physicians for hundreds of dollars have also dropped dramatically and become affordable. What's more, they can be purchased in almost any pharmacy in the country. Digital monitors are also available in department stores and through many mail-order catalogues.

Some of the fancier models actually inflate and deflate themselves and come equipped with a little printer that will provide you with a permanent record of the time of day, the date, blood pressure and pulse. We used to think that the more bells and whistles they put on these machines, the more things there were to break down. That's true, of course, but we have used such devices and confess that they are handy. Having a permanent record that you can plot on a graph or just show your doctor is very useful. The easier and more convenient something is, the more likely it will get used.

There are lots of blood pressure devices on the market. We have been especially impressed with the Omron and Marshall brands. The testers for *Consumer Reports* also gave these machines top rating for ease of use and reliability.[88] These monitors have gone through an evolutionary process and can be ordered with large-size cuffs. They come in a variety of models, from sophisticated "fuzzy logic" types, to wrist devices, to self-storing compact machines. For order information contact Omron Healthcare, Inc., 300 Lakeview Parkway, Vernon Hills, IL 60061. Phone number (800) 231-3434 or (708) 680-6200.

What Does It Mean?

Once you know the range of your blood pressure readings and have transmitted that information to your physician, how do you interpret the readings? How high is too high? In the old days, doctors usually did not start to worry unless the pressure reached l60/95. These days most U.S. physicians are far more aggressive. But there is still controversy within the medical community as to when a patient should be considered hypertensive, and treatment started. It used to be that diastolic pressure was the only thing that concerned doctors, but lately they are paying careful attention to both systolic and diastolic.

A systolic pressure below 130 and a diastolic pressure below 90 is normal, whatever that means. If you are over forty and have a blood pressure of 130/90 or less, you should consider yourself lucky because you must be doing something very right. A systolic pressure between 130 and 140 accompanied by a diastolic pressure between 90 and l00 is no reason for panic. It is reason to keep an eye out and monitor the pressure frequently, especially if you are under forty-five. These days most U.S. experts "recommend treatment above a daytime average ambulatory level of 140/90 mm Hg; few recommend treatment below 135/85 mm Hg."[89]

But physicians in other countries are somewhat more flexible. They often take age and a variety of issues into account and do not look at blood pressure as anything more than one additional risk factor. In New Zealand, for example, many people 40 to 60 years of age might not be treated until their systolic blood pressure was above 150.[90]

There has also been a growing awareness that lowering blood pressure too far may actually be hazardous. Some studies suggest that "lowering diastolic blood pressure below 90 mm Hg in patients with coronary heat disesae may have adverse effects."[91,92] Texas investigators surveyed the medical literature (13 studies involving 48,000 subjects) and noted that "The beneficial therapeutic threshold point was 85 mm Hg. We conclude that low treated diastolic blood pressure levels, i.e., below 85 mm Hg, are associated with increased risk of cardiac events."[93]

Ultimately you will have to rely on your physician's good judgment. Do keep in mind, though, that doctors vary. Some believe you must vigorously treat even mild high blood pressure. To them anything over a diastolic reading of 85 is considered a problem and they often start prescribing drugs to keep it down as close to 80 as possible. Other doctors worry about side effects from blood pressure medication. They fear that an older person who becomes dizzy and unsteady from a medicine will be at greater risk of a fall. Such physicians tend to be more conservative. They may wait till the pressure climbs above 90 or 95 diastolic before starting therapy.

Nondrug Approaches

Let's assume that everyone is in agreement. You have high blood pressure and it is time to get it down. What to do? Most physicians would start with nondrug approaches. Step one in a program of blood pressure control is often weight reduction. Overweight is well established as a contributing factor in the elevation of blood pressure, and getting rid of those love handles tends to lower blood pressure.

There is a growing belief that extra calcium, magnesium, fiber, and potassium could also help lower blood pressure.[94] High-potassium foods include apricots (dried), avocados, bananas, cocoa, dates, figs, fish, molasses, peaches (dried), peanuts, pecans, potatoes, prunes, raisins, squash, sunflower seeds, wheat germ, and brewer's yeast.

Another important nondrug approach for hypertension is physical activity. There is substantial evidence that exercise is beneficial, but this must be done under careful medical supervision. Too much or inappropriate exertion can be counterproductive (see page 186). And don't forget relaxation. There is evidence that psychological stress, anxiety, and tension can contribute to high blood pressure.[95] So learn how to relax. Biofeedback is one way to accomplish this. Relaxation tapes are another. We highly recommend Dr. Emmett Miller's audio tapes (available from The Source, P.O. Box W, Stanford, CA 94305; telephone toll-free 1-800-52-TAPES).

Medicine for Hypertension

We used to think that getting blood pressure down with drugs was by definition a good thing. Then along came MRFIT (the Multiple Risk Factor Intervention Trial). This huge study cost in excess of $100 million, took more than 10 years to complete, and involved 12,000 recruits. The trouble was that the people who got special intervention (in particular, blood pressure medications) seemed to die faster than the men who received no medicine at all.

A recent analysis in *The New England Journal of Medicine* reveals the difficulty. "Unexpected findings from the Multiple Risk Factor Intervention Trial, a trial of primary prevention of coronary heart disease, suggested that treating hypertension with high doses of thiazide diuretic drugs might increase the risk of sudden death from cardiac causes."[96] The problem was that high doses of thiazide diuretics can deplete the body of two essential minerals—potassium and magnesium. When levels of these two minerals drop there is an increased risk of irregular heart beats and cardiac arrest.[97] The current recommendation based on the latest research is to keep diuretic doses low (around 12.5 mg with hydrochlorothiazide) or, if appropriate, add potassium-sparing drugs.

Before starting drug therapy for high blood pressure, make sure you discuss all the pros and cons with your doctor. Selecting the right medicine in the right dose is as much art as science and requires patience and persistence to ensure that the treatment won't be worse than the problem. It is essential that your physician do his or her homework on the latest thinking in this constantly evolving field.

Over the last decade we have watched as physicians have moved away from traditional blood pressure medications such as reserpine and guanethidine. These drugs often caused unpleasant adverse reactions including dizziness, sexual dysfunction, digestive-tract upset, stuffy nose, depression, and drowsiness. Then came the beta-blockers—drugs such as **Inderal, Lopressor, Corgard, Blocadren**, and **Tenormin.** They worked well and had other heart-protecting benefits. But people sometimes complained of fatigue, depression, cold hands and feet, nightmares, sexual difficulties, and problems controlling cholesterol.

In recent years calcium channel blockers **(Adalat, Calan, Cardene, Cardizem, Dilacor XR, DynaCirc, Norvasc, Plendil, Procardia,** and **Verelan)** have taken center stage along with the ACE inhibitors **(Accupril, Altace, Capoten, Lotensin, Monopril, Prinivil, Vasotec,** and **Zestril).** Calcium channel blockers have been the focus of controversy, however (see page 34).

Different people respond differently to antihypertensive medication. There have been few head-to-head tests to compare one form of treatment with another. One large study of male veterans found that **Catapres** (clonidine), **Tenormin** (atenolol), and **Cardizem** (diltiazem) "were most effective for younger whites; hydrochlorothiazide was the least effective." **Cardizem** "was most effective for younger [and older] blacks."[98] Older white men had beneficial responses from virtually all classes of medicine.

Drugs such as **Catapres** and prazosin produced substantially more side effects (almost double) than drugs such as **Capoten** (captopril), **Tenormin,** and **Cardizem.** Black patients have less success with beta-blocker medication and ACE inhibitors than white patients.[99] One study suggested that **Capoten** produced more favorable "quality-of-life" outcomes than its competitor **Vasotec.**[100] But trying to make sense out of which blood pressure pill will work for which patient requires a physician's careful attention. Ultimately you will have to work closely with your doctor to find the best treatment for you. Trial-and-error may not seem scientific, but when it comes to this kind of drug therapy, often that is the only way to proceed. For specific details on individual blood pressure medications, turn to Part V at the end of this book.

References

1. Willett, Walter C., et al. "Intake of *Trans* Fatty Acids and Risk of Coronary Heart Disease Among Women." *Lancet* 1993; 341:581–585.

2. Ibid.

3. Tzonou, Anastasia, et al. "Diet and Coronary Heart Disease: A Case-Control Study in Athens, Greece." *Epidemiology* 1993; 4(6):511–616.

4. Willett, op. cit.

5. Nestel, P., et al. "Plasma Lipoprotein and Lp(a) Changes With Substitution of Elaidic Acid For Oleic Acid in the Diet." *J. Lipid Res.* 1992; 33:1029–1036.

6. Troisi, R., et al. "*Trans*-Fatty Acid Intake in Relation to Serum Lipid Concentrations in Adult Men." *Am. J. Clin. Nutr.* 1992; 56:1019–1024.

7. Longnecker, Matthew P. "Do *Trans* Fatty Acids in Margarine and Other Foods Increase the Risk of Coronary Heart Disease?" *Epidemiology* 1993; 4(6):492–495.

8. Mensink, Ronald P., and Martijn B. Katan. "Effect of Dietary *Trans* Fatty Acids on High-Density and Low-Density Lipoprotein Cholesterol Levels in Healthy Subjects. *N. Engl. J. Med.* 1990; 323:439–445.

9. Mason, Michael. "The Man Who Has a Beef with Your Diet." *Health* 1994; May/June:53–58.

10. Willett, Walter C. and Albert Ascherio. "*Trans* Fatty Acids: Are the Effects Only Marginal?" *Am. J. Public Health* 1994; 84:722–724.

11. Schnohr, P. S., et al. "Egg Consumption and High-Density-Lipoprotein Cholesterol." *J. Int. Med.* 1994; 235:249–251.

12. Ibid.

13. Kern, Fred, Jr., "Normal Plasma Cholesterol in an 88-Year-Old Man Who Eats 25 Eggs A Day." *N. Engl. J. Med.* 1991; 324:896–899.

14. Ibid.

15. Kolata, Gina. "Heart Panel's Conclusions Questioned." *Science* 1985; 227:40–41.

16. Ibid.

17. Strandberg, T. E., et al. "Long-Term Mortality After 5-Year Multifactorial Primary Prevention of Cardiovascular Disease in Middle-Aged Men." *JAMA* 1991; 266:1225–1229.

18. Oliver, Michael F. "Doubts About Preventing Coronary Heart Disease: Multiple Interventions in Middle-Aged Men May Do More Harm Than Good." *British Medical Journal* 1992; 304:393–394.

19. Little, Linda. "Justification of National Cholesterol Program Debated." *Med. Trib.* 1992; June 11:2.

20. Wilhelmson, L., et al. "The Multifactorial Primary Prevention Trial in Goteburg, Sweden." *Eur. Heart J.* 1986; 7:279–288.

21. Multiple Risk Factor Intervention Trial Research Group. "Risk Factor Changes and Mortality Results." *JAMA* 1982; 248:1465–1477.

22. World Health Organization European Collaborative Group. "European Collaborative Trial of Multifactorial Prevention of Coronary Heart Disease: Final Report on the 6-Year Results." *Lancet* 1986; i:869–872.

23. Muldoon, M. F., et al. "Lowering Cholesterol Concentration and Mortality: A Quantitative Review of Primary Prevention Trials." *BMJ* 1990; 301:309–314.

24. Davey Smith, George, and Juha Pekkanen. "Should There Be a Moratorium on the Use of Cholesterol Lowering Drugs?" *BMJ* 1992; 304:431–434.

25. Kronmal, Richard A., et al. "Total Serum Cholesterol Levels and Mortality Risk As a Function of Age." *Arch. Intern. Med.* 1993; 153:1065–1073.

26. Ravnskov, U. "Cholesterol Lowering Trials in Coronary Heart Disease: Frequency of Citation and Outcome." *BMJ* 1992; 305:15-20.

27. Vikhanski, Luba. "Few Winners Emerge in Battle Against Restenosis." *Med. Trib.* 1994; March 10:9.

28. Ibid.

29. Fackelmann, Kathy A. "Japanese Stroke Clues: Are There Risks to Low Cholesterol?" *Science News* 1989; 135:250–253.

30. Ibid.

31. Iso, Hiroyasu, et al. "Serum Cholesterol Levels and Six-Year Mortality from Stroke in 350,977 Men Screened for the Multiple Risk Factor Intervention Trial." *N. Engl. J. Med.* 1989; 320:904–910.

32. Jacobs, D., et al. "Report of the Conference on Low Blood Cholesterol: Mortality Associations." *Circulation* 1992; 86:1046–1060.

33. Dunnigan, Matthew G. "The Problem With Cholesterol." *BMJ* 1993; May 22.

34. Davey Smith, op. cit.

35. Hulley, Stephen B., et al. "Health Policy on Blood Cholesterol: Time to Change Directions." *Circulation* 1992; 86:1026–1029.

36. Dolnick, Edward. "Le Paradoxe Français: How Do the French Eat All That Rich Food and Skip the Heart Disease?" *In Health* 1990; May/June:41–47.

37. Renaud, S. and M. De Lorgeril. "Wine, Alcohol, Platelets, and the French Paradox for Coronary Heart Disease." *Lancet* 1992; 339:1523–1526

38. Breathed, B. *Outland.* Distributed by the *Washington Post* Writer's Group, July 3, 1994.

39. Mason, op. cit.

40. Ibid.

41. "Avocado: Cholesterol's Oil of Olé?" *Men's Confidential* 1993; 9(2):1–2.

42. Jain, A. K., et al. "Can Garlic Reduce Levels of Serum Lipids? A Controlled Clinical Study." *Am. J. Med.* 1993; 94:632–635.

43. Phelps, Stacy and William S. Harris. "Garlic Supplementation and Lipoprotein Oxidation Susceptibility." *Lipids* 1993; 28:475–477.

44. Swales, J. D. "Salt Saga Continued: Salt Has Only Small Importance in Hypertension." *Br. Med. J.* 1988; 287:307–308.

45. McCarron, David A. "The Shake Out on Sodium." *Food Insight* 1994; May/June:2–3.

46. Bigger, J. Thomas, Jr. "Diuretic Therapy, Hypertension, and Cardiac Arrest." *N. Engl. J. Med.* 1994; 330:1899–1900.

47. Mason, op cit.

48. Selhub, Jacob, et al. "Vitamin Status and Intake as Primary Determinants of Homocysteinemia in an Elderly Population." *JAMA* 1993; 270:2693–2698.

49. Stampfer, Meir J., and Walter C. Willett. "Homocysteine and Marginal Vitamin Deficiency: The Importance of Adequate Vitamin Intake." *JAMA* 1993; 270:2726–2727.

50. AP. "Anger Doubles Risk of Attack for Heart Disease Patients." *The New York Times* 1994; March 19:V7.

51. Williams, Redford B. "Neurobiology, Cellular and Molecular Biology, and Psychosomatic Medicine." Presidential Address, American Psychosomatic Society, Charleston, S.C., March 5, 1993.

52. "Is Hostility Killing You?" *Consumer Reports on Health* 1994; 6(4):49–51.

53. Williams, Redford, and Virginia Williams. *Anger Kills: Seventeen Strategies for Controlling the Hostility That Can Harm Your Health* (New York: HarperPerennial, 1994).

54. Gaziano, J. Michael, et al. "Moderate Alcohol Intake, Increased Levels of High-Density Lipoprotein and Its Subfractions, and Decreased Risk of Myocardial Infarction." *N. Engl. J. Med.* 1993; 329:1829–1934.

55. Frankel, E. N., et al. "Inhibition of Oxidation of Human Low-Density Lipoprotein by Phenolic Substances in Red Wine." *Lancet* 1993; 341:454–457.

56. Friedman, Gary D., and Arthur L. Klatsky. "Is Alcohol Good for Your Health." *N. Engl. J. Med.* 1993; 329:1882–1883.

57. Fraser, G. E., and H. Babaali. "Determinants of High Density Lipoprotein Cholesterol in Middle-Aged Seventh-Day Aventist Men and Their Neighbors." *Am. J. Epidemiol.* 1989; 130:958–965.

58. Paffenbarger, Ralph S., Jr., and Wayne E. Hale. "Work Activity and Coronary Heart Mortality." *N. Engl. J. Med.* 1975; 292:545–550.

59. Lakka, Timo A., et al. "Relation of Leisure-Time Physical Activity and Cardiorespiratory Fitness to the Risk of Acute Myocardial Infarction in Men." *N. Engl. J. Med.* 1994; 330:1549–1554.

60. Haney, Daniel Q. "Study: Vigorous Exercise Raises Risk of Heart Attack." *Herald Sun* 1993; December 2:A1, A4.

61. Mittleman, Murray A., et al. "Triggering of Acute Myocardial Infarction by Heavy Physical Exertion—Protection Against Triggering by Regular Exertion." *N. Engl. J. Med.* 1993; 329:1677–1683.

62. DeBusk Robert. "The Value of Exercise Stress Testing." *JAMA* 1975; 232:956–958.

63. Lichstein, Edgar, et al. "Diagonal Ear-Lobe Crease Prevalence and Implications as Coronary Risk Factor." *N. Engl. J. Med.* 1974; 290:615–616.

64. Kirkham, N., et al. "Diagonal Earlobe Creases and Fatal Cardiovascular Disease: A Necropsy Study." *Br. Heart J.* 1989; 61:361–364.

65. Moraes, D., et al. "Ear Lobe Crease and Coronary Heart Disease." *Irish Med. J.* 1992; 85(4):131–132.

66. Wagner, A. U., et al. "Ear-Canal Hair and the Ear-Lobe Crease as Predictors for Coronary-Artery Disease. *N. Engl. J. Med.* 1984; 311:1317–1318.

67. Wilson, Peter W., and Wiliam B. Kannel. "Is Baldness Bad for the Heart?" *JAMA* 1993; 269:1035–1036.

68. Lesko, Samuel M., et al. "A Case-Control Study of Baldness in Relation to Myocardial Infarction in Men." *JAMA* 1993; 269:998–1003.

69. Fraser, G. E., et al. "A Possible Protective Effect of Nut Consumption on Risk of Coronary Heart Disease: The Adventist Health Study." *Arch. Intern. Med.* 1992; 151:1416–1424.

70. Sabate, Joan, et al. "Effects of Walnuts on Serum Lipid Levels and Blood Pressure in Normal Men." *N. Engl. J. Med.* 1993; 328:603–607.

71. Moore, Thomas J. "The Cholesterol Myth." *The Atlantic* 1989; 264(3):37–70.

72. Bell, Larry, P., et al. "Cholesterol-Lowering Effects of Psyllium Hydrophilic Mucilloid." *JAMA* 1989; 261:3419–3423.

73. Anderson, J. W., et al. "Cholesterol-Lowering Effects of Psyllium Hydrophilic Mucilloid for Hypercholesterolemic Men." *Arch. Intern. Med.* 1988; 148:292–296.

74. Conner, Paul L., et al. "Fifteen-Year Mortality in Coronary Drug Project Patients: Long-Term Benefit with Niacin." *J. Am. Coll. Cardiol.* 1986; 8:1245–1255.

75. Lasagna, Lois. "Over-the-Counter Niacin." *JAMA* 1994; 271:709–710.

76. McKenney, James M., et al. "A Comparison of the Efficacy and Toxic Effects of Sustained- vs. Immediate-Release Niacin in Hypercholesterolemic Patients." *JAMA* 1994; 271:672–677.

77. "Low-Dose Niacin: Effect on Lipid Levels." *Physicians' Drug Alert* 1989; 10(11):81.

78. Aldhous, Peter. "A Hearty Endorsement for Aspirin." *Science* 1994; 263:24.

79. Underwood, M. J., and R. S. More. "The Aspirin Papers." *BMJ* 1994; 308:71–72.

80. Moher, Michael, and Neil Johnson. "Use of Aspirin by General Practitioners in Suspected Acute Myocardial Infarction." *BMJ* 1994; 308:760.

81. ISIS-2 (Second International Study of Infarct Survival) Collaborative Group. "Randomised Trial of Intravenous Streptokinase, Oral Aspirin, Both, or Neither Among 17,187 Cases of Suspected Myocardial Infarction." *Lancet* 1988; 2:349–360.

82. Patrono, Carlo. "Aspirin As an Antiplatelet Drug." *N. Engl. J. Med.* 1994; 330:1287–1294.

83. Mancia, Giuseppe, et al. "Effects of Blood-Pressure Measurement by the Doctor on Patient's Blood Pressure and Heart Rate." *Lancet* 1983; 2:695–698.

84. Pickering, Thomas G. "Blood Pressure Measurement and Detection of Hypertension." *Lancet* 1994; 344:31–35.

85. McKay, D. W., et al. "Clinical Assessment of Blood Pressure." *J. Hum. Hypertens.* 1990; 4:639–645.

86. Friedman, E., et al. "The Effects of Normal and Rapid Speech on Blood Pressure." *Psychosom. Med.* 1982; 44:545–553.

87. Pickering, op. cit.

88. "Blood Pressure Monitors." *Consumer Reports* 1992; 57(5):295–299.

89. Pickering, op. cit.

90. Jackson, R., et al. "Management of Raised Blood Pressure in New Zealand: A Discussion Document." *BMJ* 1993; 307:107–110.

91. Jackson, op. cit.

92. Cruikshank, J. M., et al. "Benefits and Potential Harm of Lowering High Blood Pressure." *Lancet* 1987; 1:581–584.

93. Farnett, Lisa, et al. "The J-Curve Phenomenon and the Treatment of Hypertension: Is There a Point Beyond Which Pressure Reduction Is Dangerous?" *JAMA* 1991; 265:489–495.

94. Clinical Investigation: "A Prospective Study of Nutritional Factors and Hypertension Among U.S. Men." *Circulation* 1992; 86:1475–1484.

95. Markovitz, Jerome H., et al. "Psychological Predictors of Hypertension in the Framingham Study." *JAMA* 1993; 270:2439–2443.

96. Siscovick, David S., et al. "Diuretic Therapy for Hypertension and the Risk of Primary Cardiac Arrest." *N. Engl. J. Med.* 1994; 330:1852–1857.

97. Bigger, J. Thomas, Jr. "Diuretic Therapy, Hypertension, and Cardiac Arrest." *N. Engl. J. Med.* 1994; 330:1899–1900.

9

Allergy:
From a Medical Quagmire
to a Quiet Revolution

O nce upon a time it may have been beneficial to have our bodies mobilize against invading armies of microscopic particles. Perhaps it forced our forefathers to change their location at certain times of the year to avoid molds, pollen, and other nasty environmental attacks. But these days it seems like a cruel joke our bodies play on us.

Allergies send tens of millions of people running to medicine chests, pharmacies, and doctors' offices seeking relief . . . some relief, any relief . . . from the miserable combination of symptoms that signals the body's reaction to invasion by something it doesn't think should be there. We shell out roughly $500 million each year on over-the-counter allergy products in an effort to stem those sniffles and sneezes.[1] Hundreds of millions more are spent on doctor's visits and prescription drugs.

Whether you call it "allergy," "hay fever," or "allergic rhinitis," this maddening

98. Materson, Barry J., et al. "Single-Drug Therapy for Hypertension in Men: A Comparison of Six Antihypertensive Agents with Placebo." *N. Engl. J. Med.* 1993; 328:914–921.
99. Ibid.
100. Testa, Marcia A., et al. "Quality of Life and Antihypertensive Therapy in Men." *N. Engl. J. Med.* 1993; 328:907–913.

malady has the power to reduce the strongest of people to a quaking mass of swollen nasal tissue, red, teary eyes, and general misery. No one really knows how many allergy victims there are. One expert estimates that as many as one out of five of us is afflicted—making it the "sixth most prevalent chronic condition in the United States, outranking heart disease."[2,3] The National Institute of Allergy and Infectious Diseases reports that 35 million Americans suffer from hay fever alone.[4]

They say misery loves company. Well, if you've got allergies, you certainly have plenty of company. And we're right there with you. In our family three out of four suffer, too. We know what it's like to wake up sneezing our heads off and to try and function with stopped-up sinuses. When hay fever is really bad you can't smell or taste worth beans. Once-enjoyable sports activities turn into torture, and, when it comes to thinking, forget it. Basically you just walk around in a daze trying not to moan and groan so often that you alienate everyone around you.

Many people first try to help themselves. But most people who take over-the-counter (OTC) antihistamines in their effort to seek relief liken the experience to walking underwater as if in slow motion. You feel weak, spacey, and wiped out.

There's a very good reason why virtually all OTC allergy remedies carry some kind of caution along the lines of "Do not drive or operate heavy machinery, as this product may cause drowsiness." People who attempt to do something that requires coordination or concentration could be a menace to themselves as well as to everyone around them. In some states you could conceivably be pulled over by police for driving under the influence of allergy medicine.[5]

Decongestant nasal sprays often give wonderful temporary improvement, but if you use such products for longer than three days, you court disaster in the form of addiction. Unfortunately, allergies almost always last longer than three days. This puts the victim in a terrible double bind. It feels so good to breathe through your nose again that it can become agony to give up that kind of relief.

Cold-turkey withdrawal from OTC vasoconstrictors brings on rebound nasal congestion. When you stop spritzing your nose, the little blood vessels that were constricted by medicine go wild and begin to dilate. That leads to super stuffiness, which can be worse than the original allergy. We have met people who have remained addicted to their nasal sprays for more than 20 years. They keep a bottle by their bedside table or under the pillow, in their cars, at work, and virtually everywhere they go. Such prolonged exposure can damage the delicate tissues of the nose.

When people become frustrated with self-treatment, they often seek medical help. Today, physicians have more and better options to offer than ever before. To be honest, prescription drugs offer far more effective relief with fewer side effects than OTC remedies. Allergies may be one condition in which self-care may be counterproductive.

What *Is* an Allergic Reaction?

A llergy used to be a big black hole—a mystery ailment that left researchers almost as puzzled as the patients who were plagued with symptoms. There are still far more questions than answers, but at long last immunologists are beginning to unlock some of the secrets.

Let's get one thing straight: "allergy" is really a catchall word for the body's inappropriate responses to substances it believes are foreign. The immune system is charged with the responsibility of defending our bodies from microscopic invaders such as bacteria and viruses, and of conducting search-and-destroy missions for cancerous cells. The allergic response appears to be an overreaction: the immune system run amok. Symptoms can range from a stuffy nose caused by pollen, mold spores, smoke, dust mites, or animal dander, to hives, eczema, stomach upset, asthma, or life-threatening anaphylactic shock.

No one knows why one person reacts like crazy to ragweed pollen, while someone may be oblivious to the pollen count and respond instead to peanuts. House dust mites, animal fur, seafood, a drug, or even cold weather or strenuous exercise can trigger an allergic reaction. The list of potential "allergens" keeps growing as the list of chemicals in our environment expands.

One of the most controversial topics in medicine today has to do with multiple chemical sensitivities—a condition, many believe, in which a person's immune system is so overwhelmed that the slightest trigger can make him or her sick. Some individuals are so hypersensitive they may react to perfume, cosmetics, detergents, pesticides, tooth powders, food additives, or hundreds of other synthetic substances. The wide use of latex gloves by a variety of health professionals has led to an increasing incidence of latex allergy. For some, this has made condom use difficult. There are even cases of women who are allergic to semen. Intercourse can bring on hives, wheezing, and, in the most extreme situation, shock.

While we don't know why some people respond in this way, we are slowly beginning to understand how the reaction is triggered. Let's take a slow-motion look at the chain of events leading to allergy symptoms.

In comes pollen, or a bit of protein from certain types of seafood, or mold spores. The body says, "Ah ha, foreign substance," and starts to churn out *antibodies*. These custom-tailored antibodies (called immunoglobulin E or IgE) are a perfect chemical fit with that one particular invading substance (called *allergen*).

The allergen and antibody latch on to one another, forming a chemical "key" that fits perfectly into the "lock" on a particular kind of cell known as a mast cell. Mast cells are found all over the body, but they are especially prevalent in the nose, skin, lungs, and digestive tract. Locked up inside the mast cell are lots of little packets of a substance you've heard referred to in hay fever allergy commercials— histamine. In goes the key, click goes the lock, and out spills the histamine.

Once upon a time, we thought that histamine was the major culprit in allergic reactions. This theory had it that once freed from mast cells, histamine made its way to target cells located in the nose, eyes, and breathing passages. These target cells had special receptors just waiting for histamine to arrive. When it did, the receptors were thought to act like tiny switches that set in motion the swelling, tearing, itching, sneezing, and wheezing.

Antihistamines found in many popular allergy remedies supposedly blocked histamine from reaching the target, thereby preventing symptoms. But there was a problem with this grand theory. As many allergy victims know, antihistamines are only partially effective. That's because they don't do such a hot job blocking the *other* unpleasant chemicals released by mast cells.

We have learned that once the key (allergen/IgE antibody combo) unlocks the mast-cell lock, Pandora's box gets opened and out spills a lot more than just histamine. Kinins (pronounced KYE-nins) are chemicals that lead to the production of more nasties—prostaglandins, leukotrienes (pronounced luke-oh-try-eens), bradykinins, enzymes, and goodness knows what else.[6] These mischief makers are also good at causing sneezing, sniffling, swelling, itching, congestion, and a general spacey feeling.

All this unpleasantness happens pretty fast after exposure to an allergen—say grass or ragweed pollen. But roughly 50 percent of allergy victims also suffer a late-phase reaction to pollen.[7] Kinins and histamine send out chemical signals—a little like blood in the water—to attract cellular sharks. White blood cells (neutrophils, eosinophils, basophils, mononuclear cells) come to check out the situation. They infiltrate and inflame already sensitive tissues during this delayed-action attack, which can come on hours after the initial exposure. All in all it's a one-two punch to your nose, skin, eyes, and lungs.

How to Spot an Allergy at Twenty Paces

Now that you know what an allergic reaction is, how do you recognize it? If ragweed pollen is the trigger, identifying it is a hardy problem. Runny, itchy, stuffy nose; watery eyes; sneezing; occasional headaches; and a general case of the blahs that doesn't go away until the first good frost—these enable most people to recognize seasonal hay fever.

On the other hand, some of the symptoms can look a lot like those of a cold, so it may not strike you that allergies are the offender until you note that the problem surfaces year after year, appearing and disappearing at about the same times.

Nonseasonal allergies such as animal-dander and house-dust allergies may be harder to recognize. Just as "hay fever" has nothing to do with either hay or fever, house-dust allergies are in fact a reaction to a microscopic mite whose home is the dust in your home, or the cotton bedding and furniture stuffing. Actually it is mite feces that combine with dust to stimulate sensitivity.

Then there is mold and mildew. Wherever there is humidity, mildew is sure to follow. Air conditioning ducts, basements, and other creepy-crawly places are great breeding grounds for such stuff. And just because it seems like an inaccessible place don't assume you are safe. Invisible particles can float through the air with the greatest of ease. So can cat dander. Cat allergens are proteins that come from glands on the cat's skin. They can circulate in the air for hours and even after a cat leaves a house permanently they can be detected for months afterward.[8] Mixed together, these substances form a veritable allergy cocktail, but it's one that will leave you feeling low, not high.

Food Allergies

Some people are allergic to food. Not all food, thank goodness, but specific foods, very often those with certain protein structures. Sometimes food allergens may be so similar to pollen proteins that there is cross reactivity, e.g., "melons and bananas, with ragweed pollen; celery, with mugwort pollen; and apple, carrot, and hazelnut, with birch pollen."[9]

Food allergies can be tough to identify, since the reaction can come quite a while after the food's been eaten, and it may be hard to single out the guilty party from an entire meal. Food allergy really isn't so common as many people believe. In children the accepted incidence is from 0.3 percent to about 7.5 percent.[10] And only 1 to 2 percent of adults are truly allergic to foods.[11]

Fortunately, children often outgrow many of their food allergies as the body's immune system matures. Some babies fed on formula show signs of food allergy very early in life. A switch to a different formula, or to breast-feeding, if that is possible, usually brings relief. Human milk seems to be less likely than formula to cause this kind of problem for babies, but occasionally a breast-feeding mother will notice that a food she herself eats (including cow's milk) may produce a colicky, allergic response in her infant.

New research also suggests that exposure to cow's milk during the first year of life may predispose certain children to diabetes. Presumably this is because a protein (bovine serum albumin) from cow's milk is chemically similar to a protein on pancreatic cells. If the immune system cranks up antibodies to the foreign bovine albumin it may prime the pump for later destruction of pancreatic cells and lead to diabetes.[12] Whether this research will hold up remains to be seen. We do know that breast-feeding does seems to protect against development of insulin-dependent diabetes and can be helpful against other food allergies as well.

The symptoms of food allergy are many, and a person may experience abdominal discomfort, cramps, bloating, diarrhea, nausea, skin rash, runny nose, red eyes, swelling, and even asthma. Indeed, some rashes of undetermined nature could be due to unrecognized food allergies. In one study, 92 percent of the children with atopic dermatitis (described as "the itch that rashes") were allergic to one or more foods. When they ate the offending food, more than half the children got worse rashes.[13]

An allergist at Georgetown University discovered that food allergy may contribute to fluid accumulating in the middle ear. He tested 104 children with this condition for reactions to different foods and discovered that 78 percent were allergic. When the culprits were eliminated from the diet, 70 out of 81 children got better.

Very occasionally food allergies can provoke anaphylactic shock. This life-threatening allergic reaction should be regarded as a medical emergency. The more common foods that cause allergic reactions are eggs, dairy products, wheat, peanuts and other nuts, soybeans, and seafood (particularly shellfish and codfish).

Sometimes it's not the food itself that causes the problems but rather an unsuspected chemical that has been added either as a coloring agent or a preservative. Some years ago sulfites were used to keep old fruits and vegetables looking fresh instead of stale and soggy. But people who were allergic to this preservative could end up gasping for breath because of severe allergy. Many wines still contain sulfites and must be shunned by those who are sensitive.

Artificial colors such as tartrazine (FD&C Yellow No. 5), which is found in a wide variety of prepared foods on supermarket shelves, can also bring on allergic symptoms such as hives and wheezing. People with asthma are especially vulnerable. They have a hard time coping with their ailment without having to worry about the food they eat. But until the FDA decides to do something about the hidden additives in food, people with asthma and those sensitive to sulfite and tartrazine will have to be extra cautious anytime they eat out or buy packaged food.

Finding the Culprit

I t should be apparent by this point that there are literally hundreds, if not thousands, of substances to which you can become allergic. Even drugs can cause serious allergic reactions. Dermatologists have estimated that as many as 10 percent of the patients in American hospitals suffer drug-related skin reactions. Aspirin, **Advil, Aleve**, amoxicillin, ampicillin, **Bactrim, Butazolidin, Clinoril**, doxycycline, erythromycin, **Feldene, Indocin, Lodine, Motrin IB, Nalfon, Naprosyn, Nuprin**, penicillin, and **Septra** are just some of the medications that can cause eruptions resembling hives.

And lest you think such skin reactions are merely annoying, we know of cases where they have led to tragedy. A child put on a sulfa antibiotic died a horrible death when the physician did not recognize the gravity of his symptoms. A man we met on *Oprah!* told a story of how his skin peeled off his body and he bled so much it penetrated his mattress and puddled onto the floor. The doctors gave him up for dead but through a miracle he survived. Fortunately, such severe reactions are extremely rare. But they point up the fact that allergic reactions can range from merely annoying all the way up to life-threatening.

With so many allergens to choose from, how can we isolate the ones responsible for your individual misfortune? Allergy specialists stress the importance of "a thorough patient history."[14] A bit—or a lot—of sleuthing is usually in order. Trying to match symptoms with an offending allergen is a little like combining the skills of Dick Tracy, Sherlock Holmes, and Agatha Christie.

The doctor will want you to try and match symptoms with exposure. So if you start sneezing and coughing after walking past freshly cut grass, that is an important clue. If your nose gets stuffy every time you go down in a friend's basement, that could mean allergy to mold. If your eyes get red and itchy when you visit grandmother's house, maybe her cat is setting you off. And if you wake up every morning with a dry mouth, congestion, and postnasal drip you might be allergic to the mites that make a home in your mattress and get on your bedclothes.

When all else fails, skin testing can add clues. This is an impressive-looking procedure, to say the least. The test is done by placing a large number of extracts of likely suspects on small areas of exposed skin—usually the back or forearm. The skin is then pricked with a needle, allowing the extracts to get into the skin. The test is "positive" when the skin that has been pricked with the extracts turns red and itchy.

Unfortunately, there are times when skin testing can be unreliable. Allergy specialists have noted that, "Positive skin tests to an allergen may be found in individuals who disclaim symptoms to that allergen."[15] In other words, there may be false-positive results. Even with such drawbacks, skin testing can be useful when done by a skilled allergy specialist who knows the inherent weaknesses of the procedure. As long as the data that is collected is put into perspective with the all-important allergy detective work it can add pieces to the puzzle.

Nondrug Remedies for Allergies

O kay, let's assume that your detective work has paid off. You and your doctor have figured out together that you are allergic to mite feces, feathers, ragweed, certain grass pollens, and Bill, the feline companion. Before rushing to the pharmacy for antihistamines or signing up for expensive desensitization shots, there are some basic steps worth following.

Avoid the Allergen

Allergists always emphasize " allergen avoidance." Pick up any allergy review article and that will always head the list of therapeutic options.[16,17,18] Remember, it is the combination of the allergen and antibody to form a key that is the first step in opening the lock. Once the door is open, all hell breaks loose. Well, if you can prevent the key from forming in the first place you will avoid activating the lock.

Allergen avoidance has lots of advantages over all other treatments. First, it is cheap. Compared to allergy shots or prescription drugs this can be a bargain. Second, it is highly effective. Third—and this is really important—it has no side effects.

But getting rid of whatever it is that irritates you (allergies now, not coworkers or family members) is not so easy as it sounds. Even if you know that Bill, your loving cat, makes you sneeze, you may be unwilling to give him up. Mold can be hard to eliminate from the basement or air-conditioning ducts. And pollen is everywhere. The only way to avoid that pesky problem is to stop breathing and we've always felt such a step was rather an extreme way to deal with allergy symptoms.

There are, however, techniques that can cut down on your allergen exposure and they can be surprisingly effective. Because the air you breathe is so important in the overall scheme of things, anything you do to improve air quality will be a blessing. If you could schedule an ocean cruise or a trip to the mountains during hay fever season, that would be a good tactic. More realistically, try to keep windows closed and air conditioning on in the summer. This is a fairly effective filtering technique, especially if you have central air conditioning with an electrostatic filter. Dehumidifiers can also cut down on dust and will help discourage mold.

Filter Your Air

Speaking of filters, we are especially fond of HEPA (high-efficiency particulate arresting) cleaners. These filters look a little like a pleated accordion. They are made of fibers that have been packed together to form a dense collecting surface. Huge industrial HEPA filters are used in hospitals and computer "clean rooms" where dust must be kept to an absolute minimum.

You can now buy HEPA filters for your home. Most heating and air conditioning installers will know how to put one on your central air flow. We have been very happy with **Space-Gard** (from Research Products Corp. of Madison, Wisconsin). Another option would be to use a portable air purifier. *Consumer Reports* gave good ratings to **Cloud 9 300, Heponaire HP-50, Vitaire H200, Enviracaire EV1**, and **Cleanaire 300**.

As long as you are trying to improve your air quality, you will want to think about your vacuum cleaner. Actually, you would be better off not thinking about vacuuming. Get someone else to do it for you and clear out of the house or apartment for a couple of hours while it is being done. The reason is that most vacuum cleaners only trap the big stuff in the bag. Small allergens can be spread all around the rooms for an hour or so after vacuuming.

There are vacuum cleaners that are less likely to spew dust particles into the air. Some, like **Nilfisk Dustless HEPA**, come with small high-efficiency filters built in. It is also possible to retrofit your existing vacuum cleaner with a somewhat more effective filter. National Allergy Supply, Inc., in Duluth, Georgia (800-522-1448), can provide you with an array of allergy equipment.

Master the Mites

Mites create misery for millions of allergy victims. The fecal pellets are highly allergenic. Unfortunately, mites love mattresses, pillows, upholstery, and other cotton stuffing materials. Mite-proofing your home is extremely difficult but worth a try. First, try encasing your mattress and box spring in plastic. Allergy Control Products in Ridgefield, Connecticut (800-422-DUST) is one supply company that carries such products. You should also be able to find them from department stores or surgical supply houses. You may also want to order a hypoallergenic pillow.

Wash your sheets, blankets, and bedspread frequently in hot water or send them to the cleaner. Mites live on dry flakes of human skin. Periodic washing will kill the mites and get rid of their food supply. There are also commercial products on the market that contain tannic acid and benzoate that will kill mites. Ask your doctor for recommendations.

Pharmacological Solutions for Allergies

The first stop will be almost inevitably antihistamines. There's strong agreement among medical people that antihistamines are the drugs of choice to relieve mild to moderate allergy symptoms. The way they work is quite fascinating. A bit earlier in this chapter we discussed how the irritating antigen and antibody produced by the body's immune system cling together and act as a key to fit in the lock on a mast cell and release histamine, which then goes to target cells and causes those all-too-familiar allergy symptoms. As its name implies, an *anti*histamine works against histamine, blocking it from reaching the target cell and thus blocking all those unpleasant consequences.

Think of these drugs as you would bubblegum that's been stuck in a lock. Our antihistamine bubblegum fits in the histamine receptor lock and jams it so that circulating histamine can no longer do its usual dirty work.

OTC Antihistamines

But which antihistamine should you use? There are hundreds of brands on the market alone and in combination with decongestants, pain relievers, cough suppressants, and goodness knows what else. Antihistamines are notorious for their tremendous variability in both effectiveness and side effects. No one, including your doctor, can predict with assurance how someone will react.

The most common side effect encountered with over-the-counter antihistamine therapy is drowsiness, and the elderly may be particularly affected. As everyone should know by now, driving under the influence of an antihistamine can be lethal since attention and motor coordination may be seriously hampered. That also goes for work requiring attentiveness. Fortunately, some people are more resistant to this lethargic, unpleasant, underwater-type feeling. But for those of us who are susceptible, it becomes necessary to experiment until we discover the product producing the least amount of drowsiness.

In many cases, the drowsy feeling will become much less noticeable after you take the medication for a week or so. For best results, antihistamines should be taken around the clock, not just when you feel stuffy.

Even though people vary in the drowsiness they feel with the different antihistamines, certain ones are notorious for their sleepmaking ability—so much so that they're now used as ingredients in over-the-counter sleeping pills: diphenhydramine (**Compoz Nighttime Sleep Aid, Nervine Nighttime Sleep-Aid, Nytol, Sleep-Eze 3, Sleepinal**, and **Sominex 2**) and doxylamine (**Doxysom Nighttime Sleep-Aid, Unisom Nighttime Sleep-Aid**). Makers of pain relievers have been so impressed with the "nighttime" market they have started adding antihistamines to products like **Aspirin Free Anacin P.M., Bufferin AF Nite Time, Extra Strength Tylenol PM, Quiet World**, and **Sominex Pain Relief**. Many people report to us that antihistamines leave them feeling groggy in the morning and it takes them awhile to get going. We are not convinced that such drugs are ideal sleeping pills.

Of most other over-the-counter antihistamines, chlorpheniramine and clemastine seem to be among the least sedating. Chlorpheniramine is found in dozens of generic house brands as well as **Aller-Chlor, Chlorate, Chlor-Trimeton, Coricidin**, and **Teldrin**. Combination products containing chlorpheniramine and a decongestant are too numerous to mention. Some of the most familiar brands include **Allerest 12 Hour, A.R.M., Contac Maximum Strength 12 Hour**, and **Triaminic 12**.

Clemastine is another excellent OTC option that is available in relatively inexpensive generic house brands. It is also sold by itself as **Tavist-1**. Combined with the decongestant phenylpropanolamine it is marketed as **Tavist-D**.

The great advantage of OTC antihistamines is price and convenience. You save a trip to the doctor and you don't pay an arm and a leg for new prescription products. But as we have said over and over—the tradeoff is drowsiness and fuzzy-headedness. If you need to work, drive, think clearly, or otherwise attempt to act intelligent, perhaps you need to see a doctor.

Nonsedating ℞ Antihistamines

There has been a quiet revolution in antihistamine treatment. It all started in May 1985 when **Seldane** (terfenadine) was launched. By 1991 more than 16 million prescriptions were being filled annually and **Seldane** dominated the allergy market. Since that time there has been competition and controversy.

Other nonsedating prescription antihistamines have joined the marketplace. **Hismanal** (astemizole) and **Claritin** (loratadine) have both cut into **Seldane**'s market share. The newcomers have a slight advantage over **Seldane** in that they offer convenient once-a-day dosing.

The new prescription antihistamines, although very expensive, have been welcomed by physicians and patients alike. At last there is allergy relief without feeling like a zombie. You can drive, work, and make love without worrying that you might fall asleep or make a fool out of yourself.

Sounds great, but there are several problems that you need to be aware of. First, **Seldane** and **Hismanal** can interact dangerously with a number of other medications. When combined with the antibiotic erythromycin (**E.E.S., E-Mycin, ERYC, EryPed, Ery-Tab, Ilosone, PCE,** etc.), or clarithromycin (**Biaxin**) or the antifungal medicines ketoconazole (**Nizoral**) or itraconazole (**Sporanox**), blood levels can rise dangerously high and possibly lead to serious irregular heart rhythms.[19] Even something as simple as grapefruit juice may increase blood levels of **Seldane,** so water or some other beverage would be preferable when dosing.

No one should ever take **Seldane** or **Hismanal** without checking first with a physician and pharmacist about any other dangerous drug interactions that may have been reported since this chapter was written.

Claritin, fortunately, does not seem to produce any heart rhythm disturbances, even in higher doses. That is a big relief, but before you relax completely, there is one other worry. The question has been raised: "Do Antihistamines Spur Cancer Growth?"[20] A study published in the *Journal of the National Cancer Institute* demonstrated that **Hismanal, Claritin,** and **Atarax** (hydroxyzine, another antihistamine) could stimulate tumor growth in rodents.[21] Now, none of these drugs actually caused cancer in animals. The researchers came up with an unconventional test in which they injected two different kinds of cancers (melanoma and fibrosarcoma) into mice. They had previously tested the antidepressants **Prozac** (fluoxetine) and **Elavil** (amitriptyline) using the same methodology. What they found was that all these drugs stimulated malignant growth after cancer cells were injected.

What does it mean? No one, especially not the folks at the Food and Drug Administration, seems to have a clue. This kind of cancer testing is unorthodox, follows no standard rules, and has everyone kerfloozled. The drug companies say the research is too preliminary to be meaningful. The FDA says it will look into the matter. (Don't hold your breath.)

An accompanying editorial from Dr. Douglas Weed in the Preventive Oncology

Branch of the Division of Cancer Prevention and Control at the National Cancer Institute (NCI) poses the question, "What, if anything, should be done?" He answers, "In this particular instance, the best answer is to wait."[22] The researchers respond, "We believe it possible that chronic consumption of many prescription and nonprescription drugs with tumor-growth-promoting properties may represent a previously unrecognized, and therefore insidious, environmental risk factor for cancer growth."[23]

So where does this leave you? Well, we agree with Dr. Weed at NCI. We are waiting and watching. More research is essential. That is an unsatisfactory answer, we know, but it is the best we can do for now. Occasional use of such drugs should not pose a problem. We do not have any idea what, if any, danger may exist with long-term use. Stay tuned for more data. And check out these drugs in Part V at the back of this book for more details.

Steroid Sprays

There is another way to get relief from allergy symptoms. Don't let the word *steroid* scare you. Yes, we know that steroids are strong substances that have a wide range of effects on body systems. They're particularly effective at reducing swelling, and for many years it's been no secret to doctors that steroids were effective against allergy symptoms. The problem is that the steroids are powerful drugs with an imposing list of very severe side effects. That hardly makes them candidates for treating a runny nose that's annoying but far from life-threatening. You don't shoot ants with an elephant gun.

Enter the nasal-spray version. Researchers discovered that applying steroids directly to the source of the problem allowed the drugs to do their good work without spreading extensively through the body and wreaking the havoc caused by more traditional oral corticosteroids.

Vancenase and **Beconase** (beclomethasone dipropionate), **Flonase** (fluticasone), **Nasalide** (flunisolide), and **Rhinocort** (budesonide) are all available as nasal sprays, and the evidence is strong that they really do help get you unstuffed.

Dexacortin Turbinaire (dexamethasone sodium phosphate) is another, somewhat older, steroid nasal spray. However, it is not as active topically and may have more side effects associated with its use.

Up to 85 percent of hay fever sufferers and almost as many persons with year-round allergic rhinitis get excellent relief using these sprays. The only side effects are an occasional nosebleed, sneezing, and temporary itching and burning.

The sprays do not seem to be absorbed into general circulation, so the body doesn't alter its other functions in response to the outside source of steroid. The potential for trouble is there, however, if you overuse the sprays. There have been several reports of cases in which a hole developed in the septum, the cartilage between the nostrils. Check with your doctor periodically to make sure you aren't getting into trouble.

If none of the above works, don't despair—at least not yet—because there remains at least one more alternative: **Nasalcrom** (cromolyn sodium) nasal spray. Whereas antihistamines block the effects of histamine after it has been released into the circulation, cromolyn actually keeps those specialized cells from releasing the histamine in the first place.

Although there may be some temporary stinging, sneezing, burning, or irritation, many good studies show that cromolyn works to lessen "mouth breathing, stuffy nose, runny nose, postnasal drip, and sneezing."[24]

One other absolutely safe option involves over-the-counter saline sprays such as **Afrin Saline Mist, Ayr Saline, Breathe Free, Dristan Saline Spray, HuMist Nasal Mist, NāSal, Nasal Moist, Ocean**, and **SeaMist**. Such products can eliminate crusting around the nose and are nonaddicting. They won't counter congestion, but some people say they are very soothing.

What Lies Ahead?

We anticipate other long-acting, nonsedating antihistamines will soon be available worldwide. For example, certirizine (**Zirtek**) has done quite well in Europe but is not yet available in the United States. And there is a new antihistamine nasal spray under development called levocabastine (already available in eyedrops). There are also more steroid nasal sprays undergoing testing that may be as good if not better than allergy shots.

Perhaps even more exciting are the compounds that will affect all those other nasty chemicals liberated during an allergy attack. Antileukotrienes, for example, are a hot area of pharmaceutical investigation.

So there you have it. There have been great strides in allergy treatment over the last two decades. But success depends to a great extent on each person taking an active role in his or her own therapy. First comes the detective work—finding out what is causing the misery in the first place. Then comes avoidance, if at all possible. Finally, selecting the right drug at the right time will require careful collaboration with a physician. But there are lots of options and we hope you discover some real peace come next hay fever season.

References

1. Bird, Laura. "Gesundheit! As Allergy Season Blooms, Snifflers Take Whatever Promises Relief." *The Wall Street Journal* 1994; April 21:B1,B6.
2. Naclerio, R. M. "Allergic Rhinitis." *N. Engl. J. Med.* 1991; 325:860–869.

3. National Center for Health Statistics, Collins, J. G. "Prevalence of Selected Chronic Conditions, United States, 1983–85. Advance Data From Vital and Health Statistics." No. 155 Hyattsville, MD: Public Health Service, 1988. (DHHS publication no. [PHS] 88–1250.)

4. Bird, op. cit.

5. Fish, Nancy. Allergy Council of America, February 1990.

6. Naclerio, op. cit.

7. Ibid.

8. Anderson, M. C., et al. "A Comparative Study of the Allergens of Cat Urine, Serum, Saliva, and Pelt." *J. Allergy Clin. Immunol.* 1985; 76(4):563–569.

9. Sampson, Hugh A., and Dean D. Metcalfe. "Food Allergies." *JAMA* 1992; 268:2840–2844.

10. Buckley, Rebecca H., and Dean D. Metcalfe. "Food Allergy." *JAMA* 1982; 248(20): 2627–2631.

11. Ibid.

12. Alberti, K. G. M. M. "Preventing Insulin Dependent Diabetes Mellitus." *BMJ* 1993; 307:1435–1436.

13. Sampson, Hugh A. "Role of Immediate Food Hypersensitivity in the Pathogenesis of Atopic Dermatitis." *J. Allergy Clin. Immunol.* 1983; 71(5):473–480.

14. Bernstein, Jonathan A. "Allergic Rhinitis: Helping Patients Lead an Unrestricted Life." *Postgraduate Medicine* 1993; 93:124–132.

15. Norman, P. S., et al. "Diagnostic Tests in Ragweed Hay Fever." *J. Allergy Clin. Immunol.* 1973; 52:210–224.

16. Kaliner, Michael, and Robert Lemanske. "Tinitis and Asthma." *JAMA* 1992; 268:2807–2929.

17. Naclerio, op. cit.

18. Bernstein, op. cit.

19. Woosley, Raymond L., et al. "Mechanism of the Cardiotoxic Actions of Terfenadine." *JAMA* 1993; 269:1532–1536.

20. Fackelmann, K. A. "Do Antihistamines Spur Cancer Growth?" *Science News* 1994; 145:324.

21. Brandes, Lorne J., et al. "Enhanced Cancer Growth in Mice Administered Daily Human-Equivalent Doses of Some H1-Antihistamines: Predictive In Vitro Correlates." *J. Natl. Cancer Inst.* 1994; 86:770–775.

22. Weed, Douglas L. "Between Science and Technology: The Case of Antihistamines and Cancer." *J. Natl. Cancer Inst.* 1994; 86:740–741.

23. Fackelmann, op. cit.

24. "Cromolyn Sodium Nasal Spray for Hay Fever." *Medical Letter* 1983; 25:89–90.

10

Contraception:
New Options

So you don't want to make a baby. What you *do* want is a simple, safe, and effective means of contraception. Good luck! Despite the advances of the past quarter century, no one has yet discovered anything that resembles an ideal method of birth control.

Even with the addition of several new methods, questions and controversies remain. Controlling fertility involves a highly complex physiological system in a cultural context that gives any decision strong social, moral, and religious overtones. The battle surrounding RU486 (mifepristone) is a good example.

This drug may be one of the most controversial compounds in the world. French doctors prescribe it to terminate pregnancy. Doctors in Sweden are testing it as a once-a-month contraceptive. In addition, the drug may offer hope to women trying to become pregnant. It is being studied as a treatment for endometriosis, a painful condition associated with infertility. Some researchers believe that if RU486 were not associated with abortion, it would be hailed as a breakthrough.

But because of this association, the FDA's decision whether to allow testing or keep it out of the United States became highly politicized.

Rather than enter the fray, we'll let you decide which contraceptive technique, if any, is acceptable to you. What we'll do is describe the options currently available, with the advantages and disadvantages of each. Unfortunately, there are some drawbacks to almost any contraceptive technique you might choose, so it makes sense to know as much as possible before you make your choice.

The first criterion, undoubtedly, is effectiveness. There is no point in using a technique unless it works. As you can see from the table below, there is a fair bit of variation in how well the major methods prevent pregnancy.

Effectiveness of Contraceptive Techniques[1,2,3]	
Technique	**Number of pregnancies per 100 women per year**
Vasectomy	less than 1
Female sterilization	less than 1
Depo-Provera injection	less than 1
Norplant implants	less than 1
Combination Pill (oral contraceptive)	less than 1, up to 3
Mini-Pill (oral contraceptive)	less than 1, up to 3
IUD (intrauterine device)	less than 1, up to 3
Condom and foam	less than 1, up to 5
Condom alone	3 to 36
Contraceptive sponge	9 to 16
Diaphragm	2 to 20
Cervical cap	6 to 18
Jelly and cream spermicides	4 to 36
Foam spermicides	2 to 25

Female condom	5 to 26
Rhythm method: temperature	less than 1, up to 20
Rhythm method: mucus	1 to 25
Rhythm method: calendar	14 to 47
Withdrawal	4 to 25
No contraception (for comparison)	60 to 85

As you can see, some of these methods have a pretty wide range of effectiveness. While condoms, diaphragms, and the rhythm method *can* be almost as effective as sterilization or the Pill, they have to be used properly, consistently, and conscientiously. Used haphazardly or casually, they may end up being only a bit better than taking your chances with nothing at all.

Please remember that none of these methods is absolutely foolproof. Even sterilization sometimes fails. British doctors estimate that vasectomy may lead to a subsequent pregnancy in about 1 case out of 2,000—pretty good odds, unless you happen to be that one![4] We heard of one couple, Fran and Moe Casto, who decided two children was enough. She had a tubal ligation and was astonished to find, some time later, that she was pregnant. After the baby was born, Moe had a vasectomy, but once again Fran became pregnant. To say they were surprised would probably understate the situation.[5] This story, which you may have read in Ann Landers' column, is highly unusual, but it illustrates that nothing is completely guaranteed when it comes to contraception.

While we can tell you the technical details, nobody but the people involved know what the varying risks of pregnancy mean to them. Some might prefer to postpone pregnancy awhile but would not be unhappy should they conceive; others would have their lives devastated by an unwanted pregnancy. Because all these factors interact, it's impossible to point at any one method of birth control and say, "Use that, it's the best thing." We'll tell you about lots of options so you can make up your mind.

The Pill

T he first big revolution in contraception came with the discovery of oral contraceptives—the Pill. This new concept seemed like the answer to everyone's prayers. It was unobtrusive, easy to use, didn't interfere with anyone's pleasure or spontaneity and, best of all, it worked remarkably well. If a woman just remembered to take the thing each day, she had contraceptive protection that was anywhere from 5 to 500 times more reliable than other reversible options.

As usual, initial reactions to the Pill had more to do with people's ideas of morality than with medical reality. Some hoped that this new effective contraceptive would be liberating enough to change the double standard of American sexual mores. Others feared the Pill would turn American youth into degenerate sex maniacs bent on wrecking society. As it became clear that neither outcome was imminent, medical worries began to arise.

A series of studies in the late 1960s and early 1970s linked the oral contraceptives (OCs) to all sorts of maladies, including thrombophlebitis (a painful irritation of a vein caused by formation of a blood clot), pulmonary embolism (a clot that breaks loose and lodges in the lungs), gallbladder disease, noncancerous liver tumors, visual problems, a higher risk of some types of cancer, and an increased risk of heart attack and stroke.

For years, proponents of the Pill dealt with these issues by pointing out that the excess risk for any given healthy woman is quite small. (But let's not forget that even a small risk multiplied by 8.5 million women taking oral contraceptives could add up to a considerable toll.) Anyway, the Pill people used to counter, it is far safer to use OCs than to get pregnant.

By the late 1970s, though, that was no longer true. With lower rates of death during pregnancy and childbirth, a woman would run almost as much risk of dying while on the Pill as she would if she got pregnant. And if she were over 35, her risks with oral contraceptives would be measurably higher.

On the other hand, the Pill can protect women, in large measure, against several major health problems such as iron-deficiency anemia, benign breast disease, ovarian cysts, and pelvic inflammatory disease.[6] All of these protective benefits have shown up in multiple studies of large numbers of Pill users. Evidence from smaller studies also suggests that the Pill may help protect against endometrial (uterine lining) and ovarian cancer.[7] Preventing these cancers is particularly beneficial since screening and treatment for them leave a lot to be desired.

The trouble is, the hormones contained in the Pill have many different effects throughout the body, and the consequences may vary with a woman's age. Dr. Malcolm Pike and his colleagues at the University of Southern California have reported an increased risk of breast cancer among women under 25 who had used the Pill for five years or more.[8] Although these results were publicly questioned and criticized,[9] they have been bolstered by a meta-analysis of many studies on this topic. The researchers found that the overall risk of breast cancer for all women using oral contraceptives is not affected, but that young women who take the Pill for ten years or more, especially those who begin using birth control pills before they first give birth, have a significant 46-percent increase in their risk of premenopausal breast cancer.[10]

By now, the picture that is emerging is obviously not black nor white; birth control pills are neither "good" nor "bad," and the risks for any individual woman may be hard to sort out. We urge you to have a complete discussion with your health care provider before you make up your mind whether the Pill is right for you. If you believe you are or may be pregnant already, you'll need to steer clear of the Pill until that issue is resolved. The DES (diethylstilbestrol) debacle proved that developing fetuses should not be exposed to estrogens.

Other reasons not to choose oral contraceptives include past or current breast cancer, active liver disease, abnormal vaginal bleeding that hasn't been diagnosed, or a history of high blood pressure, stroke, heart attack, a deep blood clot in the lung (pulmonary embolism). Any of these could mean the Pill is too dangerous for that woman. Any woman over 35 who smokes is also at greater risk of clotting problems (including stroke or heart attack), and doctors aren't supposed to prescribe birth control pills for her.[11]

As we shall see, a number of factors may influence the effectiveness of the Pill as well as its safety. More recent formulations differ from the original Pill, and timing may be more critical. Drug interactions may also interfere with the effectiveness of oral contraceptives.

How the Pill Interacts with Other Drugs

For the most part, drug interactions with birth control pills have not received as much attention as they probably should have. The big exception is nicotine, and rightly so, since OCs and cigarettes make a potentially disastrous combination. Smokers on the Pill multiply their chances of a stroke about 22 times over that of women who neither smoke nor take oral contraceptives. The risks of cardiovascular problems due to the Pill really soar when you start adding other risk factors, such as obesity, diabetes, or hypertension.

There are certain drugs that reduce the effectiveness of oral contraceptives, however. The anticonvulsant **Dilantin** (phenytoin) and others in the same category (**Mesantoin, Peganone**) rev up the liver enzymes that process contraceptive hormones. As a result, they don't last in the body as long as expected—which could mean a woman would not be protected. The same sort of interaction is documented with barbiturates and the tuberculosis drug rifampin. Sure, these are old-fashioned drugs, but with TB once again rearing its ugly head across the land, rifampin is being prescribed. And although barbiturates are not usually the first choice for preventing seizures, they are occasionally the best option. But a woman is more likely to encounter barbiturates in the prescription headache pills **Fiorinal** and **Fioricet** and their generic equivalents, particularly since oral contraceptives can sometimes trigger or aggravate migraines. The last time we wrote that taking one of these medications in combination with birth control pills could lead to an unexpected pregnancy, we were assured by the manufacturer that there were no cases of such an untoward interaction in company files. That's good, but we'd still rather have a woman be extra cautious and use additional contraception when she needs these painkillers rather than end up sorry.

We also worry about mixing certain antibiotics with the Pill. Penicillins (including ampicillins), tetracyclines (including doxycycline), and even the antifungal drug griseofulvin (**Fulvicin, Grifulvin, Grisactin, Gris-PEG,** etc.) can speed elimination of the oral contraceptive from the system. The potential consequences might include spotting, breakthrough bleeding, or unintended pregnancy. This kind of surprise you don't need. Better to use a backup method for extra protection if you must take one of these medicines.

This particular drug interaction could be an accident just waiting to happen to some women. The Pill is definitely the contraceptive method young people between 15 and 24 years old seem to prefer, with half of sexually active women that age relying on it.[12] While the Pill offers excellent protection against pregnancy, however, it affords none against various sexually transmitted infections. A young woman using oral contraceptives with multiple partners is definitely at risk of contracting gonorrhea, *Chlamydia,* or syphilis, not to mention HIV. Treatment of these infections (other than HIV) often requires tetracycline, doxycycline, or penicillin. If she is not warned to use additional contraception during treatment, such a woman could risk pregnancy even though she continued taking her birth control pills.

How the Pill Has Changed

How do oral contraceptives work? Basically, the Pill provides synthetic versions of the hormones the body uses to regulate its reproductive cycle. In the process they shut down the brain machinery that gives the ovaries the signal to release an egg. No egg, no baby. The Pill also causes changes in the lining of the uterus that make it an inhospitable place for an egg to take up residence were one to in fact be released and fertilized, and may also make the cervical mucus thicker and harder for sperm to traverse.

When oral contraceptives first came along, they contained relatively large doses of estrogen and progestin or progestogen, synthetic versions of the hormone progesterone. This chemical sledgehammer seemed necessary to ensure getting enough of the hormones into circulation. But when red flags began going up about problems, researchers began looking for ways to cut the dose of hormones, particularly the estrogen component, which was believed responsible for much of the circulatory-related problems. This was done, and very successfully.

The watershed amount of estrogen in a pill is 50 micrograms (50 millionths of a gram). Anything above that is a high-dose Pill; anything below qualifies as a low-dose Pill. The lower limit is around 20 micrograms, at which level many women experience breakthrough bleeding (bleeding at some other point in the cycle besides the regular menses).

Low-dose Pills now in use include **Lo/Ovral, Loestrin Fe 1/20, Brevicon, Modicon, Norinyl 1+35, Ortho-Novum 1/35** and **Ovcon-35,** although there are others. The low-estrogen Pills appear less likely to lead to heart attacks, strokes, or blood clots in the legs or lungs. They may even be less guilty of causing such common Pill side effects such as nausea and vomiting, breast tenderness, cramps, change in weight, breakthrough bleeding, depression, intolerance for contact lenses, or loss of interest in sex.

But we promised drawbacks for every method, and here's the downside of low-dose Pills: they're a little less effective than higher-dose Pills. When a woman takes a 50-microgram Pill like **Nelova 1/50 M** or **Ovral,** she may forget one occasionally and still might have enough of the artifical hormone circulating in her system to avoid pregnancy. Not so with the low-dose version. Miss a single little Pill and the chances of experiencing either breakthrough bleeding or even pregnancy do go up. Ideally, the Pill is taken at the same time every day, and if a pill or two is missed, the woman uses a backup method such as a condom. The riskiest times to miss a Pill are very early in the cycle, just starting a new packet, or late, as you are finishing a packet.[13]

This may come as a tremendous shock, but experts estimate that "one million unintended pregnancies are related to OC [oral contraceptive] use, misuse or discontinuation. . . . We estimate that approximately 697,000 unintended pregnancies could be avoided if all women used OCs properly."[14] We found this number almost unbelievable, and yet we keep meeting women who tell us that they became pregnant while taking birth control pills. For some it was because they were also taking another medicine (such as an antibiotic) that reduced contraceptive effectiveness. Others told us that they delayed taking their Pill by only a few hours. Apparently some of the low-dose brands are so tricky that even a few hours' variation from the usual schedule may be a problem for some women.

In addition to low-dose or high-dose combination Pills, there are now also biphasic and triphasic Pills. In these, the dose of progesterone-like hormone varies in the course of the cycle. **Tri-Levlen** and **Triphasil** also have a bit more estrogen in the second phase. These products provide the hormones on a schedule that mimics the woman's natural cycle more closely.

The Mini-Pill

By the way, just to clear up a bit of confusion, the "mini-Pill" is not just a low-dose combination pill. Mini-Pills such as **Micronor, Nor-Q.D.,** and **Ovrette** are progestin-only Pills. These Pills are somewhat less effective than combination Pills. Women on the mini-Pill are also more likely to experience breakthrough bleeding, variations in menstrual cycle length, or a lack of menstrual periods. But women differ in their responses to these hormones, and if estrogen gives you troublesome side effects, the mini-Pill might not.

Long-Acting Contraceptive Hormones

T wo other techniques for delivering contraceptive hormones have become available to American women in the past few years. Neither is exactly new, as they have both been used in other parts of the world for a long time before the Food and Drug Administration approved them in the U.S. Both use progesterone-like hormones, and both have the advantage that the woman relying on one of them does not have to remember to take a pill every day. She doesn't have to count the days between cycles, either, as she must with some birth control pills. She still gets highly reliable contraceptive protection in a method that is not intrusive at the moment of intercourse. Let's take a look at both of them.

Depo-Provera

Depo-Provera (medroxyprogesterone acetate) is an option for the woman who prefers to deal with contraception only four times a year. It is given as a shot once every three months. The injection site shouldn't be rubbed or massaged afterwards, because that will spread the medication around, causing the body to take it up more quickly and use up the contraceptive protection more rapidly.[15]

Since there are no pills to take, there's no need for backup contraception if the injection is given within five days after the period starts. There's no need for a woman to worry about contraception between shots, and there's no way for anyone besides her doctor to tell that she is using contraception, if that privacy is important. In addition, because **Depo-Provera** keeps eggs from maturing and thins the lining of the uterus, it helps lower the risk of ovarian and endometrial cancer. It may even reduce endometriosis, a potentially painful condition associated with menstrual periods. On **Depo-Provera,** most women find that periods become irregular, scanty, and eventually stop altogether.

Approval of this form of contraception was long delayed by the FDA because of a concern that it might cause cancer. Early studies in female beagles showed an increased incidence of breast nodules and a few cases of cancer. Experts seem to feel that these dogs were an "inappropriate animal model" because epidemiological studies in other countries where **Depo-Provera** has been used have not shown an increased risk in humans.[16]

The prescribing information now warns doctors that while there is no increase in the overall risk of breast cancer, there is a 219 percent higher risk of this cancer in young women (under 35) who first used **Depo-Provera** in the preceding four years.[17] A more-than-200-percent increase sounds like a lot, but in actuality women under 35 rarely get breast cancer. **Depo-Provera** increases the risk for a 30- to 35-year-old woman from approximately 27 out of 100,000 to about 58 cases per 100,000. Is that enough to worry about? You be the judge. Keep in mind, though, that a woman who has already been diagnosed with breast cancer should not use **Depo-Provera.**

Depo-Provera contraception is usually, though not always, reversible. You may have to be patient, though. The average time it takes between the last contraceptive shot and a pregnancy is about 10 months. There is a catch-22 here, though. Women who weigh less conceive sooner after discontinuing **Depo-Provera** than heavier women. The catch? Weight gain is a common side effect of this method. The average weight gain for the first year of use was just over 5 pounds, while women who used **Depo-Provera** for six years gained an average 16½ pounds.[18] It seems that the longer a woman uses this technique, the longer it may take her to get pregnant after she quits.

We did mention disadvantages to every technique, didn't we? Like the Pill, **Depo-Provera** does not protect a woman from sexually transmitted infections. Some women experience side effects from this medicine, including nausea, dizziness, headaches, depression, hair loss, and decreased interest in sex. Although pregnancy occurs only very rarely in women using **Depo-Provera,** when it does it may implant outside the uterus in a potentially life-threatening condition known as ectopic pregnancy. One long-term side effect that could be serious for some women is a loss of bone mineral density. That could contribute to osteoporosis (weakened bones) with the potential of spinal and hip fractures in later years.

Women who have blood clot problems (thrombophlebitis, pulmonary embolism, etc.), liver disease, abnormal vaginal bleeding that hasn't been diagnosed, or a history of heart attack, stroke, or breast cancer should not use **Depo-Provera.** Before administering the injection, the doctor or nurse will want to make sure the woman is not pregnant; this may require a pregnancy test.

Norplant

Like **Depo-Provera, Norplant** is a long-acting progesterone-type contraceptive. Instead of being injected every three months, however, it is contained in six thin, flexible little tubes that are implanted under the skin on the inside of the upper arm. The implants gradually release the hormone, levonorgestrel, over the course of five years. It is an extremely effective form of contraception, with a very low rate of unexpected pregnancy. Effectiveness is highest for women of low weight (under 110 pounds) and becomes lower for heavier women (over 154 pounds). If the system fails and a woman becomes pregnant, there is a small risk of ectopic pregnancy, although there is less of a risk than if no contraceptive is used.

Norplant does not, of course, protect against diseases transmitted by sexual contact. However, because it keeps the lining of the uterus from thickening with each cycle, it may reduce the risk of endometrial cancer.

Norplant has been promoted as the ultimate form of birth control for women who don't want to have to take pills every day or even think about contraception for five years. The up-front costs are high, ranging from $450 to about $750 to have the tubes implanted. As the company points out, once this initial cost is paid, the benefits can stretch as long as five years, working out to around $90 to $150 per year. That's less than some oral contraceptives. There is also a Norplant foundation that can help callers find an insurance company that will pay for **Norplant,** as some do not. To contact the foundation, call (703) 706-5983.

About a third of women on **Norplant** find that it changes the pattern of menstrual bleeding. Especially during the first year, many women experience breakthrough bleeding between regular periods, or they may find that periods last longer or are heavier than they used to be. Other women lose their periods. If you have a concern about menstrual irregularity, it should be discussed with the health care provider. For most women, menstrual periods usually stabilize in a normal pattern within two years.[19]

Norplant can cause weight gain. It may also cause nausea, hair loss, headache, lowered sex drive, dizziness, nervousness, or depression. If side effects are intolerable, the implants need to be removed. Be forewarned, however, that not all health care providers trained to implant the tubes can remove them gracefully. They are more difficult to remove than to place, requiring special skills and equipment. Ask your doctor how many **Norplants** he or she has removed. If your provider is not experienced, ask for a referral to someone who is.

Women who have clotting disorders such as thrombophlebitis or pulmonary embolism should not receive **Norplant.** Other conditions that will keep doctors from implanting the capsules include pregnancy (a test may be required), liver disease, abnormal undiagnosed vaginal bleeding, and breast cancer. The anticonvulsants **Tegretol** (carbamazepine) and **Dilantin** (phenytoin) can interfere with the effectiveness of **Norplant,** resulting in unplanned pregnancy.[20] Barbiturates, such as phenobarbital, and the tuberculosis medicine rifampin are also suspected of reducing the efficacy of this contraceptive.[21]

The Intrauterine Device (IUD)

A t one time, there were many different forms of IUD available in the United States, but owing to controversy over the Dalkon Shield device, which became embroiled in multimillion-dollar litigation, only two are currently on the market. Both are T-shaped; one releases a progesterone-like hormone to bolster its efficacy, while the other contains copper.

The intrauterine device has a long history. Rumor has it that Arab nomads, not wishing their female camels to be with burdened with camel kiddies while crossing the deserts, would insert small stones into the animal's uteruses and thus prevent conception. Current IUDs are higher tech, but the principle hasn't changed.

The IUD has its advantages. There's no messing or fussing about at the time of intercourse, so spontaneity need not suffer. It doesn't alter a woman's normal menstrual periods, but, like **Norplant** and **Depo-Provera,** it is also a long-term method. While the **Progestasert** (progesterone-releasing device) is good for a year, the copper-containing **ParaGard T 380A** can stay in place up to eight years. And it is relatively inexpensive, competing with condoms as a cost-effective contraceptive method. Effectiveness compares well with that of the Pill, and once it is removed women usually have no trouble becoming pregnant.

There are, of course, disadvantages. The IUD does a good but not perfect job of preventing pregnancy, particularly the **Progestasert,** which is a little less effective than the **ParaGard T 380A.** If a woman does become pregnant with this device in place, there is a risk of ectopic pregnancy. In some women, an IUD may come out, or it may cause menstrual cramping and heavier periods. Backaches and pain during intercourse have also been reported. Perforation of the uterus is a rare but very serious potential side effect.

Like the other methods we have already discussed, IUDs do not offer any protection against sexually transmitted diseases (STDs). Indeed, there appears to be an increased risk of pelvic inflammatory disease (PID) for women using this method of contraception.[22] Women who have already experienced a bout of PID should not consider the IUD an option for them.

The problem with PID is not just that it's produced by serious infections, though that's bad enough. It can also have nasty aftereffects, because the infection may scar the fallopian tubes. As a result, women who have had PID sometimes have difficulty conceiving at a later time, and may run a risk of a dangerous ectopic pregnancy.

This contraceptive method is potentially dangerous for women who must take the blood-thinning drug **Coumadin** (warfarin). Any woman with a **ParaGard** in place should avoid medical procedures involving microwaves or short waves. The IUD is most appropriate for the woman who has already had at least one child and is in a monogamous relationship, therefore at low risk of any STD.

Any woman wearing an IUD needs to know the early signs of pelvic infection so she can get medical attention promptly—and we do mean pronto, *not* next week. The warning signs include bleeding between periods, skipping a period, an exceptionally heavy period, unusual vaginal discharge, any abdominal pain aside from typical menstrual cramps, fever, or pain during intercourse. Early treatment of an infection may reduce the risk of later complications.

Another caution we'd recommend: if any doctor starts talking about "medical diathermy," make *sure* he or she knows you have an IUD in place. This therapeutic use of heat often employs microwaves, and metal on an IUD, just like metal in a microwave oven, can attract more than its share of heat, and possibly burn the uterus.

So there you have it . . . advantages, disadvantages, cautions, and precautions pertaining to the IUD. By now it's surely clear why contraception is still not a simple, one-size-fits-all kind of decision.

Barrier Methods

J ust about the only contraceptive methods that offer protection against the truly horrible infections that can hop from one sexual partner to another, wreaking havoc in their path, are the barrier methods. Principal among these is the condom, also known as prophylactic, rubber, sheath, skin, etc., and long promoted for the prevention of disease transmission. The old-fashioned "venereal diseases" that the Armed Forces worried about during World War II are nasty, but they're not so scary as HIV, the virus that leads to AIDS. After all, syphilis and gonorrhea (which are on the upswing) can be cured with antibiotics, while we have no medicines that can cure AIDS. Prevention is paramount.

How good are condoms against HIV transmission? If they are used consistently and correctly, "using latex condoms substantially reduces the risk for HIV transmission."[23] In one study, 123 couples in which one partner was infected and the other was not, used condoms consistently; none of the uninfected partners became infected. In the same study, 12 partners from 122 other couples who used condoms sometimes, but not every time, caught the virus.[24]

Latex condoms can also reduce a person's chances of catching herpes, gonorrhea, genital ulcers, hepatitis B, and *Chlamydia*. Women are less likely to come down with PID (pelvic inflammatory disease) if their partners use condoms.[25] It's no surprise that if they are used conscientiously (that is, correctly and consistently), condoms also have a pretty good record on pregnancy prevention. Check the lower number in the table on page 219. But many men don't use the device as carefully as they should, nor do many couples take advantage of the considerable extra contraceptive protection afforded by combining the condom with a sperm-killing vaginal foam.

Condoms are relatively inexpensive and don't require a doctor's prescription. There are relatively few medical conditions that would interfere with condom use, primarily latex allergy. Natural-membrane devices, an alternative that might appeal to those who are allergic to latex, can protect against pregnancy, but not against viral transmission. A new condom material, a thin polyurethane, is now on the market under the brand name **Avanti**.[26] This may help those few couples whose problem is latex allergy, but can it overcome the condom's image problem?

It appears that one of the major disadvantages of condoms is that people perceive condom use as interrupting lovemaking, interfering with spontaneity, and wrecking romance. A dedicated couple can learn to incorporate the condom into their erotic rituals, but this is probably an acquired taste. Social norms may be changing, but it could be a few years—or more—before the good-looking guy who forgets his condoms is condemned as a hopeless dork.

The woman who wants protection from infection as well as pregnancy but whose partner won't wear his rubbers now has recourse to a condom of her own. The **Reality** female condom is a polyurethane sheath with rings at each end. Inserted into the vagina like a diaphragm, it provides a barrier against semen and microbes. Used correctly and consistently, it would allow pregnancy in approximately 5 out of 100 women; the label will carry the much higher 26-percent failure rate for more typical use.[27] Another drawback to **Reality** is its price: introduced at $2.50 apiece, it could add up to quite a tab over the course of a year for regular use.

Other female barrier methods, the diaphragm and the cervical cap, are, like ordinary condoms, reasonably effective at preventing pregnancy *if* they are used consistently and in combination with the appropriate spermicidal jelly. They keep sperm out of the uterus and away from the eggs to prevent fertilization. They don't protect a woman's vulnerable vaginal membranes from anything else that might be swimming around in her partner's ejaculate, though, so they can't be considered effective barriers to infection. Spermicides such as nonoxynol-9 can reduce the risk of catching gonorrhea or *Chlamydia,* but do not eliminate it.[28] A spermicide-soaked vaginal sponge (similar to **Today**) had little if any effect on the transmission of HIV.[29]

Vasectomy: The Men's Turn

I t certainly isn't fair, but the major burden for contraception has traditionally fallen on the woman. Some women have suggested that because most researchers and drug company executives are men, there's a bias in favor of developing contraceptive drugs and devices that work on the opposite sex.

There may be some truth to that, but it could also be that it's just plain easier to find a way to foil a single ovum once a month than it is to totally eliminate the millions of potentially impregnating sperm that go forth with each ejaculation.

Right now the only effective male techniques of birth control remain the condom and vasectomy. Since the condom depends to a great extent upon the motivation of the user in order to be effective, its batting average is not so impressive as that of other forms of contraception. That leaves vasectomy, a simple surgical operation in which the doctor makes a small incision to cut and tie off the tubes carrying sperm from the testes. The operation is simple and sure. It produces no change in hormones, and no alteration of a man's sex drive unless he somehow psychologically feels "castrated" by the surgery. Some men apparently do, or may have when the technique was still fairly new and not very widespread, as evidenced by reports in the medical literature of psychological disturbances[30] following vasectomy.

When the first edition of *The People's Pharmacy* was written, there was considerable concern about the possibility that men who'd had vasectomies would suffer a significantly higher rate of coronary heart disease. This was thought to be an outcome of their bodies producing substances to fight off the millions of sperm which were now being dumped into the system, and were being detected as a "foreign" substance by the immune system. Some researchers feared this immune response would end up yielding chemical substances that could damage the walls of arteries and make the men more likely to have heart trouble.

These concerns were founded on the results of animal studies in which vasectomy does seem to produce such results. We're happy to report, though, that several long-term studies in humans clearly show no increased health risk of any kind to men with vasectomies.

There are hints, however, that vasectomy may be linked to a higher risk of prostate cancer.[31] Two studies, one following thousands of health professionals,[32] and the other considering the spouses of women in the Nurses Health Study,[32] found that men who had undergone vasectomies were 1.6 or 1.7 times more likely to be diagnosed with prostate cancer than men who had not. The risk increased with years passed since vasectomy, so that men whose operation was at least 20 years ago had more than 80 percent more likelihood of developing prostate cancer.

An editorial in the *New Zealand Medical Journal* notes these results, observes that New Zealanders volunteer for vasectomy more frequently than men elsewhere, and concludes, "It is still too early to judge whether the scare about vasectomy and prostate cancer will prove to be another false alarm, like those about hormonal function and atherosclerosis."[34] The take-home message for men who have already had a vasectomy is: Be conscientious about prostate screening, both the physical exam and the PSA (prostate specific antigen). And for men contemplating a vasectomy, a good chat with the doctor may be in order. As this research evolves, it may be possible to narrow down risks a little better and determine if vasectomy is a good choice for you.

Vasectomy continues to have one major drawback—it must be considered permanent. Men are told the operation is nonreversible and that restoration of fertility is practically impossible. At this stage of the game, that must be considered true, and no man who has any question in his mind about wanting to father children should undergo a vasectomy thinking it can be undone if he changes his mind. The surgical techniques have been developed to reverse vasectomies, but it is difficult, specialized surgery and by no means is it always successful.

Future Options for Contraception

S uppose you're not ready for anything quite as permanent as tubal ligation or vasectomy, and not too crazy about the Pill or the IUD? Well, take heart. First off, you've got plenty of company. And second, drug companies *are* scrambling hard to come up with better methods. After all, they're quite capable of counting up the numbers of people who need effective, acceptable birth control. There are enough to make research worthwhile.

There are some new contraceptives on the horizon, awaiting further research or clinical confirmation on their safety and effectiveness. For example, scientists at the University of California, San Diego, have produced a man-made version of a brain hormone that looks promising as a once-a-month birth control drug. The natural hormone has the tongue-twisting name of luteinizing hormone-releasing hormone—mercifully abbreviated to LHRH. The lab version is 140 times as powerful as the natural stuff. In small doses, it corrects a specific infertility problem experienced by a small percentage of women. In larger doses, paradoxically, it works as a contraceptive.

Synthetic LHRH does its job through tinkering with the timing of the complex hormonal and physical apparatus of conception. Normally a woman's cycle consists of two approximately equal phases, with the midpoint being ovulation. When women are given the super-LHRH, though, they have a very long pre-ovulation phase and a very short post-ovulation phase. So what? Well, the uterus continues on its old schedule, and is thus all primed and ready to receive an egg when there isn't one. About the time the ovum *does* arrive, the uterine lining is already starting to break down in preparation for a menstrual period.

One of super-LHRH's inventors, Dr. Samuel Yen, is the first to recognize the difficulties facing the substance. "The whole world is waiting for a better birth control pill," he says, "but it is not going to come easily."

Many others are working on pills, injections, or implantable devices that would permit drugs to be taken either less often, or continuously but in much smaller doses. University of Alabama researchers have embedded a contraceptive dose of the drug norethindrone in microcapsules that can be injected, providing up to several months' protection from pregnancy as the drug is slowly released from the "tiny time pills." It's still too early to tell what side effects this may produce.

And of course there is mifepristone, or RU486. Although it has been used for some time in Europe, it is just going into tentative early trials in the United States. Because the antiprogesterone hormone keeps the fertilized egg from implanting in the uterus, it faces considerable political opposition. The European research indicates that it could be effective as a "morning-after" pill, but it may be acceptable here only in extreme circumstances, such as following rape.

For now, however, we're left with some difficult choices. The methods now available all have disadvantages. As we warned you at the outset, there is no one "right" answer. In deciding on contraception, each person must balance the risks of pregnancy against the risks of each birth control method, and then decide where the balance lies.

We feel strongly that any such choice is difficult enough that people deserve as much information as possible on the true risks and benefits. In addition to the material in this chapter, anyone facing the birth control decision should search diligently for knowledgeable help in reviewing the choices. That help might come from a family-planning center, a nurse-practitioner, or a physician. Make certain you connect with someone who's prepared to give you all the information, rather than push their answer on you. It's a mighty serious decision, with tremendous implications for your health and happiness. There's no more important time to demand all your rights as a consumer than when deciding about birth control.

References

1. Olin, Bernie R., ed. *Facts and Comparisons.* St. Louis: Facts and Comparisons (A Wolters Kluwer Company), 1994. p. 2406.

2. *Physicians' Desk Reference.* Montvale, NJ: Medical Economics Data Production Company, 1994, p. 2414.

3. Rudavsky, Shari. "Female-Condom Maker to Introduce 'Reality' in Sober Packages This Fall." *Wall Street Journal,* July 5, 199, p. B2.

4. Smith, J. C., et al. "Fatherhood without apparent spermatozoa after vasectomy." *Lancet* 1994; 344:30.

5. Landers, Ann. "Baby born after tubal ligation and vasectomy." *Herald Sun,* Durham, NC, July 10, 1994, p. E8.

6. Ory, Howard. "The Noncontraceptive Health Benefits From Oral Contraceptive Use." *Int. Fam. Planning Perspectives* 1982; 8(3):93–95.

7. Mastroianni, Luigi, Jr., and J. Courtland Robinson. "Contraception in the 1990s." *Patient Care* 1994; 28:107.

8. Pike, M. C., et al. "Breast Cancer in Young Women and the Use of Oral Contraceptives: Possible Modifying Effect of Formulation and Age at Use." *Lancet* 1983; ii:926–929.

9. Horwitz, Nathan. "Canadian Expert Panel Pans Pike Pill Study." *Med. Trib.,* February 15, 1984, p. 7.

10. Romieu, I., et al. "Oral Contraceptives and Breast Cancer: Review and Meta-Analysis." *Cancer* 1990; 66:2253–2263.

11. Mastroianni and Robinson, op cit., p. 120.

12. "Teens' Preference for Oral Contraceptives Increases Their Risk for STDs." Press release, American Social Health Association, June 17, 1994.

13. Potter, Linda, and Martha Williams-Deane. "The Importance of Oral Contraceptive Compliance." *IPPF Medical Bulletin* 1990; 24(5):2–3.

14. Rosenberg, Michael J., et al. "Unintended Pregnancies and Use, Misuse and Discontinuation of Oral Contraceptives." *J. Reprod. Med.* 1995; 40:355–360.

15. Mastroianni and Robinson, op. cit., p. 107.

16. Ibid., p. 109.

17. "Depo-Provera." *Physicians' Desk Reference.* Montvale, NJ: Medical Economics Data Production Company, 1994, p. 2414.

18. Ibid., pp. 2414–2415.

19. Mastroianni and Robinson, op cit., p. 113.

20. Olin, op. cit., p. 389.

21. Mastroianni and Robinson, op. cit., p. 117.

22. Olin, op. cit. p. 392.

23. "Update: Barrier Protection Against HIV Infection and Other Sexually Transmitted Diseases." *MMWR* August 6, 1993; 42(30):589–597.

24. Ibid.

25. Ibid.

26. "Condom Campaign Fails to Increase Sales." *Wall Street Journal,* June 23, 1994, p. B3.

27. Rudavsky, op. cit.

28. Niruthisard, Somchai, et al."Use of Nonoxynol-9 and Reduction in Rate of Gonococcal and Chlamydial Cervical Infections." *Lancet* 1992; 339:1271–1375.

29. "Update: Barrier Protection Against HIV Infection and Other Sexually Transmitted Diseases," op. cit., p. 590.

30. Ziegler, F. J. "Vasectomy and Adverse Psychological Reactions." *Ann. Int. Med.* 1970; 73(5):853.

31. Altman, Lawrence K. "New Caution, and Some Reassurance, on Vasectomy." *New York Times,* February 21, 1993.

32. Giovannucci, Edward, et al. "A Prospective Cohort Study of Vasectomy and Prostate Cancer in U.S. Men." *JAMA* 1993; 269:873–877.

33. Ibid., "A Retrospective Cohort Study of Vasectomy and Prostate Cancer in U.S. Men." *JAMA* 1993; 269:878–882.

34. Skegg, David. "Vasectomy and Prostate Cancer: Is There a Link?" *N. Zealand Med. J.* 1993; 106:242–243.

11

Drugs and Kids:
Pregnancy to Puberty

Kids Are Not "Little Adults"

C hildren, it's been said, should be seen and not heard. When it comes to prescription medications, children are neither seen nor heard because few of the medications handed out by the doctor have been properly tested on the pediatric population.

According to an American Academy of Pediatrics report to the FDA, "possibly as many as three quarters of the drugs used in hospital pediatric practice are not officially approved for the purpose for which they are commonly employed.[1] Indeed," the report continues, "if the drugs marketed prior to 1962 are included, an even greater number of agents in current usage will be shown to lack substantial evidence of safety and efficacy." A casual glance at the prescribing information in the *Physicians' Desk Reference* will reveal that although there is a heading for "Pediatric Use," all too often the information appearing under that rubric is: "Safety and effectiveness in children have not been established."

As you have learned, the process of testing new drugs is a long and tedious one at best. Drug companies are not usually eager to extend their financial (and legal!) liabilities by going to the trouble of testing every new compound on children. The financial return would be extremely small, since most children are basically healthy and don't require much medicine except, perhaps, the occasional antibiotic for an ear infection. Even where there might be a rationale for testing a medication in kids, as in the case of **Zovirax** (acyclovir) against chicken pox, there may be a lot of discussion and controversy about whether the benefits are strong enough to balance any potential risk in otherwise healthy children.

Rigorous testing in hundreds or thousands of children would be required before the manufacturers could get labeling approval to say the drug worked on kids. Obviously, it's a whole lot easier, cheaper, and safer simply to say "safety and dosage have not been established for pediatric use." Such a disclaimer is called CYA (Cover Your A**). It is a colossal cop-out because it absolves the drug company of all blame, yet leaves the conscientious doctor hanging in limbo.

This might appear to be a very simple matter. Any drug that has not been proved safe just should not be used. But in the real world it doesn't work that way. As the American Academy of Pediatrics report so candidly states, "With few exceptions, marketed drugs find their way into widespread use and are, in fact, administered to pregnant women, infants, and children, despite disclaimer statements in the package insert."

After all, even though most children are healthy most of the time, kids do get sick. And when they contract an infection, need an operation, or, heaven forbid, come down with cancer, they need medicines that will kill the germs, ease the pain, and help them recover. Pediatricians may be well aware the drug they need to prescribe isn't approved for use in children. But imagine this difficult dilemma: Jenny Jones, age nine, has suffered for five weeks with a severe ear infection and none of the antibiotics tried so far has helped. The infection is worsening, Jenny is in intense pain and dizzy, and her mother wants something done and done quickly.

The doctor knows of a drug that should kill the resistant bacteria causing Jenny's infection. The medication has been used for more than six years in adults with excellent results and few side effects. But the drug label says that "safety and dosage have not been established for pediatric use." What would you do if you were the doctor making this decision?

Not so easy or obvious a choice is it? Now you understand some of the problems faced by patients, doctors, and drug companies when it comes to medications for kids. In many cases, Jenny Jones will get a prescription for that antibiotic, but the doctor will be more or less guessing at the right dose and the side effects she might experience.

We often have a tendency to see children as simply "little big people." If the doctor knows that a 150-pound person gets 15 milligrams of "Magicillin" to cure a certain infection, simple logic tells him that 5 milligrams of the same medicine should do the job for a 50-pound child with the same infection. Unfortunately, though, simple logic isn't always right. When it comes to drugs, children are definitely not just smaller versions of adults. Their immature organ systems often deal with drugs far differently than their grown-up systems will in just a few years. The differences can lead to unexpected reactions, ranging from uncomfortable to deadly.

Here's just one example (of the weird, rather than deadly variety): the *British Medical Journal* some time ago reported three cases in which children suffered "severe and disturbing" visual hallucinations after taking small doses of **Actifed,** which contains the antihistamine triprolidine and the decongestant pseudoephedrine.

Case 1: ... Six hours after receiving a single dose [5 ml Actifed; a three-and-a-half-year-old girl] presented screaming and unconsolable complaining of seeing crabs, snakes and spiders. She said that insects were biting her and that a crocodile was making a hole in her back.... When examined she was pushing invisible objects off herself and stamping on other invisible objects on the floor....

Case 2: A three-year-old girl received two 5-ml doses of Actifed during the night. The following day she suddenly developed episodes of uncontrollable terror complaining of seeing spiders and insects. On examination she was intermittently pushing and brushing away invisible objects and also hitting out and stamping....

Case 3: A two-year-old boy with ... frequent coughs and fevers was given Actifed and Actifed Compound in 5-ml doses at night whenever he was feverish. He was described as always being delirious when ill, seeing spiders and insects in bed and pushing them away. This was initially thought to be due to fever but when promethazine (Phenergan) was substituted for Actifed there were no further episodes despite his fever.[2]

The doctors reporting these cases suggested that pseudoephedrine was probably the culprit and that "it may produce visual hallucinations in children even when administered at the usual clinical dose."[3] In this instance, the medication that caused trouble was an over-the-counter remedy, but it illustrates quite well how unexpected reactions may crop up and be difficult to trace. The British physicians note that:

Visual hallucinations are uncommon in young children and their occurrence leads to considerable alarm if the cause is not recognized. Many parents do not regard Actifed and other decongestants as drugs when bought over the counter. . . . In addition we have anecdotal evidence of an increased incidence of nightmares, night terrors and behavior problems in children taking Actifed, but this is difficult to evaluate as these problems are common among children.[4]

In other words, we don't have any idea how common drug-induced psychological problems are in children. Doctors are quick to blame nightmares and other unusual disturbances on the illness rather than the treatment. No adult would think to blame a nice simple OTC medicine such as **Actifed, Sudafed, NyQuil** or **Robitussin-PE** since grown-ups rarely have difficulty with these medications.

Unfortunately, parents hate standing by and doing nothing while their children cough, sneeze, or run a fever. A national study of preschool children determined that more than half of the three-year-olds in the sample had been given some kind of OTC medicine during the previous month.[5] The most commonly given medicines were **Tylenol** and cough or cold remedies. Preschoolers *do* come down with a lot of colds. But nowhere is it written that they must be given OTC drugs for their symptoms. In fact, there is little evidence that the products sold for adults are really helpful in relieving children's distress.[6] The pediatrician who commented on this study for the *Journal of the American Medical Association*, Dr. Anne Gadomski, worries about the toxicity of these medicines in children and cautions doctors:

Until convincing data become available on the efficacy and safety of cough and cold medicines in young children, the *primum non nocere* ["first, do no harm"] approach to management of the common cold in children should be followed. Although they may be annoying or worrisome to the parent, the signs of upper respiratory tract infection, particularly cough, may not be distressing to the child, in which case it is truly the parent administering the OTC medication who is being "treated." In place of cough and cold medications, simple and safe remedies can be explained and instructions given as to when to return or call if the child fails to improve. For centuries, coughs and colds have been treated with home remedies, few of which have been formally studied. These remedies include tea with lemon and honey, chicken soup, hot broths, herbal teas, and, in developing countries, guava juice, cinnamon concoctions, and fish liver oil. Remedies such as tea with lemon and honey are primarily soothing, but they are also simple, safe, inexpensive, and readily available in the home.[7]

So that's the advice from a pediatric expert: Don't be too quick to reach for OTC medicines when your child has a cold or a cough. These drugs, by and large, have not been well tested in kids, they often don't do any good, and they may produce unpleasant and troubling side effects. If you feel you must do *something*, give the child a home remedy. But use your good judgment and don't give the youngster anything that might be harmful, such as alcohol.

Alcohol Is Bad for Kids

Alcohol is another problem that might easily be overlooked. Almost everywhere in the United States, you have to be at least eighteen years old to buy booze. Many states won't allow beer, wine or other alcoholic beverages to be sold to anyone under twenty-one. Yet a child can walk into almost any supermarket or drugstore in the country, plunk down a couple of bucks, and legally walk out with a bottle containing anywhere from 5 to 8 proof alcohol. In fact, many kids are actually given medicine with high alcohol content by their unsuspecting, well-intentioned parents.

Many of the most popular cold and cough remedies contain whopping doses of alcohol. **NyQuil Nighttime Cold/Flu Medicine** is 50 proof. **Contac Severe Cold & Flu Nighttime Liquid** and **Medi-Flu Liquid** are about 38 proof, while **Comtrex Liquid** and **Vicks Formula 44M Cough and Cold Liquid** check in at 40 proof. That's quite a bit of booze. Though it would hardly bother most adults, children are more sensitive to alcohol. Small amounts can have a proportionately larger effect on the nervous system. And it may also trigger hypoglycemia, or low blood sugar, in children. Alcohol keeps the liver from making glucose, the simple sugar that fuels the body. This is especially a problem when children have not had much to eat, a common situation when they are ill. Because children use up glucose quickly, it doesn't take a lot of alcohol to cause hypoglycemia.

Another area where children can get into trouble is with mouthwash. No adult would ever consider drinking **Scope** or **Listerine,** but according to the FDA children may not realize the purpose or the danger of mouthwash.

The bright colors and pleasing flavors of these products make them particularly tempting to youngsters. The bottles, usually without childproof caps, are easily accessible in the family bathroom. Persuasive television advertising depicts people smiling happily after using that minty green liquid, but they are never shown spitting it out. A young viewer might think the product is supposed to be swallowed.

Whether it is this mistaken notion or some other reason that prompts them to take a swig of mouthwash, children have been accidentally poisoned by these pretty liquids, some of which contain more alcohol than beer or wine.[8]

So next time your child has a cold or a cough, do look twice before passing the liquid cold medicine. In fact, before giving your child any medication, why not read the label and make sure there's no alcohol in it? If there's no children's dose given, you ought to think twice about guessing. And while you're reading labels, you may want to think twice before giving your very young person **Actifed, Sudafed,** or any other cold remedy with a decongestant. Preparations that contain ingredients such as pseudoephedrine or phenylpropanolamine (PPA) may cause insomnia or nightmares, not to mention other unpleasant psychological reactions.

Getting the Right Dose for Your Child

Sometimes even doctors make mundane mistakes in the directions on prescriptions for kids. You know, "Shake well, take one teaspoon three times a day with meals." In a study of more than 2,200 prescriptions for 70 of the drugs used most frequently with children, doctors at Los Angeles County–University of Southern California Medical Center found that only 5 percent of those prescriptions "contained no errors or omissions."[9]

Now, that's incredible! We're talking about a major health center, with top-notch pediatricians and residents. Yet most of the prescriptions they wrote were incorrect in one way or another. Although many of the mistakes were relatively minor, "more than one-third of the prescriptions with dosage specified contained an error."[10] In light of this, the researchers concluded that "the chance of a patient's receiving sufficient medication to maintain a therapeutic blood level is about 1 in 30."[11] The kids might be better off taking their chances at the gambling tables in Las Vegas!

It is no wonder that there were problems getting the dose right. A doctor practically needs a calculator to figure a child's dose of certain medications. The doctor needs to divide the child's weight in pounds by 2.2 (the number of pounds in a kilogram), multiply that number times the appropriate dose (in mg/kg), then divide all of that by the number of doses in a day—three? four? It may not be higher math, but as one physician points out, "This calculation can be cumbersome. Rounding off at each step may lead to an incorrect final dose."[12]

One tip before we leave the issue of dosing: Getting liquid medicine into a reluctant toddler can be a significant parental challenge. Using a teaspoon out of the kitchen drawer makes this even harder. What if you spill some? Then the child won't get enough medicine. If you give another teaspoon, it might be too much. What's more, a medical teaspoon is exactly 5 ml. Hardly any ordinary flatware is made to those specifications. Don't take a chance on the dose you give your child. Instead, use an oral syringe (no needle, just for squirting an accurate dose into a baby's mouth) or a medicine spoon, which has a hollow test-tube-like handle measured out in milliliters and teaspoons. When our kids were little, they liked a medicine spoon shaped like a little alligator.

Drugs and Pregnancy

E veryone agrees that the process of pregnancy and birth is something of a miracle. And yet we often meddle with the delicate cellular process taking place in a mother's body by administering powerful chemicals during the nine months of gestation. Nearly half of pregnant women take a prescribed medicine at some point during the pregnancy; the proportion using over-the-counter medicines is unknown but probably even higher.[13]

Stop and consider for a second what happens in pregnancy. Starting with just two cells, an indescribably complex series of events takes place that allows those cells to multiply and differentiate until there's a baby with trillions of cells and dozens of organs. Billions of biochemical reactions take place during those nine months. Disruption of just one may mean deformation, disability, or death for the growing fetus.

Nevertheless, some pregnant women continue taking drugs that have never been proved safe for use in pregnancy. In fact, because of the ethical considerations involved, it is unlikely there will be clinical testing of very many drugs on pregnant women. So anything a woman takes while pregnant should be considered an experiment unless there is evidence to the contrary.

This is tacitly acknowledged in the FDA's classification of drugs for use in pregnancy. The categories run from A, in which controlled studies in women did not show any harm to the fetus in the first three months of pregnancy, through B, C, D, to X, a category of drugs contraindicated during pregnancy because human or animal studies have demonstrated serious problems for the fetus.[14] Categories A and X are nice, clear, unambiguous pigeonholes that tell doctor and patient exactly where they stand with a given compound. As you might guess, relatively few drugs fall into these categories. Instead, most of the compounds a doctor might want to use could be described as "We don't think there's a problem, but we're not sure" (Category B), or "This might be a bad idea but take it if you really need it" (Category D), or, of course, the catchall Category C, in which there are no studies, or the studies conflict, and we really don't have a clue. (Our characterizations of these categories have not been approved by the FDA.)

We would think that after the thalidomide tragedy, women and doctors would have learned to be cautious. Unfortunately, that doesn't seem to be the case. A study done when the memory of thalidomide was still fresh was published in the *British Medical Journal*. It revealed that of 1,369 women, 97 percent took at least one medication during their pregnancy.[15]

Other reports have revealed comparable—or worse—numbers. A study of middle- and upper-class women in Houston, Texas, found that the women had used an average of ten different drugs during pregnancy, with antibiotics and antacids heading the list. One woman took 25 aspirin tablets daily during her pregnancy. When asked about it she said, "If I'd known aspirin was a drug I wouldn't have taken it."[16]

Aspirin

But aspirin *is* a drug. Because of its potential to cause excessive bleeding, aspirin should be taken during pregnancy *only* under the strict supervision of the doctor in charge. The label on the bottle warns against taking it during pregnancy, particularly during the third trimester. Some obstetricians are now prescribing low doses of aspirin to women at high risk of pregnancy-induced hypertension. A meta-analysis of six studies found that "low-dose aspirin reduces the risks of PIH [pregnancy-induced hypertension] and severe low birth weight, with no observed risk of maternal or neonatal adverse effects."[17] This does *not* mean women should be treating themselves with aspirin. Pregnancy-induced hypertension is a life-threatening condition, and aspirin should be used to treat it only upon the physician's prescription. This shows how complex the question of drug treatment during pregnancy can get.

Many other nonprescription medications that women often take for granted are better avoided during pregnancy. For example, cold medicines treat only symptoms and don't cure anything. Brompheniramine, an antihistamine that is found in some cold-and-flu mixtures, has been associated with birth defects.[18] "On theoretical grounds," obstetrics experts argue, "cold medications should be absolutely avoided during the first trimester."[19]

What about the other chemicals that so many people commonly consume? Alcohol, nicotine, laxatives, vitamin A, lithium for manic-depressive disorder, and tranquilizers such as **Valium** (diazepam) or **Xanax** (alprazolam) might all affect the unborn baby. Everything the doctor prescribes is a drug, but so are over-the-counter remedies. Not only the type of drug, but also the time of pregnancy it is taken will have an important impact on whether it leads to serious problems in the fetus.[20]

An embryo is most susceptible to birth defects during the first few weeks of pregnancy. A woman could inadvertently expose her baby to a hazardous drug even before she realized she was pregnant. That's why any woman who might possibly become pregnant should be careful not to use any drug—prescription, over-the-counter, or otherwise—unless it's necessary to her health and she knows that she is not pregnant.

Although an expectant mother should ideally avoid all drugs and other chemicals as much as possible, no one expects her to live on just bread and water for nine months. Obviously, a lot of women have gotten pregnant and had healthy babies even though they took prescription or nonprescription medications, or continued drinking or smoking. On the other hand, we would all like to improve the odds as best we can. Let's take a look at some of the chemicals that could pose potential problems.

Alcohol

This substance is so ubiquitous in our society that too often it's not even recognized as a drug. That little glass of white wine at lunch or a scotch and soda after work seems so innocuous. Yet in sufficient quantity alcohol can cause something terrible called Fetal Alcohol Syndrome (FAS).

Babies born with FAS suffer severe birth defects. They are smaller than normal at birth and continue to be underweight; they have characteristic facial abnormalities, heart problems, and kidney complications as well as irregularities of the fingers. Mental retardation and attention deficit disorders are not uncommon with this syndrome.[21]

Most of these problems are the outcome of heavy drinking, and most pregnant women aren't alcoholics. The scary question is: How much effect does a modest alcohol intake have? Unfortunately, we don't have a good answer to that one. But we are admittedly biased toward lowering risks. One group of investigators concluded that "infants exposed to alcohol in utero even in moderate amounts appear to suffer from a spectrum of developmental mental and motor delays. Severe problems typically present early, while the more subtle changes may become apparent only when the children enter school."[22] We don't know any parents who would willingly handicap their children, so why take any risk? Saying no to alcohol for nine months seems a small price to pay to have the healthiest baby possible.

By the way, that recommendation might also apply to prospective dads. Researchers at Washington University School of Medicine were interested in whether a father's exposure to alcohol might have an impact on fetal development. Naturally, it wouldn't be ethical to run this experiment on humans, so they injected male rats with enough ethanol to bring blood alcohol concentration to about 0.2 percent—way over the legal limit if rats could drive. Then they mated the males with females that had not been exposed to alcohol, planning to keep tabs on the litters as the pups grew up. To their surprise, however, relatively few of the females became pregnant. Repeating the experiments confirmed that a single large dose of alcohol, a paternal rodent "binge," reduced fertility by about 50 percent.[23] We still don't know if there's any carryover to human beings, but it seems like a good idea for men to exercise moderation, at the very least, when they're trying to start a family.

Smoking

It's certainly no secret that smoking isn't good for you. Everyone except the tobacco industry agrees on that. But some people don't seem to think about how maternal smoking affects the developing baby. Nicotine and other by-products of smoking enter the fetal circulation and have a wide range of effects. As far back as the 1930s, doctors reported that fetal heart rate was altered when mothers smoked.

Fifty years later, investigators from the Maryland School of Medicine reported the results of a study into the effect of smoking on birth weight.[24] Birth weight is an important measure of how well an infant will do during the first months of life. Generally speaking, low-birth-weight babies have more problems, and mothers who smoke have about twice the risk of giving birth to an infant weighing less than 2,500 grams (about 5.5 pounds).

Knowing this, the Maryland researchers divided 935 pregnant smokers into two groups. One group continued smoking. The other group received all kinds of support and encouragement to cut down or quit. Chemical testing shortly before birth showed that the intervention group had indeed significantly reduced their smoking habit. In fact, 43 percent had quit entirely. And the babies benefited. Infants born to the low-smoking group were on average both heavier and longer (as measured head to toe) than those born to women whose smoking was not reduced.[25]

In summing up the evidence on smoking and pregnancy, two reviewers conclude that:

A relationship exists between maternal smoking and low birth weight, decreased length, spontaneous abortion, fetal, neonatal, and postnatal deaths, prematurity, abruptio placenta, stillbirth, placenta previa, premature rupture of the membranes, delayed crying time, decrease in fetal breathing time, impaired reading attainment, and hyperkinesis.[26]

That's quite a burden to place on a baby just so that its mother can enjoy the pleasure of smoking. We second the American Cancer Society's longtime plea: "Pregnant mothers, please don't smoke."

Coffee and Caffeine

We know, it's beginning to sound as though everything you like is bad for your baby. Unfortunately, very high levels of caffeine (from tea and cola drinks as well as coffee) have been linked to a higher incidence of abortion and prematurity.[27] Women who consume the most caffeine may also have more difficulty conceiving. Moderate caffeine consumption—a few cups a day—may not be a big problem, but the real coffee compulsives, the ten-cup-a-day people, might be well advised to give themselves and their babies-in-waiting a break by cutting back.

Prescription Drugs

In general, drugs are available by prescription because they are powerful chemical substances that can cause almost as many problems as they cure. It's only logical that some of these medications could cause trouble for the developing fetus. Pregnant women should be the world's most reluctant consumers of prescription medication and the last to insist that the doctor give them a prescription for every ache and pain.

While many medications can cause complications when used during pregnancy, certain categories of drugs have proved particularly troublesome. Let the doctor know you are pregnant and ask about safety for the fetus if he or she starts talking about prescribing you any medication. This is especially true for cancer drugs, antithyroid medicines, antianxiety drugs (benzodiazepines), drugs that suppress the immune system, blood-thinning drugs such as **Coumadin** (warfarin), and lithium, which is often prescribed to control manic-depressive swings.[28]

Tetracycline antibiotics can cause discoloration of the teeth that will later emerge, and may also be responsible for impaired bone growth. Anticonvulsants pose a particular dilemma, since they have been linked to birth defects—but uncontrolled seizures could also harm the fetus. **Dilantin** (phenytoin) has been found to affect children's intelligence and language ability after they are exposed to the drug in the womb.[29] The epileptic woman will need a very good working relationship between her obstetrician and her neurologist.

At least one antihistamine, brompheniramine, has been linked to birth defects,[30] although the research is by no means definitive. Questions have also been raised about doxylamine, an antihistamine found in the over-the-counter sleeping pill **Unisom**. This was one of the ingredients in the morning-sickness pill, **Bendectin**, which was withdrawn from the market although it was never proven that the drug caused birth defects.[31] The point here is not that pregnant women should be paranoid, but that they should be extra cautious, both about prescribed medication and over-the-counter remedies. Information on OTC drugs is often inadequate in this regard. The best rule for the pregnant woman is to check with the doctor before taking *any* drug.

Drugs and Breast-feeding

The newborn baby is not safe from dangerous side effects after delivery. Far from it. Because of the consensus that breast milk is the best nutritional option for infants, women are being encouraged to breast-feed if at all possible.[32] But many drugs are secreted in breast milk, and the baby could be exposed to medication the mother is taking.

Fortunately, awareness of this problem has grown since we wrote the original

People's Pharmacy. The *Physicians' Desk Reference* now carries information on whether the medications discussed appear in breast milk. Doctors realize that they must weigh the benefits of the drug they plan to prescribe not only against the risks to the patient, but also against the risks to the nursing infant. To protect your baby from untoward effects, make sure that all the physicians who treat you know that you are breast-feeding your baby and be sure to ask if the prescribed medicine will be passed in the breast milk. Determining the benefit/risk ratio is not a routine exercise. It needs to take your particular health concerns into account, and also your dedication to breast-feeding, the baby's age, and his or her ability to thrive on a substitute for breast milk.

Cautions for Kids

Once a newborn baby survives all the pitfalls and dangers of the first few months of life, you would think a parent could begin to relax. One of the things parents learn as the children grow older is that it doesn't get easier—but the challenges change. This is also true when it comes to protecting a child from the hazards of drugs.

While the parents of a young baby need to keep baby powder out of baby's reach (if accidentally inhaled, it could cause serious harm, including breathing difficulties or pneumonia), the parents of toddlers need to be concerned about hiding all household poisons—and that does include prescription drugs, OTC remedies, and even herbs, as well as cleaning supplies. When the child gets to middle school or high school, one of the challenges will be to keep him or her from abusing drugs. That will be far more feasible if the tone has been set in the home all along that drugs are to be used cautiously, not casually. (Don't forget that kids learn best by example.)

Aspirin and Reye's Syndrome

Parents have sometimes been guilty of administering incorrect or hazardous medicines to their children. A study conducted by Georgetown University in 1975 revealed that as many as 20 percent of kids under two received potentially dangerous nonprescription drugs. Something as simple and seemingly harmless as aspirin can be quite hazardous to a youngster if given in the wrong dose or under the wrong circumstances. By now, you have probably heard of Reye's syndrome (pronounced like *rye* bread). But you may not realize how long it took for early warnings about this problem to be recognized fully.

There is no longer any reasonable doubt that aspirin poses a risk of Reye's syndrome when taken by children or teenagers who have chicken pox or influenza. Although Reye's is rare, it can be fatal in up to 30 percent of cases. It may also leave survivors with permanent brain damage. The symptoms of Reye's include irritability, personality changes, vomiting, lethargy, delirium, and ultimately, coma.

Every bottle of aspirin now comes with a clear warning about Reye's, but from the label there is no indication how controversial this issue was when it first surfaced. Some doctors as well as members of the drug industry disputed the connection, and the FDA waited a long time before deciding that a warning on the label was needed.

According to epidemiological researchers Devra Lee Davis and Patricia Buffler, 1,470 young people may have died needlessly during the five years (1981 to 1986) that the Food and Drug Administration debated the warning.[33] Once cautionary language about Reye's syndrome appeared on aspirin bottles, the incidence of this potentially deadly disease dropped dramatically.

The trouble is that it may be hard to tell if children have the flu or just a bad cold. Chicken pox starts out with a mild fever, and it may take a few days before the skin rash appears. Because early diagnosis can be difficult, the safe thing to do is give kids acetaminophen or ibuprofen for a fever instead of aspirin, unless a doctor specifies aspirin.

This little bit of pharmaceutical history illustrates some of the pitfalls of giving even familiar drugs to youngsters. So shape up, Mom and Dad! You should be at least as cautious about the medicines you give the kids as you are about the ones you take yourself. And we hope that by now you're very careful about those.

Common Childhood Problems

Parents of young children may sometimes feel their kids bounce from one health crisis to another. If it's not an ear infection, it's a sore throat, a stomachache, or a runny nose. Naturally, any parent wants to help a child feel better as soon as possible. But while it doesn't make sense to delay treatment, it's important not to overreact and possibly make matters worse.

Diarrhea

With day-care centers becoming a part of everyday life for American families, epidemiologists (those who study the pattern of disease in the population) have noted a rise in the reported incidence of childhood diarrhea. A bit of detective work soon made it clear that infections were being spread at child-care centers when hurried workers failed to wash their hands carefully after diapering infants. Their hands, sometimes contaminated with fecal bacteria, then became the vehicle for spreading the bacteria to other youngsters.

Diarrhea may seem more an annoyance than a life-threatening disease. That's generally true, but you should be aware that the risks are greater for children. It's pretty easy for a small child to become dehydrated or to lose large amounts of the electrolytes (sodium, potassium, chloride, etc.) that are responsible for keeping the proper cellular rhythms going. For that reason diarrhea in a child should always be taken seriously. Double the dose of caution when you're talking about an infant.

In most cases the cure will consist simply of withholding food for a while, during which the child is given clear liquids. Normally we encourage parents to banish soft drinks from the home, but there are times when we break down and actually suggest a cola beverage or ginger ale if it will tempt an under-the-weather child to take a few sips. If you want to use what the pediatricians recommend you will look for something like **Pedialyte** or **Ricelyte**. These special liquid supplements are designed to replenish electrolytes in the proper balance. Check with the doctor about the proper use of these solutions for your child.

Adult diarrhea medicine, whether it's prescription or OTC, is not a good idea. Diarrhea that doesn't go away by itself in 24 hours usually deserves medical attention.

Ear Infections

If there is one classic disease of childhood it would certainly be otitis media—middle-ear infections. Little kids especially often have a hard time escaping them.

Chronic ear infections are uncomfortable for the child, distressing for the parents, and potentially dangerous. Yet there remains tremendous controversy over what to do about the garden-variety ear infection.

Some doctors favor aggressive drug therapy; others opt for insertion of a tiny tube to aid in drainage of infected material, and still others give minimal treatment and just wait for the child to outgrow the problem. But though each of these approaches has its proponents, the proper course has become murkier lately. Leaving ear infections untreated runs the risk that a child will experience hearing damage. Yet the research showing the benefits of antibiotic treatment for otitis media has been called into question. In addition, overenthusiastic doctors have apparently inserted more ear tubes than are, strictly speaking, called for. Current guidelines restrict appropriate ear-tube surgery to children for whom antibiotic treatments have not been completely successful.

On top of that, selecting the right antibiotic has become somewhat of an art form. The problem is drug resistance. It used to be that simple penicillin would clear up most ear infections. But today there are all sorts of beasties roaming around and many seem capable of withstanding drugs such as penicillin, ampicillin, and amoxicillin. Pediatricians often have to resort to newer and ever more expensive medications. Obviously, treating ear infections needs close coordination and communication between parent and pediatrician. That's especially true because some of the broad-spectrum antibiotics can have rare but potentially fatal side effects and must be treated with respect. A grandmother who read our newspaper column wrote to report the following tragedy.

> Last year our 6-year-old grandson was put on Septra for a month because of ear problems. He took the prescribed medicine for three weeks when he developed a severe rash, terrible itching and hemorrhaging under the skin. His doctor sent him to an allergist. He was admitted to Children's Hospital with Stevens-Johnson syndrome and died soon after. His liver, they said, was totally destroyed. Please warn other parents and spare some other child the agony he went through.

What a heartbreaking story. We have no way of knowing for sure whether the drug really was responsible in this case. But there are instances in the medical literature of such severe symptoms occurring. Once again we are reminded that even "safe" drugs can occasionally cause severe or life-threatening reactions. The FDA reports a number of deaths in children associated with these kinds of medications. Side effects have ranged from devastating damage to the skin, to blood and liver damage. Parents must be especially vigilant when giving medicine to children. ANY unusual behavior or side effects (especially skin rash) should be reported to the physician immediately!

Bedwetting

The doctor calls it "nocturnal enuresis." To the parent it's bedwetting. And to the child it's mortifying, distressing, and sometimes psychologically disabling. Parents of bedwetters may fail to realize that many children just don't have the physical maturity to have complete bladder control until they're a bit older. While many make it by age five, about one-fifth won't. Becoming anxious, angry, demanding, or demeaning (or sometimes all of those) compounds the physical problem by adding a psychological one and usually helps neither child nor parent.

It's estimated that 20 million American youngsters over the age of five are bedwetters. In our society where we often expect instant relief for everything that bothers us, it's no surprise that both doctors and patients (actually parents of patients) are quick to look towards drugs as the magic solution. But there are options that ought to be tried first.

Just living patiently with the problem for a while will often be the cure. You may be able to speed the process along by offering encouragement and prizes for dry nights, but not in such a way as to create too much pressure. The child should have the responsibility for keeping a chart of dry and wet nights and should receive lots of praise, accompanied with gold stars and a special treat for each success.

The young person should also have the responsibility for changing wet sheets and seeing that they are placed in an appropriate place for washing. In this way the idea is transmitted without punishment that the child is responsible for his actions. It may also be of some benefit to cut down on fluid intake well before bedtime, and have Mom or Dad wake up the child at various intervals throughout the night.

For those who must intervene, a variety of alarm systems that help the child help himself have proved relatively effective over the years. Products with hokey names such as **Wet-Stop** and **Wee-Alert** are effective conditioners and help about 70 percent of children. The battery-operated apparatus sounds an alarm when a small amount of urine touches two electrodes and closes a circuit. If placed under the child's sheet, it will wake him up at the first sign of wetting. The child should be encouraged not to wear pajama bottoms to maximize the alarm's effectiveness.

Lots of reassurance should be provided in the beginning because kids can be frightened by the mystery or complexity of the thing. Each child should be taught how to set the alarm himself and what is expected—that whenever the buzzer goes off he or she is expected to get up and go to the bathroom and then reset the alarm. Mom and Dad should be prepared to wake the child up at the sound of the ring during the first few weeks of treatment until he gets the hang of things. If the conditioning process is continued for about a month after a cure is established, the chances of relapse may be significantly reduced.

For a child who needs short-term help so she can go to camp or he can stay at a friend's house, there is now an effective prescription medication with a reasonable side-effect profile. Desmopressin, under the brand name **DDAVP**, helps children's bodies make more antidiuretic hormone (ADH) at night while they are sleeping. This is the normal rhythm for this hormone in most people, especially adults, but it seems that many bedwetters don't have a normal increase of ADH at night and go on making urine as if it were daytime.

DDAVP has benefited up to 80 percent of the children who used it in studies,[34] and at least one researcher suggests that continuous use of the medicine for at least three months can reduce the rate of relapse. **DDAVP** is not a pill, but rather available in a nose spray. If your nondrug approaches haven't worked and your patience is wearing thin, you might ask the doctor if this medication would be appropriate.

Now that **DDAVP** is available, doctors are much less likely to prescribe the old standby for bedwetting, an antidepressant. In our opinion, that is a very good thing. Medications such as **Tofranil** (imipramine) have many side effects in young people and are very dangerous in overdose. It is difficult to justify them being used for a problem as minor as bedwetting, and we're pleased to see they are rarely prescribed for this anymore.

ADHD: Attention Deficit Hyperactivity Disorder

This is a really hot potato. We have rarely seen such emotion and controversy about a pediatric health issue. Some doctors argue that attention deficit disorder is being overdiagnosed and overtreated. They worry that normal kids who are overly enthusiastic or easily bored by dull classroom routines are being falsely labeled as hyperactive. Experts in the field counter that children who cannot focus their attention get labeled as lazy or disruptive, fall behind in school, develop poor self-esteem, and become trapped in a downward spiral of failure.

Unquestionably, most children and many adults will demonstrate some characteristics of attention deficit disorder or hyperactivity. People who learn best by touching and doing are going to have a hard time sitting still while a teacher talks or writes on the blackboard. Who hasn't daydreamed during a particularly boring class? We know lots of extremely successful grown-ups who fidget and are impatient. They have many other ADD symptoms; they may be disorganized, easily distracted, impulsive, restless, or high-energy people. But they are also creative and have learned to handle these potential disadvantages and turn them into assets.

In a child, ADHD can lead to an almost constant fever pitch of motion. This can hurt the child's ability to concentrate in school, interact with his playmates, get along at home, and fit into most situations. Although there are undoubtedly children misdiagnosed as "hyperactive" or as having ADHD, the problem is real. The child suffers, siblings suffer, and the parents suffer. While some children simply outgrow the problem by early adolescence, the havoc wrought on the family and the victim is great. And in other cases, a bad start may be linked to behavior problems that continue into adulthood. It is no wonder that parents, teachers, and health professionals keep searching for ways to deal with this disorder.

That's why many parents and doctors resort to powerful drugs, such as **Ritalin** (methylphenidate), **Cylert** (pemoline), and **Dexedrine** (dextroamphetamine). These stimulant drugs paradoxically calm kids with ADHD and can make a tremendous difference when they are used appropriately. Children who formerly faced only frustration at school can suddenly attend and get their work done. They can sit still long enough to play with other children, eat dinner, and lead a relatively normal life. But to work, the medications must be administered carefully and supervised by a doctor who will adjust the dosage properly.

The drugs do not work for every child. In some cases, they are ineffective. In others, side effects are more than the child or the family can tolerate. They can cause insomnia, reduced appetite, weight loss, and growth difficulties. Stomachache, skin rashes, headache, irritability, and even hallucinations may be associated with such therapy. And since long-term effects are uncertain, many parents worry about committing a child to a 10- or 15-year diet of stimulants.

While the medications used to treat ADHD can be extremely helpful for some children, they need to be used within the context of a full treatment program. That means proper diagnosis and periodic evaluation by experienced professionals. The family needs to be involved in the process. We have found no better book than *Driven to Distraction: Recognizing and Coping with Attention Deficit Disorder from Childhood through Adulthood,* by Edward M. Hallowell and John J. Ratey (New York: Simon & Schuster, 1994).

Drs. Hallowell and Ratey have some excellent suggestions for families coping with ADD in one or more members, including educating the family and making it clear that ADD is nobody's fault. They provide lots of wonderful coping strategies for children as well as adults whose lives are made difficult by this disorder. They also describe some new approaches to pharmaceutical management, including antidepressants such as **Wellbutrin** (bupropion), **Norpramin** (desipramine), and **Prozac** (fluoxetine).

We still don't understand what causes ADHD and we appear far from a cure. Our best hope is that continuing research into this condition will eventually yield clues that allow us to replace the current drug treatments with something both more specific and safer.

Children and Drug Safety: Poison Protection

Medicine can be a valuable tool in the fight against childhood illness. It can also turn in an instant from savior to killer.

It's difficult to say anything about childhood drug poisoning that parents don't know. Yet in spite of the obvious dangers and obvious solutions, more than three million children under the age of five will be poisoned this year, many of them on drugs left within easy reach.

Childproof caps have helped cut the toll, but to be effective they have to be used. Sometimes people with children in the house request non-childproof caps on their prescription medications for convenience. They *are* easier to get open. For anyone—and that's the problem.

A surprising number of poisonings happen because somebody leaves the cap off the medicine and/or leaves it within easy reach. Keep in mind that to a child the pills may look like candy, being brightly colored as they often are. In one recent incident, eight children between the ages of two and four were poisoned when they found half a dozen discarded bottles of rheumatism and heart medications in a garbage can. They thought the tablets were candy.

Children are also great imitators. They learn to walk and talk by seeing adults do those things so we shouldn't be surprised when they take a pill just like they've seen their parents do. It's impossible for a young child to understand that the pill Mom or Dad just took with impunity could be a fatal overdose for her.

We'd hate to think any of our readers will ever suffer the agony of having their child poisoned on medications intended to relieve discomfort. The best defense is a good offense. To help prevent drug poisoning in children do the following:

Do a drug audit—Go through the medicine chest right now. First, properly dispose of any drugs that aren't current and needed (we'll talk about proper disposal in a moment). Think of every drug in your medicine chest as a poisoning opportunity for a child.

Second, check and make certain that each and every drug is stored in a child-proof container. While many parents think the tricky caps are more adultproof than childproof, the evidence is overwhelming: Childhood poisoning incidents have decreased considerably since the safety caps were mandated.

Third, consider putting a lock on the medicine cabinet or moving medications to someplace where they can be kept under lock and key. It may seem like an inconvenience, but remember there is no limit to either the curiosity of a child or to his or her ability to get into things when your back is turned. By the way, that goes double for household chemicals like cleaning fluids, detergents, drain cleaners, paint thinners, fuels, or whatever. NEVER store them under the sink or in an accessible cupboard. That's just asking for trouble!

Dispose of drugs properly—In the case we just mentioned, children wound up in danger because someone just threw unwanted drugs in the trash rather than disposing of them carefully.

By carefully, we mean seeing that the liquids are poured down the drain, capsules emptied of their contents, and pills crushed into powder and flushed. "Crush and flush" is a good rule to remember and an easy one to follow. It will take only seconds to render your potent medication truly childproof. If this approach is not practical or ecologically desirable, return old medicines to the pharmacy and ask the pharmacist to dispose of them.

Do some drug education—Keep in mind that children want more than anything to please. So let them know you'll be most pleased if they understand how carefully we must all use pills and how they themselves should never take *anything* unless an adult is there to help them.

For the very young you might agree on a danger symbol such as a red X or a Mr. Yucky face and then put that on pill bottles. Make it a rule that the child may not even touch anything marked in that way.

In spite of everyone's best efforts some children will still manage to poison themselves, if not on drugs then perhaps on common household substances. Every household with a child in it should be stocked with the basics to treat poisoning.

First on the list is the telephone number of the local Poison Control Center. Next comes ipecac syrup. Properly administered, this will cause the child to vomit. In many cases this is the best first aid, since it eliminates the vast majority of the poisonous substance from the stomach before it's absorbed. The exceptions are substances such as lye, acid, cleaning fluid, petroleum-based products, and other caustic substances that will do more damage coming back up than if remaining in the system. Don't try to guess, though. The Poison Control Center will tell you over the phone if ipecac is appropriate.

Ipecac must be given properly if it's to work. That means administering a couple of glasses of water along with the syrup and, according to one of our consultants, getting the child in motion. It seems that shaking everything together gets the job done better. The best way to do this is by gently jiggling the child, walking him, or putting him on a swing.

Riding in the car may also work (take along a bucket and some towels). This is just as well, since every case of suspected poisoning should be attended to at the hospital emergency room or the doctor's office. Poisoning is a complex problem and one where prompt, competent treatment can make the difference between life and death. This is definitely *not* a do-it-yourself job. Call the Poison Control Center nearest you no matter what. And no matter how great your young person looks after vomiting (which probably won't be all that great, to tell you the truth), get the child medical attention immediately.

References

1. "General Guidelines for the Valuation of Drugs to Be Approved for Use During Pregnancy and for Treatment of Infants and Children." A Report of the Committee on Drugs, American Academy of Pediatrics, 1974.
2. Sankey R. J., et al. "Visual Hallucinations in Children Receiving Decongestants." *Br. Med. J.* 1984; 288(6427):1369.
3. Ibid.
4. Ibid.
5. Kogan, Michael D., et al. "Over-the-Counter Medication Use Among U.S. Preschool-Age Children." *JAMA* 1994; 272:1025–1030.
6. Smith, M. B. H., and W. Feldman. "Over-the-Counter Cold Medications: A Critical Review of Clinical Trials Between 1950 and 1991." *JAMA* 1993; 269:2258–2263.
7. Gadomski, Anne. "Rational Use of Over-the-Counter Medications in Young Children." *JAMA* 1994; 272:1063.
8. Hecht, Annabel. "What's That Alcohol Doing in My Medicine?" *FDA Consumer* 1984; 18(9):12–16.
9. Wingert, Willis, et al. "A Study of the Quality of Prescriptions Issued in a Busy Pediatric Emergency Room." *Public Health Reports* 1975; 90(5):402.
10. Ibid.
11. Ibid.
12. Reynolds, Ronald D. "Accurate Dosing of Pediatric Medications." *Arch. Fam. Med.* 1994; 3:365–370.
13. Gazaway, Preston M., et al. "Cardiac and Respiratory Drugs in Pregnancy." *Patient Care,* October 15, 1993:53–66.
14. Ibid., p. 60.

15. Cohlan, S. Q. "Fetal and Neonatal Hazards from Drugs Administered During Pregnancy. *N.Y. State J. Med.* 1964; 64:493–499.

16. Rodriguez, S. V., et al. "Neonatal Thrombocytopenia Associated with Ante-Partum Administration of Thiazide Drugs. "*N. Engl. J. Med.* 1964; 270:881–884.

17. Imperiale, Thomas F., and Alice Stollenwerk Petrulis. "A Meta-Analysis of Low-Dose Aspirin for the Prevention of Pregnancy-Induced Hypertensive Disease." *JAMA* 1991; 266:261–265.

18. Gazaway, et al., op. cit., p. 62.

19. Ibid., p. 60.

20. Ibid., p. 56.

21. Gal, Peter, and Martha K. Sharpless. "Fetal Drug Exposure—Behavioral Teratogenesis." *Drug Int. and Clin. Pharm.* 1984; 18(3):186–201.

22. Ibid.

23. Fackelmann, K. A. "Male Rats Find Alcohol a Fertility Downer." *Science News* 1994; 146:6.

24. Sexton, Mary, and Richard J. Hebel. "A Clinical Trial of Change in Maternal Smoking and Its Effect on Birth Weight." *JAMA* 1984; 251(7):911–915.

25. Ibid.

26. Hill, Reba M., and Leo Stern. "Drugs in Pregnancy: Effects on the Fetus and Newborn." *Drugs* 1979; 17:182–197.

27. Weathersbee, P. S., et al. "Caffeine and Pregnancy—a Retrospective Survey." *Postgraduate Med.* 1977; 62(3):64–69.

28. Gazaway, et al., op. cit., p. 56.

29. Scolnik, Dennis, et al. "Neurodevelopment of Children Exposed In Utero to Phenytoin and Carbamazepine Monotherapy." *JAMA* 1994; 271:767–770.

30. Gazaway, et al., op. cit., p. 62.

31. "Merrell Dow Ceases Production of Bendectin—'Burden Too Heavy.' " *Med. World News* Jul. 11, 1984, pp. 55–56.

32. Stashwick, Carole A. "Overcoming Obstacles to Breast-feeding." *Patient Care,* February 15, 1994:88–112.

33. Davis, Devra Lee, and Patricia Buffler. "Reduction of Deaths After Drug Labelling for Risk of Reye's Syndrome." *Lancet* 1992; 340:1042.

34. Kaluber, George T. "Clinical Efficacy and Safety of Desmopressin in the Treatment of Nocturnal Enuresis." *J. Pediatrics* 1989; 114(4): 719-722.

Saving Money
on Medicines

Prescription drug prices are skyrocketing. At least, that's what the *Washington Post* said in a headline in 1991.[1] If you have you been to the drugstore lately, this is not news. In fact, if you've had to pay for a prescription recently, it will come as no surprise that the pharmaceutical industry is "America's most profitable business."[2]

Take the teenager with cystic acne. Her dermatologist prescribed **Accutane** (isotretinoin), which he assured her would be a miracle cure for her severe skin problem. What he didn't tell her was how much it would cost. When the pharmacist handed her a three-month supply of **Accutane** and a bill for more than $350, she almost fainted.

Mickey of Durham, North Carolina, knows what that's like. One day in 1992 he was told his antidepressant, **Prozac** (fluoxetine), was going to cost $69 for one month's supply, up from $51 the month before:

like to have had a heart attack . . . [the cashier] just said, "They went up on us, so we had to go up on y'all," and that's been the excuse for years now. . . . [Drug companies] are making too much of a profit, and it's time someone went in and said, "Y'all can't do this anymore."[3]

Watching Prices Soar

There are probably a lot of people who agree with Mickey. More and more of the new medications doctors prescribe are extremely expensive. People with arthritis may find their monthly bill runs between $50 and $80 for drugs such as **Relafen** (nabumetone), **Voltaren** (diclofenac), **Naprosyn** (naproxen), or **Lodine** (etodolac). If you also have to take high blood pressure pills, such as **Cardizem CD** (diltiazem) or **Capoten** (captopril), or medicine such as **Mevacor** (lovastatin) or **Pravachol** (pravastatin) to lower cholesterol, your monthly medicine bill might well exceed $100.

The tragedy is that older people are most likely to need more medications, and they are exactly the ones who often find it difficult to pay the tab. So many are on a tight budget and end up in a desperate situation, as this reader has:

My drug bills are ruining me. I am a widow and an insulin-dependent diabetic. I also need blood pressure pills and they are so high I have to buy them on credit. Now I have such a big bill I don't know how I'll ever pay it.

Medicare doesn't cover drugs and my doctor and hospital bills from a recent back operation are about to take everything I've got. My home is up for sale, but I haven't sold it yet. It's sad when you work hard all your life and then have to give it all away.

Other people are getting crunched by big bills, too. When cancer strikes, it may cause a financial crisis along with life-threatening health problems. Here's how hard it can be:

How do drug companies decide what to charge? My husband is on chemotherapy and must have two medicines—**Mitomycin** for the cancer and **Zofran** to control the nausea. Together they come to over $900 every time he has treatment.

Between the doctor's bills and the medicine it won't be long before our life savings are gone. It is cheaper to lie down and die. What makes these medicines so expensive?

No wonder people are calling for health care reform. Any "system" that could save a man's life but leave him and his wife with nothing to live on definitely needs some adjustment. After all, it isn't like a new car that you can decide not to buy for a few years. If you need a medicine to cure your cancer, fight a lethal infection, or overcome a heart attack, you can't wait until you've saved enough to pay for it.

We had to tell this reader that drug manufacturers can charge whatever the market will bear. There is no federal agency that regulates or controls the price of medicine, and over the last decade the cost of many pharmaceuticals has doubled or tripled. Many of you know this from personal experience, like Elizabeth who writes:

I am elderly, sick and on a fixed income. A medication for which I paid $1.25 years ago now costs $23.91. The prices those greedy drug makers charge should be rolled back to reflect only inflation. It is to be hoped that the pharmaceutical industry will soon package heart in little pills.

This small sample of chain-store price data we have collected over the past twenty years gives you an idea of what's been happening at the cash register. All prices are for 100 brand-name pills:

DRUG	1975	1980	1985	1995
Coumadin (10 mg)	$9.40	$6.13	$13.85	$86.19
Dyazide	$9.25	$10.45	$16.20	$33.69

DRUG	1975	1980	1985	1995
Flagyl (250 mg)	$20.65	—	$79.20	$148.99
HydroDIURIL (50 mg)	$5.70	$6.40	$11.83	$26.59
Lanoxin (0.25 mg)	$1.00	$1.69	$3.00	$8.59
Lasix (40 mg)	$9.73	$9.29	$8.95	$19.99
Premarin (1.25 mg)	$6.90	—	$15.95	$46.89
Valium (5 mg)	$8.99	$10.89	$20.30	$62.29

Please recall that between 1975 and 1980, especially while Jimmy Carter was in office, people complained of horrible inflation. As you can see from this table, though, drug prices didn't go up very much. They really soared, going up over 150 percent on the average, over the last ten years. During that time, economists have been telling us that inflation in the general economy has been more or less under control, but drug prices were going up three times faster than almost everything else. Doesn't it look as though the greed mentality of the 1980s captured the pharmaceutical industry? The saddest thing is that we the consumers are being held hostage. Although public pressure has held recent prescription drug price increases down a little, the price tag on many medications can still cause a lot of pain.

Drug company spokespeople don't agree, of course. They point out, quite rightly, that it costs money to discover and research new medicines. Exactly how much money is a matter of debate, it turns out. Estimates range from about $130 million (after taxes) to as much as $500 million (before taxes).[4] Such a wide discrepancy suggests that these figures aren't exactly of pinpoint accuracy.

Nonetheless, we can certainly accept that it costs a lot of money to get a new drug to market. And that, of course, is why the newest medicines are often among the most expensive, as this pharmacist points out:

> I'm a pharmacist with a lot of older customers. It broke my heart yesterday when one of them burst into tears as I handed her the refill for her blood pressure medicine. I had to tell her the price had gone up and her bill was over $30. She sobbed that they were going to cut off her lights if she didn't pay her electric bill, and it would have to be either that bill or this medicine. The electric bill won.
> Why don't doctors realize some patients can't afford the fanciest, newest medications?

Many people can't afford the latest drug breakthroughs. The cost of the anti-stroke drug **Ticlid** (ticlopidine) can exceed $80 for a month's supply. **Cognex** (tacrine), a brand-new drug for Alzheimer's disease, may cost $4 a day. This is certainly a bargain compared to nursing-home care, but for many elderly patients on fixed incomes it will take a big bite out of the budget. Then there's the just-approved medicine for multiple sclerosis. **Betaseron** (interferon beta-1b) will cost $989.40 per month. Even patients who aren't poor will have a hard time swallowing a $10,000 annual drug bill.

Even if we grant that R&D (research and development) costs have gone through the roof, resulting in astronomical prices for the latest medications, that still doesn't explain why many drugs that have been around for decades, like the ones in the table on pages 258–259, can now cost five, six, or seven times more than they did 20 years ago. If the computer industry worked this way, we'd be paying $35,000 or more for a personal computer instead of $1,000 to $2,000. Presumably the R&D bills on these old medicines were paid off long ago. But they are still making their contribution to overall pharmaceutical-industry expenses, including some pretty fancy salaries.

By the early 1990s most of the major drug firms were paying their top officers salaries of over $1 million, with millions more in stock options.[5] Many CEOs enjoyed yearly compensation packages well in excess of $5 million. It's likely these company heads do not experience pharmacy sticker shock in quite the same way our readers do.

Taking the Sting Out of Sticker Shock

If you're mad as all get-out about the way pharmaceutical prices have been rising, you may want to make your opinion known during the debate about health care reform. Contact your own senators and representatives. Let them know what you think, and what you'd like to see done.

In the meantime, there are some strategies that can help you get the best possible deal on the drugs you purchase. But you will have to work at it, and you need to start long before you saunter up to the cash register at your local drugstore.

One of the first things you'll have to do is change the way you think about drugs. You see, most of us tend to treat medicine as if it were sacred. If the doctor prescribes a specific brand, then that's what we think we must take, even though a generic version may be only a fraction of the price. And if we see an ad on television for **Actifed** or **Pepto-Bismol**, then those are the brands we look for, rather than some unfamiliar-sounding chemical name.

Attitudes must change if we're going to save any money. Many familiar medications come in several different brands, sold by a number of different companies. It's up to you, the patient, to shop around and make the best deal on the product you need.

The first obstacle, though, may be the doctor's attitude about brand-name drugs. Many physicians have been sold a bill of goods by the huge pharmaceutical firms. They are often told that generic drugs are inferior to brand-name versions. Doctors then pass the same message on to the patient and as a result people may end up paying 200 or 300 percent more for a brand-name drug. Sometimes they really can't afford it, as we heard from this unemployed factory worker:

My wife suffers from severe depression. Twice in the past five years she's tried to commit suicide. Luckily she was saved both times, but you can imagine that when she gets depressed it scares me.

Her doctor has her on a medicine called Elavil. It's been working well, but this drug really strains our limited budget. A month's supply costs over $15.

The last time we got it refilled, the pharmacist told us this drug is available much cheaper—under $6 for the same amount.

The trouble is, she can't dispense this generic medicine without the doctor's permission. But when I asked him, he said the generic does not work as well. Is this true? Saving money would be a big help, but I don't want to take a risk with my wife's life.

Slowly but surely, these prejudices are beginning to change. Some generic products now rank among the 100 most frequently prescribed medications.[6] The savings can be impressive, so that is one of the tactics we'll explore further. But first, let's take care of the people who have to sell their homes, deplete their life savings, or worry about losing a loved one in order to pay for their medicines.

Free Medicine

T he pharmaceutical industry should be ashamed that so many people find it so difficult to afford essential medicines. It is clear that most major drug companies care far more about profits and the bottom line for their stockholders than they do about people's health.

As public outrage over the cost of drugs mounted, the industry responded with a multimillion-dollar advertising campaign in an attempt to defuse the criticism. Touching photographs of grandparents and their grandchildren appeared in both medical journals and popular magazines. The message is that drug research is expensive but essential for the nation's health. The motto "Pharmaceuticals: Good Medicine for Containing Health Costs" underscores the idea that drugs are a bargain.

We'd be the first to tell you to look beyond pharmaceutical ads for real information, and that goes in this case too. The expensive ads don't mention the extraordinary amount of money the industry pours into marketing and promotion. Nor do they tell us that Americans pay more for their medicine than people in any other country. The pharmaceutical industry is one of the most profitable in the world. Even during hard times, people still need medicine. When they possibly can, they somehow manage to pay for it. When they can't, they may suffer, like these friends of Linda's:

L inda related her visit with a friend in the hospital one day after the woman had a stroke. Her friend told Linda, "I cut down on my blood pressure medication because it was so expensive." It is quite possible that the stroke was brought on due to inadequate blood pressure control.

Linda has another friend who was put on a pill to prevent cancer recurrence. "Her concern about the cost was worse than her fear that the cancer would return. Things just don't seem fair."

For many years some drug companies have had a policy of providing medications for patients who could not afford to buy them. Although these programs existed for many years, it wasn't until recently that they became well publicized. As public indignation rose and congressional scrutiny was threatened, the Pharmaceutical Manufacturers Association decided to make these "indigent programs" more visible. Whether this effort should be classified as public service or public relations, we are unsure.

Be forewarned: To benefit from an indigent program, you will need your doctor as your ally. The definition of "needy" is vague at best, and the criteria vary from one company to another. However, a doctor's interest and certification that the drug bills cause hardship goes a long way. If your drug bills are paid by insurance or public assistance, you probably won't qualify, but many plans are not limited to the poverty-stricken.

To start, ask your physician to contact the manufacturer. Your doctor can find out whom to contact at the company that makes your medicine by calling **1-800-PMA-INFO**. When he or she calls the company, a representative will describe the eligibility requirements. If you qualify for one of these assistance programs, it could make a big difference in your monthly drug bills.

Another option may be some form of public assistance. Nine states provide patient assistance programs specifically for older people who are financially strapped. Connecticut, Illinois, Maine, Maryland, New Jersey, New York, Pennsylvania, and Rhode Island have state-funded programs. Minnesota has made provisions for both children and older people on a voluntary basis. If you are fortunate enough to live in one of these states, it would be worth checking with social services. Don't overlook special programs such as PACE (Pharmaceutical Assistance Contract for the Elderly) in Pennsylvania, and PAAD (Pharmaceutical Assistance to the Aged and Disabled) in New Jersey.

Deciphering the Prescription

I t wouldn't be nearly so hard to save money on prescription drugs if the doctor knew exactly what they cost. Unfortunately, that information isn't featured in the drug reference doctors are most likely to use, and there hasn't been a lot of incentive for most physicians to learn. In one survey, 100 primary care physicians were questioned about the prices of the most frequently prescribed medications. Their guesses weren't even close.[7]

That sad state of affairs won't do you any good. We don't suggest you put the doctor on the defensive by quizzing him or her. If cost is an issue, though, be upfront about it. There's a possibility the physician will be able to suggest some non-drug approaches to try first, or maybe an over-the-counter drug, while less effective, would be worth a try. She may not realize you're interested in that kind of treatment unless you let her know.

If a prescription medicine is the most appropriate treatment, you'll need to learn to read the prescription. Not only will this help you do the homework you'll need to do to save money, it will also help you take the medicine more safely.

Although the pharmacist and the physician may use a code (often composed of Latin abbreviations), it's not too hard to figure out, especially with regard to the information required for saving money. What you need to know is the name of the drug, the form (tablets, capsules, elixir, etc.), the potency (100 milligrams, or whatever) and the amount you are to receive (40 tablets, 100 capsules, etc.). Check out the sample prescription form below and see if you can get the hang of it.

John Doe, M.D.
1801 Hytek Medical Center
Anytown, US
234-7890

Name: John Q. Public   Date: Dec. 17, 1995
Address: 123 Division Ave
West Anytown, US   Age: 43

℞:

Tagamet, 400 mg
Dispense 60 tablets
Label: Take one tablet daily at bedtime

John Doe, M.D.

Far too many physicians still specialize in writing illegibly. They may also resort to such abbreviations as *disp.*, *cap.* (easily figured out to mean *dispense, capsule*), or less comprehensible jargon such as *Sig.: 5, gtt., t.i.d., p.c.* Such abbreviations come from a dead language (Latin). That's modern medicine? The pharmacist translates this secret message to mean "label the prescription: 5 drops, 3 times a day, after meals."

If this seems a little arcane to you, join the crowd. Even the board of the American Medical Association has taken doctors to task for sloppy unreadable scrawls. They found that "medication errors are not rare events" and attributed some of them to technical causes such as "illegible handwriting, misspelling and the use of inappropriate abbreviations in written orders."[8]

It would certainly simplify life for everyone, even the pharmacist, if physicians printed out prescriptions in plain English. It would give you a chance to question the doctor about his instructions and would cut down on mistakes. Of course, if your doctor is unreformable that doesn't mean you're out of luck. Fortunately, it is not necessary for you to be able to understand all the cryptic scribbles on a prescription form since hopefully the pharmacist will write them out in English on the label. If you would like to decipher the Latin, though, there is a list of common abbreviations and their meanings on page 52.

Once you know what medication you are supposed to take, remember there can be an awful lot in a name. By now most people have heard the word *generic*, and are aware that it has something to do with reduced prices. But to take full advantage of it, you need to understand how to make generic prescribing work for you.

When a pharmaceutical manufacturing company develops a new drug in the lab, it receives a number. For months, and often years, it's known only by this number.

As it reaches the clinical testing phase the drug gets an official name. This is the generic, "scientific," or nonproprietary name. It's created by a quasi-official organization under the direction of the American Medical Association and the American Pharmaceutical Association, among others.

The drug acquires, along the way, two important things in addition to its generic name. First, a patent, which assures the drug company roughly 17 years of protection against competition, and second, a trade (also called proprietary) name. This easily promoted brand name is usually quite different from the official generic title, which may be hard to spell, difficult to remember, and practically impossible to pronounce.

Let's take a look at a few examples. **Dyazide** has long been one of the most commonly prescribed medications in the country. It is a diuretic that lowers blood pressure without depleting the body of potassium. Its ingredients, hydrochlorothiazide and triamterene, hardly come tripping lightly to the tongue. Or how about **Bactrim**? This antibacterial agent is used for everything from urinary tract infections to earaches and traveler's diarrhea. Just try to remember or pronounce its generic components: sulfamethoxazole and trimethoprim.

Even single-ingredient drugs such as **Vasotec** (enalapril), **Zantac** (ranitidine), **Darvocet N** (propoxyphene napsylate), **Xanax** (alprazolam), or **Dilantin** (phenytoin) are a lot easier to twist your tongue around in their brand-name incarnations. Is it any wonder doctors tend to stick with the snappy names they can spell and pronounce with ease? Don't forget, the drug companies put plenty of bucks into promoting these catchy names.

For the life of the patent (and even long afterwards) glossy full-color ads in medical journals will tout the drug's abilities and emphasize its trade name. The doctor will be visited by assertive drug detail reps who will bombard him with free samples, notepads, pens, rulers, calendars, and all other manner of geegaws. Each of these samples and goodies bears a drug's trade name.

This goes on for years, until the drug "comes off patent." This means that other companies, after establishing their ability to produce a chemically identical product, can manufacture the same stuff and sell it under either the generic name or under a new trade name they create.

That doesn't mean that the brand-name advertising will stop, of course. Years after **Valium** (diazepam) came off patent, there were ads in medical journals urging the doctor to prescribe **Valium** and specify "dispense as written" or words to that effect. That's to prevent the pharmacist from substituting generic diazepam. Some doctors have been misled by the industry's campaign against generics and believe that they are not as good. That is hardly ever the case, however.

Now all this wouldn't make much difference if diazepam and **Valium** cost the same. But a generic drug is almost always cheaper than its trade-name rival. After all, somebody has to pay, not only for the original research leading to the drug's discovery, but also for all that advertising, the drug reps on the road, the imprinted pencils and pads, etc. Pharmaceutical manufacturers spend over a billion dollars a year just promoting their drugs to doctors. There is, on the other hand, little incentive to advertise an unbranded generic. As we'll see in a bit, the differences in drug costs to the consumer are often unbelievable.

Generic vs. Brand Name

I t would seem that saving money on drugs should be easy. Most pharmacists will tell you generic drugs are the key to cutting costs. So you just get the generic version of the medicine and you're home free. It's almost that simple, but let's look at a few more steps.

First, even if your doctor has written you a generic prescription that doesn't mean the medicine is available generically. Many medications are available only under their trade names either because the patent period hasn't expired, or because the market wasn't large enough to entice a generic manufacturer to take up production.

But suppose your medicine is indeed available both from the original manufacturer and from generic suppliers at significant savings. Your physician can do one of three things. He can write a brand-name prescription such as **Xanax** or its generic counterpart, alprazolam. In most states that wouldn't matter since the pharmacist has the option to substitute a generic product even when the doctor writes a brand name, unless the doctor specifies that substitution isn't permissible.

It's this third option that can cost you money. When the physician writes "dispense as written" (*d.a.w.*) or "Do not substitute" (*d.n.s.*), the pharmacist has no leeway. The drug must be dispensed exactly as called for, which usually means by a specific brand name.

Why would the doctor do that? Two possible reasons: First, because he or she has read a careful, scientific study demonstrating that one company's preparation of a drug acts differently in the body than another company's. These are very rare. Or, second, because the doctor has become convinced that the brand-name drug is more effective than the generic, without any scientific information supporting that conclusion.

That wouldn't be altogether surprising. After all, the pharmaceutical industry has put a lot of time, money, and ingenuity into convincing doctors that generic drugs are inferior. Even though the FDA holds every manufacturer—brand name and generic alike—to high standards designed to assure consumers that the final product is what it's supposed to be in terms of dose, potency, and so forth, the major pharmaceutical manufacturers have figured out a way to have their cake and eat it too.

Having invested so much effort in promoting their brand-name products, the companies realize that many physicians and patients have developed a loyalty to their brand-name products. The fact that the brand-name drugs may be 30 or 40 percent more expensive than the generic is not the manufacturers' concern. Why should they worry about your pocketbook, when you're willing to improve the state of theirs?

So they continue to market drugs such as **Naprosyn, Tenormin,** and **Cardizem** at high prices. At the same time they reap profits by providing distributors with the identical drugs for resale as generics. That's right. We're talking about the very same compound made by the same company, sometimes at the same facility and on the same equipment as the brand-name product. Now, how could that be inferior? You may rest assured, however, the price differences remain. **Naprosyn,** for years one of the most popular prescription arthritis medications, can cost more than $80 for a month's supply. Now that it is off patent, most consumers can save $20 a month on generic naproxen that acts identically in the body.

The manufacturers don't really want doctors to know about this program. After all, for years they've been trying to convince physicians they can't trust generics. So they don't usually sell the generic themselves. But sometimes the generic company is a subsidiary of the pharmaceutical firm. For example, Syntex sells **Naprosyn** and Hamilton Pharma, an affiliate, sells naproxen. Marion Merrell Dow sells the highly successful brand-name blood pressure pill **Cardizem.** Its subsidiary, Blue Ridge Labs, markets a generic version, diltiazem.

Generic prescribing has become a lot more common, but unfortunately, many physicians still don't get it. Up to one-fourth of the prescriptions written for naproxen specify **Naprosyn** even though the generic is made by the same company that sells the brand name. So if you ask the doctor for a generic prescription and you are told that the brand name is better, politely ask for the data.

If your doctor is sincere and looks it up, he or she is likely to find that drug manufacturing and distribution resembles a giant shell game as much as anything else. Way back in 1975 the Council on Economic Priorities studied antibiotics and their pricing. Here's what the experts found back then:

> It is a widespread practice for one firm to manufacture a product and sell that product to different firms, which in turn sell at different prices under different brand names. For example, taking into account only the major firms, we find that Milan Laboratories manufactures final dose-form erythromycin for SmithKline, Pfizer, Parke-Davis, Squibb, and Wyeth, each of which

sells the erythromycin under its own name. Bristol Laboratories manufactures ampicillin for it-self as well as for SmithKline, Robins, Parke-Davis, and Wyeth. Beecham sells ampicillin to Pfizer, Lederle and Ayest. Not only do each of these firms sell each of these products at differ-ent prices, but small generic houses purchase final dose-form antibiotics from the same manu-facturers.[9]

It is not very likely that the drug industry has simplified, streamlined, re-formed, or otherwise altered this general state of affairs since the study was done. That's why we're puzzled. Why don't more doctors prescribe generics? Suppose you needed a new car and decided that a Ford Taurus was the model for you. If you learned that you could save $5,000 by purchasing an identical car, made on the same Ford assembly line, but without the Taurus label, wouldn't you go for it?

Selling Prescription Drugs

Make no mistake about it. Drug companies are in business and their pricing policies reflect that. Even the drug companies admit it. One Squibb Corpo-ration vice president said, "Drugs are priced to assure a cash flow, to provide the kind of return needed to support new research and to attract capital and talent."[10] Believe us, the bean-counters at these firms are among the finest in the world, but they are interested in the health of their bottom line rather than your pocketbook. There's generally little consideration for the consumer who can't afford to keep up with the "market price."

There are plenty of ways to economize when the budget is tight. Instead of steak, you buy chicken—or beans. You patch old clothes instead of buying new ones, and you learn to do without. But when it comes to medicine, everyone wants you to take it.

The public-service announcements remind you constantly that high blood pressure is the "silent killer." You are exhorted to take your medicine. If you have heart disease or asthma, the pills are your lifeline. Doing without could be like committing suicide.

That's why generic drugs could save some people's lives. A name-brand med-ication usually costs 30 or 40 percent more, sometimes even two to three times as much as a generic copy. When the brand-name antidepressant **Elavil** costs $14.79 for a month's supply, generic amitriptyline is only $4.19. That's a big savings! If it means a person can continue treatment, it might literally keep him or her from suicide.

If you want big numbers, how about these: one hundred 250-mg tablets of

Flagyl (more than anyone is likely to need at a single time, we grant you) would cost $142.79, while metronidazole, the generic, same strength, same amount, would run $31.00.

By now there should be no doubt that sometimes generic drugs can be dramatically cheaper than their brand-name counterparts. But to benefit, you must get your pharmacist to pass the savings on to you. This may not be as hard as it used to be. Although the markup on an expensive brand-name medicine can be lots more than on an inexpensive generic, competition is a powerful motivator. Most pharmacies now do a brisk business in generic drugs and are eager to pass some savings along. They fear you might take your business elsewhere if they don't. What's more, many pharmacists are caring, compassionate individuals who really want to do their best to help.

The point of all this is that with some planning on your part and some help from your doctor and your pharmacist, you should be able to get your prescription drugs at the lowest possible price.

Your Best-Priced Prescription

Imagine the doctor has done the exam, decided what you have, and is about to write a prescription. Leap into action right here or you'll lose all chance of saving money.

Step #1—Ask what drug the doctor is prescribing, and whether the drug is available generically. It is not enough to simply say, "What are you giving me, Doctor?" The answer could well be a brand name. Ask if it is. If the drug is still patent-protected, ask if there is any acceptable alternative medicine that might be available generically. Sometimes a protected brand is all there is, and the doctor can't help out any further in the quest for savings.

However, if the doctor is preparing to write a brand-name prescription for something available generically, *ask that it be written generically.* If he or she balks, calmly explain that you are attempting to keep your medical costs as low as possible.

It may be difficult to be so assertive the first time (this gets easier with practice), but remember the doctor is almost never acting on firm information when he insists that a brand-name drug is somehow superior. Ask him for the evidence. If there's good scientific data, then pay attention—but often there is none. Ask yourself—and the doctor—if it's enough reason for you to be spending two to three times as much on your prescription.

Doctors are often surprised at what drugs cost. Many are only vaguely aware of the actual cost to a patient of a particular course of drug therapy. They may not know that the price spread between brand name and generic is so substantial. Help educate them. Many become considerably more cooperative when the actual numbers are brought to their attention. More and more doctors are finally taking cost into account when getting ready to write a prescription, and the cost factor has even become a selling point in some drug company ads of late.

Be sure to let the doctor know you both appreciate and expect his or her efforts to hold down the cost of your health care.

In the table at the end of this chapter, you'll find a list of some of the brand-name drugs that are available generically. It certainly won't hurt to copy the list and take it along when you go to the doctor's office. There are literally thousands of drugs, and it's entirely possible that even the most conscientious doctor might be unaware of a drug's availability in generic form, especially if the switch has happened relatively recently. Remember, one of the reasons generics cost so much less is because they don't advertise and don't send expensive salespeople around to hawk their wares. Don't be too surprised if the doctor asks you to leave a copy of the list for his or her use.

Step #2—Ask the doctor for a free sample plus a prescription for enough medication to last a moderately long time. Quantity is the second most important key to saving money on medicines, right after buying generic when you can. As with most things, drug are cheaper when purchased in larger quantities. But you don't want to get a prescription for three months' supply only to find out after taking several pills that you are allergic to the medicine. The pharmacist won't take the bottle back and you'll be stuck with expensive pills you can't use.

If your doctor gives you a small free sample—enough to get you by for several days—you can find out if the medication agrees with you. If it does, you can take the prescription in and get it filled at substantial savings. Prices often show discounts at quantities of 50 and 100, so if the prescription can reasonably be written for one of those amounts, ask the doctor to do it. Always ask the pharmacist to put the expiration date on the label. You don't want to get so much medicine that it will go bad before you use it.

The other consideration here, of course, is cash. If the medication is expensive, you might not want to fork over a large sum of money all at once in order to save a relatively small amount per pill. If the doctor has prescribed a large quantity and you find the total tab will be more than you want to spend at the moment, ask the pharmacist to dispense a smaller amount. This should be no problem. This is also the tack to take if the doctor does not have any samples. Ask the pharmacist for just enough medicine to get you through several days, long enough to find out if you can tolerate it. Once you're sure it's okay, then you can get your large prescription filled.

Step #3—Comparison-shop. Do it by phone if you can. Yes, there are going to be times when you feel utterly miserable and just want to get the prescription as quickly as possible. It may be worthwhile to pay a higher price in exchange for your comfort, especially when the total amount involved is relatively small or when the prescription is a one-shot deal.

If you know that's the situation, you might ask the doctor to write one small prescription and a second, larger one for the balance of the drug you'll need. Get the first day or two of pills wherever it's convenient. Then, when someone else is available to shop around for you, or when you feel a bit better, fill the rest of the prescription at the best possible price.

Comparison-shopping becomes very important when you have a long-term prescription for a drug to be taken daily. This would include drugs for heart problems, high blood pressure, arthritis, and other chronic problems. The cost of some of these drugs can run to several dollars a day, and it can make a heck of a difference over the course of a year whether you pay top or bottom price.

If nothing else, shopping around by phone will yield some very interesting information about drug prices. You'll find, first of all, that some drugstores don't want to quote over the phone. Why not? Because they know once you're in the door, the chances of your marching out again are pretty small. Don't fall for it.

You'll also find that drug prices vary a whole lot more for an identical item than almost any other consumer product. Normally, competition, advertising, and other market forces in an area act to keep most retail prices pretty close from store to store. Sure, the Ritz Emporium is getting a few bucks more, the Dollarama Discount Palace a few bucks less. But I'm willing to bet the variation from store to store on a particular prescription will surprise you.

And there will be neither rhyme nor reason to it. The fanciest drugstore won't always have the highest price for everything, and the "discount" pharmacy won't always have the lowest. The store that's low on one prescription may be high on another.

Step #4—Talk to the pharmacist before the prescription is filled. Don't be bashful. Say you want the prescription filled with a low-cost generic. Also, ask if the drug is available in a nonprescription form. It may be possible to save money by purchasing OTC **Pepcid AC** instead of **Pepcid,** or **Aleve** in place of prescription **Naprosyn.** Ask the pharmacist for help in getting the dose the doctor prescribed.

Remember that generics are not all created equal when it comes to price. Often a pharmacy will stock both a brand name and a generic equivalent, and sometimes that pharmacy will stock the brand name and two or more generics. Which you get might depend on the time of day, which bottle was closer to where the pharmacist was standing, or how much the pharmacist thinks you can afford to pay. Let him know early that you're shopping for the minimum price.

Once in a great while, minimum price might even mean favoring the brand name over a generic! This is a real switcheroo, and it won't happen very often. This situation can occur because the generic is indeed normally priced higher, or it can happen because the pharmacist has gotten a particularly good deal on a batch of the brand-name drug. Maybe he purchased in a large quantity, or bought from a distributor who needed to turn over the inventory for one reason or another.

Step #5—Consider shopping by mail. This won't work if you need a one-shot prescription for some immediate illness. However, if you have have a chronic problem which requires ongoing medication, shopping by mail can save you big bucks.

The reason is that there are a number of super-discount pharmacies that operate mail-order services. Probably the largest and best known is run by the American Association of Retired Persons. You can get price information by writing to:

Retired Persons Services
500 Montgomery Street
Alexandria, VA 22314
Telephone toll-free (800) 456-4636

America's Pharmacy
6109 Willowmere Drive
Des Moines, IA 50321
Telephone (515) 287-6872

Action Mail Order
P.O. Box 787
Waterville, ME 04903-0787
Telephone toll-free (800) 452-1976

Family Pharmaceuticals
P.O. Box 1288
Mount Pleasant, SC 29565-1288
Telephone toll-free (800) 922-3444

American Preferred Plan
P.O. Box 9019
Farmingdale, NY 11735
Telephone toll-free (800) 227-1195

Medi-Mail
P.O. Box 98520
Las Vegas, NV 89193-8520
Telephone toll-free (800) 331-1458

A number of other mail-order pharmacies are also doing business and may offer an alternative, particularly if you somehow don't qualify as a "retired person." You will want to check on prices and policies, as they are likely to vary from one to the other.

Growing up as we did with the habit of going to the corner pharmacy to get a prescription filled, the notion of sending off for one's medication may seem a bit strange at first. But in reality it's a very simple, very easy process. In fact, it can be even easier than going to the local pharmacy. You just stick your prescription in an envelope (along with your name and address, written legibly, which the doctor won't have done on the prescription blank) and a check for the number of pills. Back comes the prescription, delivered to your door by the postal carrier. No muss, no fuss, and at rock-bottom prices.

Just because this is the cheapest option does not mean it's the best. There are a lot of good reasons for paying the difference and going to the handy-dandy pharmacy. In addition to immediate service, you get (or should get) the chance to consult personally with a licensed, qualified pharmacist who can provide information on the drug, how to take it, any possible adverse effects, interactions with other drugs, and so on.

You should actually shop for a pharmacist the same way you shop for a lawyer, plumber, physician, electrician, or any other service professional. After all, the pharmacist is a highly trained health professional who can provide you with crucial information about your medicine and help you avoid serious mistakes. Remember, though, the pharmacist may understandably resent being asked to provide information on the prescriptions you buy through the mail.

If you've got a prescription for a new drug, having someone knowledgeable to talk with can be especially important, and the services of a competent, patient, and interested pharmacist can be invaluable. On the other hand, if it's your fortieth refill of a high blood pressure or heart medication, you probably don't need that much counseling anymore.

The long-term medication user should definitely shop around, and do so carefully. Compare prices locally, and then compare the best of these against the mail-order places. It takes a little bit of advance planning to get the order in far enough ahead to keep yourself supplied, but the savings can be more than worth the effort.

If you've taken these five steps, chances are very good you'll walk out of the pharmacy with the best possible deal on your prescription. Whether you saved dimes or dollars, you did something else that's important—you helped impress upon the medical establishment the fact that we, as consumers, have an interest in the cost of our health care as well as its quality.

References

1. Rich, Spencer. "Prescription Drug Prices Said to Be Skyrocketing." *Washington Post*, September 24, 1991, p. A1.
2. "America's Most Profitable Business." Cover story, *Fortune*, July 29, 1991.
3. Zimmer, Jeff. "The Upward Spiral: Digging Deep to Foot the Soaring Cost of Prescription Drugs." *Herald Sun*, March 14, 1993, p. G1.
4. Anders, George. "Vital Statistic: Disputed Cost of Creating a Drug." *Wall Street Journal*, November 9, 1993, p. B1.
5. "The Highest-Paid Pharmaceutical Executives." *Medical Advertising News*, November 1992, p. 40.
6. Simonsen, Laura La Piana. "Price of Average Rx Up Only 2.9%: Top 200 Drugs of 1993." *Pharmacy Times* 1994; 60(4):18–32.
7. Ricks, Delthia. "Doctors are Writing Prescriptions with No Idea of Costs." *News & Observer*, November 21, 1993, p. F1.
8. Bristow, Lonnie R. Report of the Board of Trustees: Medication (Drug) Errors in Hospitals. Board of Trustees Report, A-94.
9. Brooke, Paul A. *Resistant Prices. A Study of Competitive Strains in the Antibiotic Markets*. New York: Council on Economic Priorities, 1975.
10. Waldholz, Michael. "Prices of Prescription Drugs Soar After Years of Moderate Increases." *Wall Street Journal*, May 25, 1984, p. 31.

Brand-Name Drugs
(Prescription and Over-the-Counter)
Available in Generic Form

Brand Name	Generic Name
Achromycin V	tetracycline
Actifed	pseudoephedrine/triprolidine
Adapin	doxepin
Advil	ibuprofen
Afrin	oxymetazoline
Aldactazide	spironolactone/HCTZ
Aldactone	spironolactone
Aldomet	methyldopa
Aldoril	HCTZ/methyldopa
Alupent	metaproterenol
Aminophyllin	aminophylline
Amoxil	amoxicillin
Anaprox	naproxen
Ansaid	flurbiprofen
Antepar	piperazine
Antivert	meclizine
Anturane	sulfinpyrazone
Apresazide	hydralazine/HCTZ
Apresoline	hydralazine
Aralen	chloroquine
Aristocort	triamcinolone
Artane	trihexyphenidyl
Ascriptin	aspirin, buffered
Asendin	amoxapine
Atarax	hydroxyzine

Brand Name	Generic Name
Ativan	lorazepam
Atromid-S	clofibrate
Azulfidine	sulfasalazine
Bactocill	oxacillin
Bactrim	sulfamethoxazole/trimethoprim
Beepen-VK	penicillin V potassium
Benadryl	diphenhydramine
Benemid	probenecid
Bentyl	dicyclomine
Blocadren	timolol
Bonine	meclizine
Bufferin	aspirin/magnesium/aluminum
BuSpar	buspirone
Butazolidin	phenylbutazone
Cafergot	ergotamine/caffeine
Calan/Calan SR	verapamil/verapamil SR
Cardene SR	nicardipine slow-release
Cardizem/Cardizem SR	diltiazem/diltiazem SR
Catapres	clonidine
Centrax	prazepam
Chlor-Trimeton	chlorpheniramine
Choledyl	oxtriphylline
Cinobac	cinoxacin
Cleocin	clindamycin
Clinoril	sulindac
Cloxapen	cloxacillin
Cogentin	benztropine
Colace	docusate
Col-Benemid	colchicine/probenecid

Brand Name	Generic Name
Combipres	chlorthalidone/clonidine
Compazine	prochlorperazine
Contac	chlorpheniramine/PPA
Corgard	nadolol
Cortaid	hydrocortisone
Coumadin	warfarin
Cyclapen	cyclacillin
Dalmane	flurazepam
Danocrine	danazol
Darvocet-N	propoxyphene napsylate/APAP
Darvon	propoxyphene
Decadron	dexamethasone
Delta-Cortef	prednisolone
Deltasone	prednisone
Demerol	meperidine
Demulen	ethinyl estradiol/ethynodiol diacetate
Depakene	valproic acid
Desyrel	trazodone
DiaBeta	glyburide
Diabinese	chlorpropamide
Diamox	acetazolamide
Diflucan	fluconazde
Dimetane	brompheniramine
Dimetapp	brompheniramine/PPA
Diprosone	betamethasone
Ditropan	oxybutynin
Diucardin	hydroflumethiazide
Diupres	chlorothiazide/reserpine
Diuril	chlorothiazide

Brand Name	Generic Name
Dolobid	diflunisal
Doriden	glutethimide
Dyazide	HCTZ/triamterene
Dymelor	acetohexamide
Dynapen	dicloxacillin
Ecotrin	enteric-coated aspirin
E.E.S.	erythromycin ethylsuccinate
Elavil	amitriptyline
Endep	amitriptyline
Enduron	methyclothiazide
ERYC	erythromycin DR
Ery-Tab	erythromycin DR
Erythrocin	erythromycin
Esidrix	HCTZ
Eskalith	lithium
Fastin	phentermine
Feldene	piroxicam
Fioricet	butalbital/acetaminophen
Fiorinal	butalbital/aspirin/caffeine
Flagyl	metronidazole
Flexeril	cyclobenzaprine
Fulvicin	griseofulvin
Furadantin	nitrofurantoin
Gantanol	sulfamethoxazole
Gantrisin	sulfisoxazole
Garamycin	gentamicin
Halcion	triazolam
Haldol	haloperidol
Hydergine	ergoloid mesylates

The People's Pharmacy®

Brand Name	Generic Name
HydroDIURIL	HCTZ
Hydropres	HCTZ/reserpine
Hygroton	chlorthalidone
Ilosone	erythromycin estolate
Imodium	loperamide
Inderal	propranolol
Inderal LA	propranolol, LA
Inderide	propranolol/HCTZ
Indocin	indomethacin
Indocin SR	indomethacin SR
INH	isoniazid
Ismelin	guanethidine
Isoptin SR	verapamil SR
Isordil	isosorbide
Keflex	cephalexin
Kenalog	triamcinolone
Kwell	lindane
Lanoxicaps	digoxin
Lanoxin	digoxin
Larotid	amoxicillin
Lasix	furosemide
Librax	chlordiazepoxide/clidinium
Librium	chlordiazapoxide
Lidex	fluocinonide
Limbitrol	chlordiazepoxide/amitriptyline
Lioresal	baclofen
Lomotil	diphenoxylate/atropine
Loniten	minoxidil
Lopid	gemfibrozil

Brand Name	Generic Name
Lopressor	metoprolol
Loxitane	loxapine
Ludiomil	maprotiline
Maalox	aluminum & magnesium hydroxide
Macrodantin	nitrofurantoin
Mandelamine	methenamine mandelate
Marax	ephedrine/hydroxyzine/theophylline
Maxzide	HCTZ/triamterene
Meclomen	meclofenamate
Medipren	ibuprofen
Medrol	methylprednisolone
Megace	megestrol
Mellaril	thioridazine
Metamucil	psyllium
Metandren	methyltestosterone
Methotrexate	methotrexate
Micro-K	potassium
Micronase	glyburide
Midamor	amiloride
Miltown	meprobamate
Minipress	prazosin
Minocin	minocycline
Moduretic	amiloride/HCTZ
Motrin	ibuprofen
Mycodan	homatropine/hydrocodone
Mycostatin	nystatin
Mysoline	primidone
Nalfon	fenoprofen
Naprosyn	naproxen

Brand Name	Generic Name
Navane	thiothixene
NegGram	nalidixic acid
Nembutal	sodium pentobarbital
Nicobid	niacin
Nicolar	niacin
Nitro-Bid	nitroglycerin SR
Nitro-Dur	nitroglycerin TD
Nolvadex	tamoxifen
Norinyl 1+35	norethindrone/ethinyl estradiol
Norinyl 1+50	mestranol/norethindrone
Norpace	disopyramide
Norpace CR	disopyramide CR
Norpramin	desipramine
Nuprin	ibuprofen
Ogen	estropipate
Oretic	HCTZ
Orinase	tolbutamide
Ortho-Novum 1/35	norethindrone/ethinyl estradiol
Ortho-Novum 1/50	mestranol/norethindrone
Orudis	ketoprofen
Pamelor	nortriptyline
Paraflex	chlorzoxazone
Parafon Forte	chlorzoxazone
PBZ	tripelennamine
Pediazole	erythromycin/sulfisoxazole
Pentids	penicillin G potassium
Pen-Vee K	penicillin V potassium
Percocet	acetaminophen/oxycodone
Percodan	aspirin/oxycodone

Brand Name	Generic Name
Periactin	cyproheptadine
Persantine	dipyridamole
Placidyl	ethchlorvynol
Plegine	phendimetrazine
Polycillin	ampicillin
Principen	ampicillin
Pro-Banthine	propantheline
Procan	procainamide
Procardia	nifedipine
Prolixin	fluphenazine
Proloprim	trimethoprim
Pronestyl	procainamide
Pronestyl SR	procainamide CR
Prostaphlin	oxacillin
Proventil	albuterol
Provera	medroxyprogesterone
Quinaglute	quinidine gluconate
Quinora	quinidine sulfate
Reglan	metoclopramide
Restoril	temazepam
Rheumatrex	methotrexate
Ritalin	methylphenidate
Robaxin	methocarbamol
Robaxisal	methocarbamol/aspirin
Robinul	glycopyrrolate
Saluron	hydroflumethiazide
Seconal	secobarbital
Septra	sulfamethoxazole/trimethoprim
Serax	oxazepam

Brand Name	Generic Name
Sinemet	carbidopa/levodopa
Sinequan	doxepin
Slow-K	potassium Cl
Soma	carisoprodol
Soma Compound	aspirin/carisoprodol
Stelazine	trifluoperazine
Sudafed	pseudoephedrine
Surmontil	trimipramine
Symmetrel	amantadine
Synalar	fluocinolone
Tagamet	cimetidine
Tavist	clemastine
Tegopen	cloxacillin
Tegretol	carbamazepine
Temaril	trimeprazine
Tenoretic	atenolol/chlorthalidone
Tenormin	atenolol
Tenuate	diethylpropion
Terramycin	oxytetracycline
Tetracyn	tetracycline
Theo-Dur	theophylline
Tofranil	imipramine
Tolectin DS	tolmetin
Tolinase	tolazamide
Toprol XL	metoprolol
Transderm-Nitro	nitroglycerin TD
Tranxene	clorazepate
Triavil	perphenazine/amitriptyline
Trilafon	perphenazine

Brand Name	Generic Name
Trilisate	choline magnesium trisalicylate
Trimpex	trimethoprim
Tums	calcium carbonate
Tylenol	acetaminophen
Tylenol w/ Codeine	acetaminophen/codeine
Tylox	acetaminophen/oxycodone
Urecholine	bethanechol
V-Cillin K	penicillin V potassium
Valisone	betamethasone
Valium	diazepam
Vancocin	vancomycin
Velosef	cephradine
Ventolin	albuterol
Vibramycin	doxycycline
Vicodin	acetaminophen/hydrocodone
Visken	pindolol
Vistaril	hydroxyzine
Wellcovorin	leucovorin
Wygesic	acetaminophen/propoxyphene
Wymox	amoxicillin
Xanax	alprazolam
Zyloprim	allopurinol

Some Brand-Name Drugs Likely to Come Off Patent Between 1996 and 2001

Brand Name	Generic Name
Activase	alteplase
Adalat CC	nifedipine extended release

Brand Name	Generic Name
Altace	ramipril
Augmentin	amoxicillin/clavulanate potassium
Beclovent	beclomethasone
Beconase	beclomethasone
Capoten	captopril
Capozide	captopril hydrochlorothiazide
Ceftin	cefuroxime axetil
Didronel	etidronate
DynaCirc	isradipine
Eldepryl	selegiline
Estrace	estradiol
Ethmozine	moricizine
Eulexin	flutamide
Fortaz	ceftazidime
Hismanal	astemizole
Humulin	insulin
Hytrin	terazosin
Inderide	propranolol/hydrochlorothiazide long-acting
Intal	cromolyn sodium
Lotensin	benazepril
Lozol	indapamide
Lupron	leuprolide
Mefoxin	cefoxitin sodium
Mevacor	lovastatin
Nizoral	ketoconazole
Normodyne	labetalol
Paxil	paroxetine
Pepcid	famotidine
Platinol	cisplatin

Brand Name	Generic Name
Primaxin	cilastatin sodium/imipenem
Prinivil	lisinopril
Prozac	fluoxetine
Relafen	nabumetone
Retrovir	zidovudine
Rocephin	ceftriaxone sodium
Rogaine	minoxidil
Sandimmune	cyclosporine
Seldane	terfenadine
Ticlid	ticlopidine
Timoptic	timolol maleate
Trandate	labetalol
Trental	pentoxifylline
Unasyn	ampicillin/sulbactam sodium
Vanceril	beclomethasone
Vascor	bepridil
Vasotec	enalapril
Zantac	ranitidine
Zestril	lisinopril
Zocor	simvastatin
Zoladex	goserelin
Zovirax	acyclovir

Part IV

Self-Treatment

13

Home Alone or Hiking in the Himalayas: What to Do When the Doctor Won't Come

This chapter is for anthropologists, adventurers, travelers, reporters, back-to-the-landers, Arctic explorers, and hermits. It is also for Mom, Dad, Grandma, Grandpa, and all the kids.

Previous editions of this book aimed self-treatment primarily at travelers. We wrote this section as a practical guide for those who may not have immediate access, or any access, to medical treatment—traveling in a foreign country where medical services may be unavailable, or even getting away from it all on a backwoods vacation.

This chapter could help alleviate some of the suffering that goes with being sick while on the road. Whether it's a strain, a pain, or a case of traveler's diarrhea, any sickness away from home is automatically worse. For those who can't find conventional medical services, we present recommendations for stocking your very own little black travel bag.

This is not meant to be a substitute for good medical supervision, when that's available and appropriate. In fact, you'll need a doctor's assistance in acquiring some of the medicines we're going to suggest. If the notion of doctoring yourself sounds radical, take solace in the fact that Grandma did it more often than not, and got along pretty well, thank you. Perhaps thinking back to the self-reliance of your forefathers (and foremothers, too) will bolster your confidence. They knew how to care for themselves, find their own dinner in the wild, and take care of most of the rest of life's necessities.

Nowadays we turn to a specialist to fix our car, do our hair, raise our food, install our plumbing, repair our appliances, and take care of us when we're sick. But just as we can learn how to get out the jumper cables when the car battery is dead, there are certain medical problems that are serious enough to treat but that might not require full-scale helicopter evacuation to the nearest hospital.

Even when you're not a hundred miles or more from the doctor's office, there may be times when self-treatment is desirable. For many of the common, everyday things that go wrong it is hardly necessary to make the trip. Why zoom off to the physician with a headache, a blister, or a temperature that's two degrees high? The headache will usually go away with two aspirin, the blister can be treated with common sense, and there's good evidence that a moderate fever serves a purpose in fighting a nonlethal infection.[1]

We're not advocating the notion that pain and suffering is somehow morally uplifting. *The People's Pharmacy* does not encourage biting bullets as a means of coping. But any number of popular medicines are either overprescribed or misprescribed, mostly because doctors feel pressured to prescribe something for the patients who come to see them.

Most doctors want very much to be helpful and to cure you of whatever nastiness is making life less than pleasant. It's hard for them to say no when you stand there insisting on a pill or potion, even when they know that what they're prescribing won't cure the problem. It's sort of a case of "Do nothing and your cold will be gone in a week, or you can take these and your cold will last seven days."

With the health care system in a crisis and expenses going through the roof, we can't afford to overutilize health services. Once, within living memory even, doctors would order all kinds of tests and put patients in the hospital for a week or more. Now, hospital stays are minimized as much as possible. Babies are delivered and gallbladders removed, barring complications, on an overnight "less than 24-hour" basis. And all sorts of experts are peering over the doctor's shoulder to keep him or her from spending too much on your care.

Believe it or not, you, even with no years of medical school and no stethoscope, are the best first line of defense when it comes to taking care of your body. Why? Because by not running to the doctor with every sniffle, and by not insisting on a prescription just because you've made a trip to the doctor's office, you'll contribute a lot to your overall health and will help to "control costs." Keep in mind, as we've discussed throughout this book, that every drug, every treatment, carries some risk of mistreatment, of adverse effects, of unexpected consequences. If something will go away by itself, let it.

Of course, part of being your own doctor means knowing when to "refer." That's good doctoring for you, just as it's good doctoring when the family physician realizes he or she needs help and calls for a specialist. Think of yourself as the "doctor" of first resort. If something seems minor, try living with it for 24 hours to see if it gets better. But be sure to draw upon your most precious resource: your common sense. Don't lie there all day with a heart attack waiting to see if it's getting better. You know your body better than anybody, so if something seems serious, get help as soon as you can.

Here are *The People's Pharmacy* candidates for do-it-yourself diseases and drugs. We'll discuss what you might take along when you're leaving home, as well as some additional medications that might usefully be added to the home medicine chest. With a bit of preparation, and some cooperation from a sympathetic physician, you'll be in pretty good shape to cope with most of life's minor ills.

Diarrhea

Traveler's Diarrhea

Let's get the number one problem for travelers out in front and solved first: diarrhea. You knew you shouldn't have eaten from that roadside stand, but the food smelled so good, and somebody said there was no danger if the stuff had been heated, and. . . .

First, stop blaming yourself. One study found that tourists who ate only in four-star hotels suffered intestinal problems just as frequently as those who foraged at will.[2] Roadside food stands have been taking a beating for years, yet they may often be innocent. It's possible that some folks succumb to the runs just because their systems don't adapt readily to the changes in food and water. It's not necessarily that the food and water harbor dreadful bugs, just that it's a different set of bugs than your intestines are used to entertaining.

A fair percentage of the time, though, there is evidence of a bacterial invader. One bacterium, *Escherichia coli,* is estimated to account for from 40 to 70 percent of the cases of traveler's diarrhea,[3] with a variety of other bacteria, viruses, and protozoans accounting for the rest. There are lots and lots of varieties of *E. coli*, and you don't have to travel to exotic places to encounter some of them. Turista is usually fairly mild, but a mutated strain of *E. coli* was responsible for an epidemic of serious illness in those, particularly young children, who ate undercooked burgers at a fast-food chain.[4]

One or more gentler strains of this bacterium are normal inhabitants of even the best-bred gut. When an unfamiliar type sets up housekeeping in your territory, though, it can run riot, producing a large quantity of toxins that cause fluid to be secreted in the intestines. It's downhill from there.

Before leaping to counterattack, be aware that most cases of diarrhea will run their course in four to seven hours. About one-third of the people with traveler's diarrhea will wind up in bed, and about 40 percent will have to change their plans somewhat to deal with their inconvenient problem.[5]

What's that? You're not going to just lie there and take it? Well then, let's try and deal with the beast in the belly.

A lot has changed in the treatment of the trots in the last few years. We now know of several things that work pretty well, though one is for prevention and the others are to be taken only if the bug strikes.

Heading the list is an old friend, bismuth subsalicylate. Don't recognize it? You would if we put it in its familiar pink trade dress. It's the active ingredient in **Pepto-Bismol**. Lots of studies show this is pretty good at preventing diarrhea, especially when the problem is *E. coli*. **Pepto-Bismol** is effective, cheap, and available over the counter. It can turn stool black—do not panic—and it shouldn't be taken by anyone who is allergic to aspirin. Otherwise it is without serious side effects for most people.

It used to be difficult to manage with **Pepto-Bismol**, especially if you were going far. In the liquid formulation it takes two ounces of liquid four times a day. That's 21 eight-ounce bottles needed for just one person over a three-week vacation. Fortunately the tablets can be substituted. (Do not, however, confuse them with **Pepto Diarrhea Control** caplets, which contain loperamide and should be used for symptomatic relief only.) The appropriate dose of **Pepto-Bismol** for prevention is two tablets in the morning, two in the evening.

Please note that **Pepto-Bismol** contains salicylate. That's awfully similar to aspirin, so anyone who is sensitive to aspirin or is taking medicine that interacts with aspirin (**Coumadin,** methotrexate, **Anturane, Benemid,** etc.) needs to steer clear. And never take aspirin at the same time you are taking **Pepto-Bismol** because that would be like doubling your aspirin dose.

One of the more recent additions to our antidiarrheal armamentarium is loperamide. This medication used to be available only under a doctor's supervision, but now can be purchased without a prescription as **Imodium A-D** (liquid or caplets), **Kaopectate II, Maalox Anti-Diarrheal Caplets,** or **Pepto Diarrhea Control**. Loperamide is one of the more effective products on the market for combating the symptoms of diarrhea. The recommended dose is two caplets when the first symptoms strike, then one after each loose stool, not to exceed eight pills daily.[6]

Loperamide works by slowing down the intestinal tract and reducing fluid loss. Be aware, though, that if you tangle with a really nasty bacterium such as typhoid, you won't want to slow it down and give it any more time in your system. As a result, don't take loperamide if you have a high fever as well, or if the diarrhea is bloody. (That could constitute a serious medical emergency, much worse than ordinary traveler's diarrhea. Get medical attention somehow.) Side effects of loperamide are rare, but constipation, nausea, vomiting, dry mouth, drowsiness, and dizziness have occasionally been reported.

If you are traveling somewhere that diarrhea is common, you may find oral rehydration solutions available in a local drugstore or grocery. If not, take care that you are getting enough fluids, but that what you are drinking is safe and not going to make matters worse.

Checking in with your doctor before you depart is always a good idea. He or she may prescribe an antibiotic for you to take along in the event of moderate or severe diarrhea. *The Medical Letter's* expert consultants report they sometimes prescribe **Cipro** (ciprofloxacin), **Floxin** (ofloxacin), or **Noroxin** (norfloxacin) twice a day until symptoms resolve (not more than three days).[7] Although most people can handle any of these medicines pretty well, they do predispose susceptible folks to a nasty sunburn. Don't even think about sitting in the sun while you're recuperating. Side effects may include nausea, vomiting, headache, rash and, paradoxically, diarrhea. Rare but serious neurological reactions have also been reported. These are heavy-duty drugs and require careful medical supervision.

Other treatments sometimes prescribed for traveler's diarrhea are **Vibramycin** (doxycycline—also prescribed in some cases for malaria prevention) or **Bactrim** (a combination of the drugs trimethoprim and sulfamethoxazole, now called cotrimoxazole and also sold under the brand name **Septra**). Both pills proved remarkably effective in trials over a decade ago, reducing the incidence of traveler's diarrhea anywhere from 50 to 95 percent.[8] In some parts of the world, however, *E. coli* and other intestinal critters have built up resistance to these antibiotics.

If your doctor prescribes **Vibramycin**, do NOT combine it with **Pepto-Bismol** on the assumption you'll kill twice as many *E. coli*. The bismuth subsalicylate decreases the availability of the doxycycline by about half. Also watch out for sun exposure if you're using **Vibramycin**. Like most tetracycline drugs, it can make you a lot more sensitive to sun, so you could get a nasty burn in a remarkably short time. Instead, cover up, use sunscreen, stay in the shade as much as possible, and don't forget your UV protective sunglasses.

Bactrim or **Septra** should be avoided by anyone who has ever had an allergic reaction to sulfa drugs. When you are discussing this medicine with your doctor, be sure to get complete information about symptoms that would indicate you should discontinue it. Serious side effects are uncommon, but could be life threatening. About 20 percent of those taking this drug for a week or more will have a skin rash. In this case the drug should be discontinued unless you are directed otherwise by a qualified doctor. Again, sunlight may increase the risk of rash, so stay inside and get well quickly.

For our money, the best bet, whether you are traveling or at home, is to swallow no antibiotics until—and only if—you get sick. Since all the drugs can cause problems of their own, and since there's a better-than-even chance you won't get even a slight case of traveler's diarrhea, why suffer the indignity of being made sick by something you were taking to stay well?

Once again we encounter the first principle of do-it-yourself medicine: Whenever feasible, do nothing in order to do no harm. However, the second principle of do-it-yourself medicine is: Be prepared. Discuss your options with your doctor before you head into strange territory.

Catching a Milky Culprit

Sometimes diarrhea has nothing to do with traveling. Our friend Philip complained that his new blood pressure medicine gave him a bellyache. His doctor said it couldn't be due to the drug, but Philip knew that whenever he took his pills he could expect gas, diarrhea and abdominal discomfort within the hour. Other people—probably some you know—experience similar problems after eating desserts like pudding, ice cream, cakes, or cookies. Some people have such problems only when they drink four glasses of milk a day as is now recommended for adequate calcium intake.

Tens of millions of Americans share this problem of lactose intolerance. Their digestive systems do not make the enzyme lactase, which is essential for digesting milk sugar. Some are so sensitive that, like Philip, they suffer even from the tiny amounts of milk sugar added to many pills as "filler."

Most people lose some lactase activity as they get older. Lactose intolerance is normally present in about three-fourths of adults of all ethnic groups except those originating in northwest Europe, who are less likely to experience this problem. Probably many of those who lack lactase learn early to avoid milk and other dairy products. If not, they may experience nausea, gas, bloating, stomach rumbles, diarrhea, or abdominal cramps in a half hour to two hours after drinking a glass of milk.

For many people, lactase-treated products provide a way to enjoy the nutritional benefits of milk without suffering from the consequences of undigested milk sugar. Lactase tablets (**Lactaid, Lactrase**) can help people like Philip who find it difficult to take needed medication and vitamins because they contain lactose as an "inactive ingredient."

Lactase breaks the milk sugar down so that it doesn't accumulate, undigested, in the intestinal tract where it can lead to trouble. The tablets are designed to be taken with meals that contain any milk or lactose, however well-disguised. They are also useful for those who react to medications containing lactose, such as **Benadryl, Calan, Dyazide, Inderide LA, Librax, Librium,** and **Premarin.** If you have any question about whether your medicine contains lactose, check with the pharmacist or doctor. The package insert, the *Physicians' Desk Reference,* or other drug information resources should list lactose if it is among the inert ingredients.

When diarrhea strikes, it helps not only to "be prepared," as we said earlier, but also to do a little detective work and find out just what is causing that gastrointestinal upset.

Urinary Tract Infections

S ince we mentioned **Bactrim** and **Septra** in the discussion of traveler's diarrhea, let's talk about urinary tract infections (UTIs). These same drugs are often prescribed for UTIs.

There seem to be two groups of women in the world—those who've had urinary tract infections, and those who are going to get them. Many women suffer repeated infections. While men are occasionally afflicted, it's a pretty rare event for a male under age 50. Susceptibility seems to have to do with the way the plumbing lines were designed. There's evidence that birth control pills further predispose some women to UTIs.

Anyone who's ever experienced the pain and discomfort of a UTI will certainly remember the experience. For those fortunate enough to remain uninitiated, a UTI can have you running to the bathroom every few minutes, with each trip a separate experience in pain.

If a UTI strikes on a trip, especially in a foreign country, it can be particularly trying. First, it can really cramp your style. Second, it may be difficult to explain the trouble to a doctor who doesn't speak your language.

What exactly has gone wrong? Just as the name says, a urinary tract infection is a bacterial infection of some portion of the urinary system. The kidneys produce urine and funnel it to the bladder, where it accumulates and passes by way of the urethra to the outside world. If the infection is way up in the kidney, you have pyelonephritis. If the infection has taken up residence in the bladder, the problem is referred to as cystitis. And if it's in the tubing leading from bladder to exit, it's urethritis. Regardless of where it is, it means pain and suffering.

The first problem is diagnosis. Not everything that causes painful or frequent urination is a urinary tract infection. You may get some help here from a handy, chemically treated strip called **Microstix-Nitrite Reagent Strips** or **Biotel u.t.i.** home screening tests. They're available at most pharmacies, and you don't even need a prescription. Dip the strip in a urine sample. If one part of the strip turns pink in 30 seconds, it's likely that a UTI lurks somewhere in the system. There are also more sophisticated sets of test strips called **Chemstrip 8** or **N-Multistix,** which cover a wide variety of other things detectable in the urine. There's no reason to get the fancier model unless you have had problems in the past that call for you to keep track of sugar, ketones, protein, or blood in the urine.

By the way, the best urine sample is one taken midstream. The first part of the urine voided will contain a fair number of bacteria that normally live in the lower and external parts of the system. With those swept out of the way, the midstream sample is a pretty good indication of what's really going on up there.

For children with frequent infections, such home tests can be helpful in alerting a parent to the need for treatment. Some doctors may not be delighted with your self-diagnosis. They'll tell you UTIs are a very complicated subject, and that can certainly be true. If you have access to medical care when pain and urgency appear, see the doctor right away. But if the problem arises while a woman is out in the boonies somewhere, some information and a start on treatment is probably better than having neither information nor treatment. And the **Microstix** has been designed so that most anybody who reads the directions and follows them can get good results.

If the problem turns out to be a UTI, the chances are good the offending organism is our old friend *E. coli*. Yes, the same *E. coli* of diarrhea fame. That's why it should come as no surprise when **Bactrim** and **Septra** again turn up as useful bacterial bashers to treat urinary tract infections.

The strategy of attack has altered. For years, doctors have tinkered with varying doses and varying periods of administration, sometimes keeping women on the drugs for weeks. There's now a definite trend toward single-dose treatment for uncomplicated infections. You swallow a couple tablets of **Bactrim DS** or **Septra DS**, or 200 mg of **Furadantin** (nitrofurantoin), or 400 mg of **Proloprim** or **Trimpex** (trimethoprim) and very often that will do the trick. All these are prescription drugs, and will require that the doctor cooperate in seeing you're properly supplied with instructions for correct dosing as well as the prescription itself.

There's something neat and tidy about being able to put **Bactrim** or **Septra** into the suitcase or knapsack and know that the drug does at least double duty, helping cure either traveler's diarrhea or UTIs. Whenever we can get two-for-one, we take it.

The *Merck Manual* says you can also ease the pain in the first day—not as a substitute for antibiotics, but along with the treatment—by taking half a teaspoon of baking soda in half a glass of water every four hours.[9] You'll want to keep a running tab with the **Microstix** test to see if the bacterial beasties have been defeated.

Keep in mind that some symptoms of UTI (including flank pain, pubic pain, frequent urination, or a sense of the need to urinate coming on very suddenly) can also be warning signs of other, more serious troubles including kidney stones and venereal disease. Also, UTIs that are stubborn and persist for long periods can cause substantial damage to the kidney tissue, so this isn't something to mess around with. If it's a simple UTI and you can zap it quickly, great. If not, rev up the sled dogs and get help.

Nausea, Vomiting, and Motion Sickness

Most of us aren't real keen on being sick to our stomachs. Sometimes it may be Mother Nature's way of saying that what you sent down for lunch wasn't acceptable. The system has a remarkable capacity for knowing its own limits, and there may be a good reason for rejects.

Very often, though, the cause of vomiting is motion sickness. Whether it's a rough plane ride, the gentle rise and fall of a ship, or a car tour over twisting mountain roads, motion sickness can strike with amazing swiftness. And when it does, it causes misery.

People who don't suffer motion sickness seem to think that those of us who do are sissies or softies. But try telling that to our astronauts. About half of those sky explorers get sick on each space shuttle mission! NASA and the astronauts were so embarrassed they renamed the problem "Space Adaptation syndrome," and now refuse to divulge who on each mission is suffering the problem. (Apparently on a billion-dollar mission nobody can get just plain old motion-sick.) But the evidence is in the bag.

If you know you're prone to motion sickness, but plan to go for a sail, a cruise, or a plane ride anyway, ask the doctor about **Transderm Scop.** It's a prescription-only adhesive patch containing the drug scopolamine, which has proved to be a pretty effective antinausea medication. You apply the patch behind your ear, and leave it in place for up to three days. The drug slowly seeps out of the patch and into your system, keeping lunches and dinners in their place.

Transderm Scop has to be applied several hours before the ship (or whatever) starts swaying. Be very careful not to get anywhere near your eyes with the patch or with your fingers after you've handled the patch. Scopolamine can dilate pupils and cause blurred vision. Even though this effect is temporary, it could be scary while it lasts.

Like most motion sickness medications, **Transderm Scop** has some side effects. About two-thirds of those using the patch will experience a dry mouth, and about one-sixth report drowsiness. Older people may be more sensitive to reactions, and the drug is not appropriate for children.

Transderm Scop may also cause difficulties for men with enlarged prostates that interfere with urination. In the worst case, a man could find his bladder full but be unable to empty it, a urinary emergency that sometimes requires catheterization. Needless to say, this is not a situation that even bears contemplation if you can't get to medical care.

We have heard some reports of withdrawal reactions. People who use **Transderm Scop** for more than three days may end up on dry land, take off their patch— and find themselves mighty seasick. If your cruise is going to last longer than three days, you might want to give yourself some days without the patch, just to reduce the risk of suffering this kind of reaction.

Before subjecting yourself to medications, you might give ginger a try. As we discussed in Chapter 6, this common household spice may provide relief from the nausea and vomiting associated with motion sickness. In one study, ginger was even more effective than the old standby **Dramamine** (dimenhydrinate).

Constipation

A mericans are hung up on bowel function. Incredible as it may seem, there are hundreds of laxatives sold in this country, and many of them sell very well. But there are real dangers lurking at the laxative counter. Regular laxative use over a period of years can actually damage the bowel and make a person dependent on laxatives. So watch out for advertisements touting laxatives with "natural ingredients." Taking a laxative isn't natural.

Whatever the state of your bowels, though, traveling can produce temporary shifts in regularity. The simultaneous change of food, drink, time zone, and place can cause the system to slow down.

The best cure? One more time—do nothing. Ignore it. No bowel movement today? Great. Maybe tomorrow. If you're on vacation, go see the sights. Otherwise, go about your normal routine. Don't worry about it. What went in will eventually come out.

We urge you to stay away from laxatives, especially local varieties. Many of these are not just laxatives, but extremely strong purgatives. Folk beliefs in many parts of the world say that a person needs a regular "cleaning out," and, believe us, some of these concoctions will really clean your closet. That can set in motion a very dangerous cycle of purge/constipation/purge. That's a merry-go-round you don't want to hop on.

Eat moderately and sensibly and let your bowels work on their own schedule seems to be the best advice.

Experts rarely recommend laxatives as a primary treatment for constipation. Instead, they suggest that people increase their intake of dietary fiber and fluids (to at least 6 cups daily). Exercise is also very important. If these approaches are not sufficient, a bulk-forming laxative such as psyllium (**Metamucil, Perdiem Fiber, Reguloid, Serutan**, etc.) or polycarbophil (**Fiberall** Tablets, **FiberCon, Mitrolan**, etc.) may be the next step. Because these products are essentially a way of adding extra fiber to the diet, they don't seem to produce dependence and bowel damage as other laxatives might.

Sunburn

R epeat after us: The sun is terrible for my skin. Dermatologists are absolutely right when they say that the quest for the perfect tan will lead to premature spotting, aging, wrinkling and drying, not to mention a significantly greater risk of skin cancer. Let's face it—youth fades fast enough, so why help it along?

Vacations and sunburn seem to go together. Perhaps people don't want to worry about anything when they step out of their daily routine. But there's a catch in that thinking. The problem, of course, is that most of us don't get a chance to lie about in the sun year-round. When opportunity knocks for a suntan, we don't just cautiously crack the door ajar—we fling it wide open. The result is usually one body baked to a brilliant, painful red.

Avoiding such problems has become considerably easier in the past decade or so. Effective sunscreens are readily available and should be a part of every home first-aid kit. Don't forget to take one along when you travel.

The FDA requires manufacturers to label every bottle of suntan goo with a rating called the Sun Protection Factor. The SPF numbers allow you to tell which suntan lotion does the best job of blocking burning rays. A wise traveler would carry a bottle of SPF 15 or higher, to use whenever he or she has already had enough exposure. The idea is to start the day outside coated with a suntan lotion appropriate to his or her particular skin sensitivity, then switch to the more potent sunscreen after a while. Those who turn dark on merely seeing the sun can get by with something with an SPF of less than 8. Those who burn anytime after dawn better stay with the higher numbers. Over 15 should provide pretty decent protection, but you can find products that go as high as SPF 50.

There has been a lot of publicity lately about the dangers of overexposure made possible by effective sunscreens that prevent burns. The trouble is that most lotions block the UV-B rays that can cause redness, but not the UV-A that probably cause more lasting damage, such as wrinkles and cancer. One chemical has recently been approved for blocking UV-A and is starting to show up in sunscreens. Check the ingredient listing for avobenzone, also called Parsol 1789. Look for it in **Shade UVA-Guard** and other products.

The best protection against too much UV-A is probably a dose of common sense, our favorite all-purpose panacea. If you're traveling in the tropics or other sunny lands, try to stay under cover during the middle of the day. Use protective clothing—and a hat!—as well as generous amounts of your chosen sunscreen. Don't be fooled by overcast weather, since a lot of ultraviolet light can penetrate those clouds, and do be cautious about water, snow, sand, and other surfaces that can reflect the light back up at you. Ever hear of someone burning the underside of their chin and nose? It happens at ski resorts around the world.

If you've slipped up and gotten burned, be cautious about using any of the creams, sprays, and lotions such as **Americaine Anesthetic, Lanacane, Solarcaine**, or **Unguentine**. We know the commercial implies you can spray away the pain, and you're lying there suffering. But these concoctions all work because they contain a local anesthetic called benzocaine, which for some people may actually irritate the skin and thereby add to their woes.

Probably the best thing to do is take a bath in cool water or apply cool compresses of **Burow's Solution** (aluminum acetate) for about twenty minutes, three or four times a day. Topical steroids such as **Cortaid, CaldeCort**, or **Lanacort** may be helpful, particularly in the one-percent strength. Moisturizers such as **Lubriderm, Nivea, Eucerin**, or **Vaseline** petroleum jelly may also be soothing. To ease the pain, you may want to take two aspirin every three to four hours, and promise yourself you won't leave home again without your SPF 15 suntan lotion.

A really bad burn probably requires oral steroids like cortisone or prednisone. Taken for only a few days such drugs can dramatically relieve the suffering with relatively few side effects. But that's not a case for self-treatment. A dermatologist must decide if the problem is so severe that it requires the heavy artillery.

Many prescription medications can either sensitize the skin, making you more vulnerable to sunburn, or can make you more subject to heat stroke. If you are taking any prescription medication, it would be a good idea to check its possible effects in the sun before venturing out. Some of the drugs that may cause such problems are listed in the chart that follows.

Drugs That Can Lead to Bad Sunburn

Brand Name	Generic Name
Accutane	isotretinoin
Achromycin V	tetracycline
Actifed with Codeine	codeine/triprolidine/pseudoephedrine
Adapin	doxepin
Aldactazide	hydrochlorothiazide/spironolactone
Aldoclor	chlorothiazide/methyldopa
Aldoril	hydrochlorothiazide/methyldopa
Altace	ramipril
Anaprox	naproxen
Ancobon	flucytosine
Apresazide	hydrochlorothiazide/hydralazine
Aquatag	benzthiazide
Aquatensen	methyclothiazide
Aventyl	nortriptyline
Azo Gantanol	phenazopyridine/sulfamethoxazole
Azo Gantrisin	phenazopyridine/sulfisoxazole
Bactrim	trimethoprim/sulfamethoxazole
Benadryl	diphenhydramine
Benylin	diphenhydramine
Brevicon	ethinyl estradiol/norethindrone

Brand Name	Generic Name
Butazolidin	phenylbutazone
Capoten	captopril
Capozide	captopril/hydrochlorothiazide
Cardioquin	quinidine
Combipres	chlorthalidone/clonidine
Compazine	prochlorperazine
Compoz	diphenhydramine
Cordarone	amiodarone
Corzide	nadolol/bendroflumethiazide
Dapsone	dapsone
Declomycin	demeclocycline
Deconamine	chlorpheniramine/pseudoephedrine
Demulen	ethynodiol/ethinyl estradiol
Depakene	valproic acid
Depakote	valproic acid
DiaBeta	glyburide
Diabinese	chlorpropamide
Diamox	acetazolamide
Dimetane	brompheniramine/phenylpropanolamine/codeine
Diucardin	hydroflumethiazide
Diulo	metolazone
Diupres	chlorothiazide/reserpine
Diuril	chlorothiazide
Diutensen	methyclothiazide/cryptenamine
Doryx	doxycycline
Duraquin	quinidine
Dyazide	hydrochlorothiazide/triamterene
Dymelor	acetohexamide
Efudex	fluorouracil

Brand Name	Generic Name
Elavil	amitriptyline
Eldepryl	selegiline
Endep	amitriptyline
Enduron	methyclothiazide
Enduronyl	methyclothiazide/deserpidine
Enovid	mestranol/norethynodrel
Esidrix	hydrochlorothiazide
Esimil	hydrochlorothizaide/guanethidine
Etrafon	amitriptyline/perphenazine
Eulexin	flutamide
Eutron	methyclothiazide/pargyline
Exna	benzthiazide
Fansidar	sulfadoxine/pyrimethamine
Feldene	piroxicam
Floxin	ofloxacin
Fluoroplex	fluorouracil
Fulvicin	griseofulvin
Gantanol	sulfamethoxazole
Gantrisin	sulfisoxazole
Glucotrol	glipizide
Grifulvin V	griseofulvin
Grisactin	griseofulvin
Gris-PEG	griseofulvin
Haldol	haloperidol
Hismanal	astemizole
HydroDIURIL	hydrochlorothiazide
Hydromox	quinethazone
Hydropres	hydrochlorothiazide/reserpine
Inderide	hydrochlorothiazide/propranolol

Brand Name	Generic Name
Janimine	imipramine
Lasix	furosemide
Limbitrol	chlordiazepoxide/amitriptyline
Loestrin	ethinyl estradiol/norethindrone
Lo/Ovral	ethinyl estradiol/norgestrel
Lopressor HCT	metoprolol/hydrochlorothiazide
Matulane	procarbazine
Maxaquin	lomefloxacin
Maxzide	hydrochlorothiazide/triamterene
Mellaril	thioridazine
Metahydrin	trichlormethiazide
Metatensin	trichlormethiazide/reserpine
Mevacor	lovastatin
Micronase	glyburide
Minizide	polythiazide/prazosin
Modicon	ethinyl estradiol/norethindrone
Moduretic	hydrochlorothiazide/amiloride
Monodox	doxycycline
Mykrox	metolazone
Myochrisine	gold sodium thiomalate
Naturetin	bendroflumethiazide
Naqua	trichlormethiazide
Navane	thiothixene
NegGram	nalidixic acid
Nelova	mestranol/norethindrone
Neptazane	methazolamide
Nordette	ethinyl estradiol/levonorgestrel
Norethin	mestranol/norethindrone
Norinyl	mestranol/norethindrone

Brand Name	Generic Name
Norlestrin	ethinyl estradiol/norethindrone
Normozide	labetalol/hydrochlorothiazide
Noroxin	norfloxacin
Norpramin	desipramine
Oretic	hydrochlorothiazide
Orinase	tolbutamide
Ornade	chlorpheniramine/phenylpropanolamine
Ortho-Novum	mestranol/norethindrone
Orudis	ketoprofen
Ovcon	ethinyl estradiol/norethindrone
Ovral	ethinyl estradiol/norgestrel
Ovulen	ethynodiol/mestranol
Oxsoralen	methoxsalen
Pamelor	nortriptyline
Panmycin	tetracycline
Perfumes	bergamot/cedar/citron/lavender/lime/musk/ sandalwood
Periactin	cyproheptadine
Pertofrane	desipramine
Phenergan	promethazine
Prinzide	hydrochlorothiazide/lisinopril
Prolixin	fluphenazine
Quinaglute	quinidine
Quinamm	quinine
Quinidex	quinidine
Quinora	quinidine
Rauzide	bendroflumethiazide/rauwolfia
Renese	polythiazide
Rheumatrex	methotrexate

Brand Name	Generic Name
Ridaura	auranofin
Robitet	tetracycline
Saluron	hydroflumethiazide
Salutensin	hydroflumethiazide/reserpine
Seldane	terfenadine
Septra	trimethoprim/sulfamethoxazole
Ser-Ap-Es	hydralazine/hydrochlorothiazide/reserpine
Sinequan	doxepin
Solganal	gold salts
Stelazine	trifluoperazine
Sumycin	tetracycline
Surmontil	trimipramine
Taractan	chlorprothixine
Tavist	clemastine
Tegretol	carbamazepine
Temaril	trimeprazine
Tenoretic	atenolol/chlorthalidone
Terramycin	oxytetracycline
Tetracyn	tetracycline
Thorazine	chlorpromazine
Timolide	hydrochlorthiazide/timolol
Tofranil	imipramine
Tolinase	tolazamide
Trandate	labetalol
Triavil	amitriptyline/perphenazine
Trilafon	perphenazine
Tri-Levlen	norgestrel/ethinyl estradiol
Tri-Norinyl	norethindrone/ethinyl estradiol
Triphasil	norgestrel/ethinyl estradiol

Brand Name	Generic Name
Trisoralen	trioxsalen
Uri-Tet	oxytetracycline
Urobiotic	oxytetracycline
Vaseretic	hydrochlorothiazide/enalapril
Vasotec	enalapril
Velban	vinblastine
Vibramycin	doxycycline
Vibra-Tabs	doxycycline
Vivactil	protriptyline
Zaroxolyn	metolazone
Zestoretic	hydrochlorothiazide/lisinopril

Bites, Stings, Rashes, and Itches

Ask any traveler and you'll find there are bugs abroad. And some of them have been working up an appetite just for a taste of you. Although they are usually not life-threatening, insect bites can be annoying and even maddening. And some of those biters do carry diseases, especially malaria. If you are going to be traveling where malaria is rampant, see the doctor before you leave. He or she may have to check with the Centers for Disease Control and Prevention in Atlanta, Georgia ([404] 332-4555), for the latest guidelines on prescription medicine to keep you from catching malaria.[10] It is very important to take the medicine as directed, since malaria is probably worse than you imagine. There is hope of a vaccine in the future, but we wouldn't suggest holding your breath or putting off your trip waiting for it to be ready.

In addition to antimalarial medicine, it's a good idea to take steps to keep from getting bitten. A mosquito net for your bed, fairly fine mesh and permethrin-impregnated, is a good idea to keep them from feasting on you while you're helpless. You can't spend all your time in the sack, though, so you'll need long sleeves, long pants, and probably a reliable repellent.

As we already mentioned in Chapter 6, diethyltoluamide or DEET has little or no serious competition as the most effective bug juice on the market. It's even garnered a vote of confidence from the United States Army. No doubt about it—it works. However, the safety of concentrated formulas has come into question in recent years. So, as we said, DEET-containing products should be used judiciously and with caution, especially on children. Spraying protective clothing with **Permanone** (permethrin) may also prevent bites with less contact of chemicals on the skin.[11] We don't know of any tests that demonstrate the safety of this approach for children, however. Don't use both together.

Of course, no insect repellent yet invented is guaranteed to keep every last critter from grabbing a piece of the action . . . in this case, you. So there you are with an itching bite, or perhaps prickly heat, or maybe the aftermath of a losing battle with poison ivy. Now what?

On the theory that less is more, try hot water, as we disussed in Chapter 6. Running some hot water on the offending area for a few seconds can give up to several hours of relief. Remember, the water has to be warm enough to be mildly uncomfortable, but not so hot that it will burn.

When itching gets out of control and becomes generalized over the entire body, it's time for something special. Add one cup of an oat-based bath powder such as **Aveeno** or **Nutra•Soothe** to a tub of lukewarm water and soak for 10 to 20 minutes. Be careful—the bathtub could become very slippery. Put a towel on the bottom to keep from breaking your neck. No sense getting hurt by the cure.

If there's no oat bath powder at hand, you may want to try cornstarch. Add one to two cups of cornstarch powder to four cups of water and mix it into a paste. Then put the glop in a tub of lukewarm water, stir thoroughly, and crawl in. A 20- to 30-minute soak is good for almost any inflammatory skin condition. It will help relieve rashes, itching, crotch irritation, or an allergic reaction. Once again, be extra careful about slipping and sliding when getting in or out of the tub.

After drying, resist the urge to slather on one of the highly promoted topical ointments. Instead, make up a Burow's Solution of aluminum acetate. Dissolve one **Domeboro** tablet (available without a prescription at the pharmacy) in a pint of water and mix it well. Loosely bandage what itches, and then dribble the mixture over the bandage little by little, keeping the dressing wet. If your patience allows, keep at it for several hours. Another thing good for itching is plain calamine lotion.

You can also use a nonprescription hydrocortisone cream. The one-percent products, such as **Cortizone•10, Extra Strength CortaGel,** or **Maximum Strength Cortaid**, are just about strong enough to do some good. If you ask your doctor nicely, though, you may be able to get a prescription for an ointment with real anti-itching power. **Aristocort** (triamcinolone), **Valisone** (betamethasone), **Topicort** (desoximetasone), **Synalar** (fluocinolone), or **Lidex** (fluocinonide) are strong steroids and should not be used indiscriminately over large portions of the body or for long periods of time. But if you want fast relief for a day or two, such drugs are extremely effective. Of course, some doctors would say that using such medications for bug bites is ridiculous, like killing flies with a sledgehammer.

We've already covered insect-sting treatment, but just as a reminder—a dab of meat tenderizer can be very effective at neutralizing the venom left behind by a bee or other stinging insect. Anyone who is severely allergic to insect stings probably knows it, and should definitely be carrying an emergency kit such as **EpiPen** or

Ana-Kit (available by prescription), which allows them to self-inject a dose of adrenaline. Such people face a life-threatening crisis when stung, and prompt treatment is absolutely vital.

Fungus Infections

Athlete's Foot

When traveling to warm, humid climes even those who've never had a fungal infection can find it amazingly easy to become a breeding ground. Some of our readers have complained that they suffer from athlete's foot every summer without fail. What starts out as slightly reddened, slightly itching skin can in short order turn into a mass of white, soggy, macerated tissue that will itch more than you ever imagined anything could.

Fungal infections are notoriously difficult to combat. That's partly because of the way in which fungi live and reproduce, and partly because there just hasn't been as much research into drugs for fighting fungi as there has been on antibacterials.

For those who've suffered a lifetime of athlete's foot, forget the old names like **Daliderm** and **Quinsana Foot Powder**. There are now several effective antifungal medicines available over-the-counter. Your choices include **Micatin** (miconazole), **Lotrimin AF** and **Mycelex OTC** (both clotrimazole), and **Aftate, Tinactin,** or **Ting** (all tolnaftate). They need to be applied twice daily while you keep the affected area clean and dry. If you can manage that, the problem should clear up in a couple of weeks.

If things are really bad, it's possible you have not just a fungal infection, but a combined fungal/bacterial duet going on between your toes. For a long time we assumed all athlete's-foot was just a fungal infection. But diligent research established that very often the fungi colonize, but are then followed by bacteria that set up housekeeping in their own territory, adding to the problem.[12] One of the reasons some athlete's-foot infections have been so treatment-resistant is that a plain antifungal can't handle a combined infection.

One answer may be to try aluminum chloride in a 20- to 30-percent solution. This is a nonprescription item any pharmacist should be able to whip up in a jiffy. This common chemical has been used for years as an underarm deodorant or antiperspirant. It may also be helpful for resistant athlete's foot. By drying the skin, it makes the area between your toes inhospitable to invading bacteria. Meanwhile, it kills the little devils at the same time.

Aluminum chloride should be applied once or twice a day until things start to look better. Never apply it after a shower or when feet are wet, since it will burn and sting. One other word of caution: Don't use aluminum chloride if your foot has open sores, since this could aggravate the irritation.

If you can't find a pharmacist who will brew up the aluminum chloride solution for you, then talk to your doctor about a prescription product called **Drysol**. This is nothing more than a 20-percent solution of aluminum chloride in alcohol, sold for people who sweat excessively.

Once you've got the athlete's-foot problem under control, you will want to keep those tootsies cool, calm, and dry to prevent flare-ups. A foot powder, cotton socks, and shoes that breathe are a good way to keep the fungi away. If you can wear sandals, so much the better.

Jock Itch

Jock itch (which is a misnomer, since it can affect men and women equally and is certainly not restricted to athletes) is nothing more than an athlete's-foot type of fungal infection in a different location. Warm, moist areas provide great conditions from a fungus's point of view, and that's why the toes and groin are prime targets.

The same treatment here will work equally well. In fact, though you'll find **Micatin** with the foot-care products at the pharmacy, read the label. It says, "Proven clinically effective in the treatment of athlete's foot (tinea pedis), jock itch (tinea cruris), and ringworm (tinea corporis)."

Ringworm plagued the son of one of our readers. The kid, who was on the high-school wrestling team, developed a rash on his arm that the trainer said was ringworm. The trainer recommended **Micatin**. The mother was worried about using an athlete's-foot remedy, but she had no need to fret. Both ringworm of the body and ringworm of the feet are caused by fungal infections—not a worm. The same medicines often work for both.

Micatin comes as an ointment, spray, and powder. Once the infection is controlled, an occasional dusting with the powder can help keep these normally moist areas dry while also killing off any fungal spores that might have notions of taking up residence.

You will also want to stick to light, loose-fitting clothing that doesn't chafe. That rules out leggings, tight jeans, or pantyhose and tips the scale for boxers vs. briefs. Anything that soaks up sweat, such as **Zeasorb Powder**, should also help prevent the condition from starting in the first place.

Cuts and Scratches

H ome treatment has long relied on the idea that if it hurts, it must be good for you. The louder a kid hollers, the better the stuff must be. A time-worn American ritual involves pouring potent antiseptics that hurt like hell over wounds and scratches. Killing germs is somehow associated with healing wounds, but that's nonsense. The truth is, minor cuts require absolutely no special attention. They should be washed carefully with plenty of mild soap and water, and that is all.

By the way, if you have a choice between soggy bar soap and liquid soap, we'd pick the liquid soap. Dr. Jon Kabara, a pharmacologist at Michigan State University, has found that used bar soaps in public lavatories can harbor a wide variety of microbes. Dr. Kabara wrote to the *Journal of the American Medical Association*:

To the Editor.—Because my research findings have become a focal point of controversy in the choice of liquid soap vs. bar soap, I feel compelled to present further information for the followers of this saga. . . .

Others have talked on the dangers of bar soap: Steere and Mallison warned, "However, bars of soap frequently remain in pools of water that might support the growth of organisms"; two experts on infection control stated, "These bar soaps (multiuser) are frequently misused and stored carelessly in contact with moisture. The resulting jelly mass is unsightly, difficult to use effectively, and, in some cases, found to harbor live pathogenic bacteria of *Staphylococcus* and *Pseudomonas* genera, which may be transferred from one user to another"; still others affirm the potential danger of bar soap, "the frequent contamination of bars of soap suggests that organisms may be obtained during the very procedure performed to prevent transfer"; and, finally a recent study has shown that "meticulous bathing with the bar soap issued by the hospital (containing triclocarbon) did not eliminate colonization and was frequently associated with the shifting of these bacteria to adjacent sites on the body."[13]

Healthy people probably don't need to worry too much about the germs lurking on bar soap. But if you are washing out a cut or a scratch, it seems only good sense to avoid contamination if possible. Remove any dirt that may have penetrated the wound but resist pouring special "degerming" junk on the tender skin. If you expect to be somewhere the soap might be as unappealing as that described above—or worse yet, where there's no soap at all—you might want to consider toting your own little squeegee bottle of uncontaminated suds.

Now, it is hard to resist temptation. If Mom painted your scratches with **Merthiolate, Medi-Quik**, or **Unguentine**, you are going to want to do *something*, if not the same thing, for your kid. If you feel that scrape needs to be "disinfected," you could use a little antibiotic ointment on the bandage, something such as **Polysporin**. In addition to helping prevent infection, this kind of goo can help keep a cut or scrape moist for rapid healing.

What happens if the skin does become infected? Again, the conservative approach is preferable. Unless the infection is serious, hot-water soaks or compresses will increase blood flow to the area and enable your own body to do the rest. Even a wet/oozy skin infection is best treated by soaks or compresses. Dermatologists have long acknowledged that "wet-to-wet" treatment will paradoxically dry out the skin lesion.

A serious or persistent skin infection calls for medical care. The doctor may prescribe either **Bactroban** (mupirocin), an antibiotic ointment that works especially well against *Staph* infections, or an oral antibiotic that will be specific for the kind of infection that you have. Red streaks leading from the wound toward the center of the body are a danger signal that mean get help fast!

Pain Relief

P ain. Headaches. Muscle aches. Arthritis. Pain is good. At least it is for the drug companies. They sell $2.6 billion worth of over-the-counter analgesics each year. With so much money at stake, the competition is heating up. First there was aspirin, then acetaminophen, then ibuprofen.

The latest entries into the pain-relief circus are over-the-counter forms of the popular prescription arthritis drugs **Naprosyn** (naproxen) and **Orudis** (ketoprofen)—**Aleve**, **Actron,** and **Orudis KT,** respectively. And if past history is any indication, they should be popular. Often consumers are impressed and intrigued when a drug previously obtainable only by prescription is made available without a doctor's ℞.

Medicines such as ibuprofen or naproxen may be great for menstrual cramps. But you say you have a headache? What do you do?

Take two aspirin.

That's the best possible prescription. Aspirin is really a wonder drug. It provides an incredible amount of pain relief, at a virtually invisible price if you buy only what you need—plain USP aspirin, no additives, no fancy brand name.

In the event of a genuine "my head is splitting open" episode, a good backup would be a few tablets of **Empirin with Codeine**, or, if your doctor prefers, acetaminophen with codeine. This last is perennially high on the list of most frequently prescribed drugs, especially if you lump it together with the brand-name **Tylenol with Codeine.** Either acetaminophen or good old aspirin with a bit of codeine should take care of almost any kind of pain you'd tolerate without going to the hospital emergency room.

We don't quite understand why doctors seem more likely to prescribe acetaminophen instead of aspirin these days. After all, aspirin has benefits **Tylenol** can't even aspire to. But it has taken a long time for medicine to recognize its merits. The story begins with a doctor, a family-practice physician in Glendale, California, who urged his friends and patients to take an aspirin a day to reduce the risk of heart attacks and strokes. That may not sound so radical in these days and times, but back in 1948 Dr. Craven's recommendation was revolutionary.

Dr. Lawrence Craven came up with the idea of using aspirin to prevent blood clots in the late forties. He routinely supplied each of his tonsillectomy patients with **Aspergum** and instructed them to chew one stick, with 3.5 grains of acetylsalicylic acid, a half hour before each meal and bedtime. While the pain was usually relieved, several of his patients had serious postoperative bleeding.

From this seemingly unrelated observation, Dr. Craven concluded that aspirin interfered with blood clotting and could be "of value as a preventive of vascular thrombotic conditions."[14]

If only other doctors had paid attention to this old doc's advice! Dr. James E. Dalen, editor of the *Archives of Internal Medicine*, believes that "if his rule of 'an aspirin a day' had been adopted by Americans in 1950, hundreds of thousands of myocardial infarctions [heart attacks] and strokes might have been prevented."[15]

In 1989, the American College of Chest Physicians finally agreed. A study carried out on more than 22,000 American doctors demonstrated convincingly that one aspirin every other day could reduce the risk of heart attack by 44 percent.[16]

As a result of this research, many physicians are now prescribing aspirin for those at risk of heart attack. What is still uncertain is the optimum dose. A study from Texas suggests that as little as 10 milligrams or even 3 milligrams a day might be enough to provide anticlotting benefit without risk of stomach irritation.[17] We point out that 3 milligrams is only one one-hundredth of a standard aspirin tablet. At this time, there is no convenient way for American consumers to take such a low dose.

When it comes to treating headaches, of course, it still takes two aspirin tablets. And it is definitely possible to overdo. One of the country's leading headache experts, Dr. Joel Saper of Ann Arbor, Michigan, tells us that he sees many patients who have treated themselves into a tormented vicious cycle. Using any over-the-counter pain reliever more than twice a week for recurrent or chronic headaches is a sign that medical attention is needed. In many instances, people experience horrible headaches when they stop taking aspirin or acetaminophen painkillers. They need help weaning off these medicines.

Aspirin also has side effects. At analgesic and especially at anti-inflammatory doses, aspirin can cause stomach upset and ulcers. Some people experience bruising, ringing in the ears, allergic reactions, asthma attacks, and nasal polyps. And many common drugs can interact adversely with aspirin. The moral here is, be informed. If aspirin will be dangerous for you, with your health conditions and other medications, choose acetaminophen or another pain reliever.

Sometimes people get headaches from nasal congestion, particularly when they've been on airplane flights with the numerous changes of cabin pressure. If the headache is a long-lasting one that seems to arise in the facial area, you may be more in need of a decongestant than anything else. If so, **Neo-Synephrine** or any one of the dozens of short-acting nasal-spray decongestants should do the job. Continued use, however, runs the risk of rebound nasal congestion. An oral decongestant such as **Sudafed** is another alternative, as long as you don't suffer from high blood pressure, heart trouble, diabetes, or thyroid disease.

At times, flying is associated with a different kind of pain. Rather than a headache, extreme ear pain afflicts some passengers as the plane descends. One of our readers wrote to tell us she had found a great solution:

> I n 1992 I purchased two plastic units called Ear Ease which work unbelievably well. I have used them for at least ten landings and now never fly without them. Before descent I ask the attendant for hot water to fill the units. They work great.
>
> The only drawback is the price. They cost $24 per pair plus postage. Too bad the airlines do not provide them or rent them like they do movie earphones. Hope this helps.

We don't know of any studies that show **Ear Ease** is effective, but if you're interested, you can check with the mail-order company Solutions at (800) 342-9988. As of this writing, they have lowered the price to $10 each or $18.50 per pair.

Another reader came up with a similar solution. Hers has one advantage—it is free:

> A sk the flight attendant to bring you two Styrofoam coffee cups stuffed with very hot wet paper towels. You put the cups over your ears before descent begins. You can't carry on a conversation and you feel kind of dumb but it works.

Be careful not to get burned by the hot water. This remedy may not work for everyone, but it's possible that the heat opens the eustachian tubes to equalize pressure and relieve pain.

Sniffles and Sneezes

S peaking of nasal congestion, there's nowhere in the world where you can escape from the common cold. We once spoke with a couple who'd just returned from a wonderful trip to China, marred only by the nasty chest cold they both caught. Wherever chicken soup is available (and it is almost as ubiquitous as the cold), that would be our recommended remedy.

For advice on using OTC cold medicines, see Chapter 5 on over-the-counter medicines. Don't be tempted to try the cold remedies you may encounter in other places. One reader sent us a gold foil packet and wrote:

> I recently traveled to Tokyo on business. I was coming down with a cold and the flight attendant offered me a cold remedy. It helped, but I was a little worried about taking it since I couldn't read the Japanese writing on the packet. Can you tell me what was in this medicine?

We got some help with the translation and discovered that basically this was the kitchen-sink approach. We often complain about all the unnecessary ingredients in American cold remedies. There were nine different compounds in that foil packet from Japan.

The powder he downed contained acetaminophen (the ingredient in **Tylenol**), ephedrine (a decongestant and asthma medicine), dihydrocodeine (a narcotic pain reliever), noscapine (a narcotic cough suppressant), guaiacol (an expectorant), and carbinoxamine (an antihistamine). In addition, it had caffeine and several B vitamins.

We wouldn't suggest you take a potpourri like this even at home. Combining cough suppressants and expectorants is illogical, and taking so many narcotics with an antihistamine could make you groggy. That might be okay on a long flight over the Pacific, but not so good on the ground.

Remember that a cold will generally go away by itself. It is also the quintessential self-treatment condition, because there is nothing the doctor can do for an uncomplicated cold that you can't do for yourself. If, on the other hand, the flu is on the rampage and you feel like you were hit by a truck, don't wait. Do see a doctor as promptly as possible. There are now two antiviral prescription medicines, amantadine and **Flumadine** (rimantadine), that can be very effective against influenza A if they are taken early enough in the course of the illness.

Vitamins

"**D**on't waste your money on vitamins," said the doctor. "You'll just end up with expensive urine."

For years conventional medical wisdom has resisted supplements. Physicians were convinced that any amount of vitamins beyond the minimum needed to stave off scurvy or beriberi would be discarded by the body.

The American public doesn't seem to agree, though. One out of four are taking supplements, just as this woman is:

> **M**y wife is convinced that vitamins keep her healthy. She takes a fistful every morning. The kitchen table is littered with vitamin C, beta-carotene, folic acid, zinc, vitamin E and goodness knows what else.
>
> I don't take a thing and feel great at 68. I eat healthy food and walk two miles every day. She keeps pushing her health food publications at me and wants me to take vitamins too. I think the whole thing is a waste of good money. Please tell her to ease up.

We'd hate to step into the middle of this argument. Although we think he's doing well to get his exercise and eat healthy food, he still might want to consider a multiple vitamin and mineral supplement. A Canadian study, published in *The Lancet*, found that healthy older people given a nutritional supplement had stronger immune systems, as measured by several laboratory tests, than an identical group given a placebo. Most important, the supplement group came down with only half as many infections during the year.[18]

Over the last several years, researchers have uncovered a wide range of potential benefits from certain vitamins. As the evidence mounts, more and more nutrition scientists are taking vitamins themselves. Jeffrey Blumberg, associate director of the Human Nutrition Research Center on Aging at Tufts University, believes that nutrients at adequate levels may help prevent some chronic diseases.

"I recommend that people take a multivitamin-multimineral supplement at one to two times the RDA as nutritional insurance," he told the Center for Science in the Public Interest. He admitted that he takes vitamin E "because of the studies that suggest that antioxidants reduce the risk of heart disease, cataracts, and cancer." He points out that simply delaying such diseases by only ten years could save billions of dollars in medical costs.

Scientists believe that antioxidants protect the body from chemical deterioration and may have anti-aging properties. They include beta-carotene, vitamin C and vitamin E, among others. Beta-carotene, a substance the body uses to make vitamin A, occurs naturally in orange or green fruits and vegetables, such as carrots, cantaloupe, or collard greens.

But while some excellent research, such as the Physicians' Health Study, indicates that beta-carotene may reduce the risk of stroke, heart attack, and death, a Finnish study published in the *New England Journal of Medicine* in 1994 cast doubt on the value of this supplement in reducing the risk of lung cancer in smokers. Further research reported early in 1996 supports the Finnish findings on beta-carotene failing to prevent cancer. Despite disappointment with this supplement, though, no nutrition scientist we know of would tell people to limit their intake of fruits and vegetables.

Doctors and dietitians worry about toxicity. Some vitamins (including vitamins A and D, niacin, and B_6) can be dangerous in high doses. Too much vitamin

A (more than 50,000 international units daily) can quickly lead to toxicity, with side effects such as dry cracked lips, brain disorders, bone abnormalities, hair loss, itching, and liver problems. This vitamin is also dangerous during pregnancy, as high doses may lead to malformations. Beta-carotene, a natural building block of vitamin A, may interact with alcohol to increase the risk of liver damage.[19]

Heart disease and cancer are complicated processes, with no single causes or solutions. Common sense dictates that exercising, avoiding smoking, and eating a diet high in fruits and vegetables and low in meat and fat should be helpful. But have you had your three to five servings of vegetables and two to four servings of fruit today? Only one in ten of us have. The rest might consider some vitamin insurance.

Multipurpose Medicines

L et's take a quick look at some drugs whose biggest virtue is that they will do several jobs. That makes them the ideal choice when you've got to travel light, yet want to be prepared to cope with as many problems as possible.

We've already seen how the trimethoprim/sulfamethoxazole (co-trimoxazole) combination sold as **Bactrim** or **Septra** can be of help in fighting both traveler's diarrhea and urinary tract infections. We'd have to say such double-duty capability could earn it a spot in many world travelers' kits. (Obviously, if you have ever taken it and learned it makes you break out in a rash, it will do you no good. Leave it home.)

Another must-take would be aspirin. Nothing else can give so much relief for so little cost. Not only will it relieve pain, but it is also effective in reducing fever and inflammation. And if you suspect that you are having a heart attack you could pop half a pill on your way to the E.R.

If sentenced to life on an island, and given just one drug to tote, though, we'd probably opt for codeine. It's an excellent painkiller, relieving the agony of everything from a backache to a tooth with a cavity. Codeine is also effective against diarrhea at a dose of around 15 milligrams every four to six hours.

Codeine also is an excellent cough suppressant. In fact, codeine is the standard to which all other cough preparations are compared. If you have a really nasty, painful cough, codeine is your drug. A dose of 15 to 30 milligrams should do nicely.

On top of all that, codeine has a little sedative action, so it can help put you to sleep if that cough, or painful tooth, is leading to a loss of slumber time.

If codeine is so great, why isn't it used more often? Actually it is. Compounds such as **Tylenol with Codeine** are high on the list of most-prescribed drugs. Codeine is rarely prescribed by itself, even though it would be far cheaper that way, perhaps because the FDA makes it harder for doctors to prescribe pure codeine than a codeine combination. Apparently codeine by itself is seen as a drug with abuse potential. In reality, the likelihood it would be abused is low when the drug is given in the small doses needed for the uses we're discussing here.

You will have to ask the doctor for codeine. Ten tablets of 30 milligrams' potency will get you through most short-term medical emergencies. It would be very difficult to become much of a big-time addict on that, so the doctor shouldn't be too reluctant. For diarrhea or cough, divide each 30-milligram tablet in half and you'll have an adequate dose. As long as the physician realizes that you need only a small quantity to get you by during an emergency he shouldn't have a problem providing such a prescription. Skip the codeine if you are among the people who suffer nausea or vomiting from it.

Recommended Reference Material

D octors always have lots of diplomas on their walls and lots of books on their shelves. We can't help your doctoring with any diplomas, but there are a few books the aspiring do-it-yourselfer should have at hand, in sickness and in health.

First, of course, we do hope you'll take a look at one of our other books, such as *Graedons' Best Medicine* (New York: Bantam, 1991). If it's not in your local library, you can request an order form by writing to: The People's Pharmacy, Dept. PP-3, P.O. Box 52027; Durham, NC 27717-2027. This order form also lists a number of helpful brochures (including our Guides to Home Remedies, Drug and Food Interactions, and Drugs That Affect Sexuality), and audiotapes from our syndicated public radio show as well as other books. We're especially proud of *The People's Guide to Deadly Drug Interactions* (New York: St. Martin's Press, 1995) and think it serves as a useful reference to this vital topic. Please don't overlook the information in Part V of this *People's Pharmacy*, either. It summarizes the most important information about a number of popular prescription products.

Before purchasing anything else, you will probably want to invest a few bucks in a paperback medical dictionary. This will help in translating to English the complicated words medical writers seem to favor. Don't get hung up trying to render every last word. A few of the big ones will usually be enough to help you figure out what they're trying to say.

The one book we would definitely take to that isolated island is *The Merck Manual of Diagnosis and Therapy*, which is now in its 16th edition. *The Merck Manual* is a phenomenon, a book originally published and intended for physicians, which has grown to be a popular best-seller. Within its 2,800 or so tissue-paper pages you'll find a description of just about everything imaginable (and quite a few things unimaginable) that can go haywire with the human body, and what can and can't be done about each. The descriptions are concise, precise, and useful. The index alone is a virtual medical education, and it provides quick access to the material. It's very helpful, especially in alerting you to a potentially serious situation that shouldn't be treated on your own. We anticipate an easy-to-read consumer edition soon.

For drug information in a dictionary form we would recommend *The Pill Book*, edited by Harold M. Silverman, Pharm. D. Now in its 6th edition (copyright © 1994), it is available in paperback from Bantam Books. That really should be enough, but if you feel you really have to have a "doctor's reference," we'd suggest the *PDR* (*Physicians' Desk Reference*), *PDR Generics* (Montvale, NJ: Medical Economics) or *Physicians' GenRx* (Smithtown, NY: Data Pharmaceutica, Inc.). While probably few households need such references on a regular basis, public libraries should be encouraged to include them in their holdings.

As long as we're in the library, we might mention a few other references that are too large and expensive for most home bookshelves, but are sometimes useful for specific questions. We check the latest edition of the *Handbook of Nonprescription Drugs* (Washington, D.C.: American Pharmaceutical Association) for questions on over-the-counter products. And for the increasingly popular herbal remedies, our favorite resource is *The Lawrence Review of Natural Products* (St. Louis: Facts and Comparisons).

References

1. Mackowiak, Philip A. "Fever: Blessing or Curse? A Unifying Hypothesis." *Ann. Int. Med.* 1994; 120:1037–1040.

2. Steffen, Robert, et al. "Epidemiology of Diarrhea in Travelers." *JAMA* 1983; 249(9):1176–1180.

3. Cook, G. C. "Traveller's Diarrhoea—An Insoluble Problem." *Gut* 1983; 24:1105–1108.

4. "Update: Multistate Outbreak of *Escherichia coli* O157:H7 Infections from Hamburgers—Western United States, 1992-1993." *MMWR* 1993; 42:258–263.

5. Ibid.

6. "Advice for Travelers." *The Medical Letter on Drugs and Therapeutics* 1994; 36:41–44.

7. Ibid.

8. Weiss, Barry. "Traveler's Diarrhea Update." *Am. Fam. Phys.* 1983; 27(4):193–195.

9. Berkow, Robert, ed.-in-chief. *The Merck Manual of Diagnosis and Therapy*, 16th ed. Rahway, NJ: Merck Research Laboratories, 1992, p. 1719.

10 "Advice for Travelers," op. cit., p. 43.

11. Ibid., p. 44.

12. Leyden, J. L., and A. M. Kligman. "Aluminum Chloride in the Treatment of Symptomatic Athlete's Foot." *Arch. Dermatol.* 1975; 111:1004–1010.

13. Kabara, Jon J. "Bar Soap and Liquid Soap." *JAMA* 1985; 253:1560–1561.

14. Craven, Lawrence L. "Acetylsalicylic Acid, Possible Preventive of Coronary Thrombosis." *Annals of Western Medicine* 1950; 4:95–99.

15. Dalen, James E. "An Apple a Day or an Aspirin a Day?" *Arch. Intern. Med.* 1981; 151:1066–1069.

16. Steering Committee of the Physicians' Health Study Research Group. "Preliminary Report: Findings from the Aspirin Component of the Ongoing Physicians' Health Study." *N. Engl. J. Med.* 1989; 318:262–264.

17. Lee, Makau, et al. "Dose Effects of Aspirin on Gastric Prostaglandins and Stomach Mucosal Injury." *Ann. Intern. Med.* 1994; 120:184–189.

18. Chandra, Ranjit Kumar. "Effect of Vitamin and Mineral Supplementation on Immune Responses and Infection in Elderly Subjects." *Lancet* 1992; 340:1124–1127.

19. Leo, M. A., et al. "Interaction of Ethanol with Beta-Carotene: Delayed Blood Clearance and Enhanced Hepatotoxicity." *Hepatology* 1992; 15:883–891.

Part V

People's Pharmacy Guide to Popular Prescription Drugs

What follows is a compendium of commonly prescribed medications. We have also tried to list some of the up-and-comers—those new drugs that we believe will soon become popular with physicians. This list is not complete, because there are thousands and thousands of prescription drugs and there just isn't room to cover them all.

The instructions, side effects, drug interaction information, and other precautions that you will find on the following pages do not detail every reported problem for each medication. We tried to hit the highlights so you could use this information as a starting point to establish good communication with your physician. If you suspect you or someone you know is experiencing a side effect or interaction, contact your physician as soon as possible.

Remember, balancing benefits against risks is a tricky process. We hope the following data is useful in helping you maintain your good health.

acetaminophen with codeine

APAP with Codeine

Capital with Codeine

Margesic

Phenaphen with Codeine

Tylenol with Codeine

Overview: Acetaminophen and codeine is an excellent analgesic combination for mild to moderate pain relief. It can ease the discomfort of a bad toothache or the aftermath of minor surgery, as well as a wide array of other situations that call for pain management. One of the most commonly prescribed brand-name preparations is **Tylenol with Codeine**. It is also available as **Margesic** and **Phenaphen with Codeine**. The number on the formula represents the amount of codeine the formula contains. No. 1 has 7.5 mg of codeine; No. 2, 15 mg; No. 3, 30 mg; and No. 4 contains 60 mg of codeine.

Special Precautions: Like any narcotic, codeine may make you drowsy. Do not drive or attempt any activity that requires coordination and judgment. Older people may be more susceptible to this reaction. Light-headedness or dizziness could make walking dangerous. Never stand up suddenly, as it may make you feel faint.

Long-term use of acetaminophen and codeine has drawbacks since codeine may be habit-forming if you take it regularly. Do not increase the dose on your own in a quest to achieve greater pain relief. But don't play the hero by skipping doses during an acute crisis. Pain is more easily managed if it can be nipped in the bud instead of trying to play catch up when it has gotten out of control.

Taking the Medicine: Some people react to codeine with nausea or vomiting. Taking it with food may reduce stomach upset. Nausea, dizziness, and other common reactions may be less troublesome if you lie down for a while.

Side Effects and Interactions: Other than dizziness, drowsiness, and nausea, side effects may include constipation, loss of appetite, headache, sweating, and euphoria. Some people experience shortness of breath, especially if they have asthma. Other less common reactions include an allergic rash, disorientation, dry mouth, and urinary difficulties. Report any such symptoms to your physician promptly.

Acetaminophen may cause liver or kidney problems in large doses or over long periods. Your physician should evaluate your need for this combination pain reliever periodically.

If you are taking any other medicines, check with a physician or pharmacist about compatibility. Alcohol as well as many over-the-counter and prescription drugs can add to the sedative effect of this analgesic and should be avoided. Antihistamines, antianxiety agents, and sleeping pills may require extra caution. Both tricyclic and MAO-type antidepressants may interact with this analgesic to cause greater toxicity, and the anticonvulsant **Dilantin** may increase the risk of liver damage.

Ambien

zolpidem

Overview: **Ambien** is the first in a new class of sleeping medicines. It is prescribed for the short-term treatment of insomnia. Studies indicate that the stages of sleep approach normal in patients on **Ambien**, and there is a low incidence of next-day hangover.

Special Precautions: Older people are more sensitive to **Ambien** and usually require a lower dose.

Insomnia often occurs as a result of physical or psychological illness. While **Ambien** can shorten the time it takes to fall asleep, and lengthen the time a person sleeps, it can't help correct any underlying problems, which should be diagnosed and treated appropriately.

Although there is no evidence that **Ambien** produces physical dependence or addiction, anyone with a history of substance abuse should be monitored carefully while on this or any other sleeping pill.

Taking the Medicine: **Ambien** works very quickly. It should be taken on an empty stomach immediately before going to bed.

Side Effects and Interactions: People on **Ambien** may experience daytime drowsiness, dizziness, diarrhea, nausea, vomiting, or headache.

Other side effects reported include lethargy, weakness, drugged feelings, amnesia, dry mouth, constipation, allergy, and sinusitis. Because this medication is still quite new, some rare reactions may not yet have shown up. Be sure to report any symptoms to your physician promptly.

Relatively few studies have considered **Ambien** in combination with other medications. **Ambien** interacts with alcohol, which should generally be avoided by everyone taking sleeping pills. Antianxiety medicines such as **Xanax** and other sleeping pills, such as **Dalmane** or **Halcion**, might magnify the effects of **Ambien**. This sleeping pill can reduce peak blood levels of **Tofranil** (imipramine) by 20 percent and decrease alertness. Increased impairment has also been reported when **Thorazine** is combined with **Ambien**. Check with your doctor and pharmacist to make sure **Ambien** is safe in combination with any other drugs you take.

amoxicillin

Amoxil   **Trimox**

Larotid   **Wymox**

Polymox

Overview: Amoxicillin is the most commonly used medicine in the United States. Frequently prescribed under the brand name **Amoxil**, it belongs in the penicillin class of antibiotics. Other versions of amoxicillin include **Larotid, Polymox, Trimox,** and **Wymox**, among others.

The extraordinary success of amoxicillin is due in large part to its broad-spectrum activity against a large number of bacteria. It is effective in fighting infections in many places in the body including the urinary tract, lungs, ears, throat, skin, and genital tract.

Special Precautions: Because it is related to penicillin, anyone allergic to this class of antibiotics must generally avoid amoxicillin like the plague. Symptoms such as breathing difficulty, wheezing, sneezing, hives, itching, and skin rash require immediate emergency treatment. Life-threatening anaphylactic shock may produce an inability to breathe, and cardiovascular collapse can occur within minutes of exposure. If you experience a serious reaction and you ever have to go into the hospital, make sure a sign is placed over the bed alerting hospital personnel to penicillin allergy.

Taking the Medicine: The most effective way to swallow amoxicillin is probably on an empty stomach and with a full eight-ounce glass of water. That usually means at least one hour before eating or two hours after food. There is some disagreement among health professionals on this matter, however, and if the drug upsets your stomach it can be taken with meals without losing potency. Ask your pharmacist to check on the particular formulation dispensed and get a specific recommendation on how to take it.

Side Effects and Interactions: The most common side effects of amoxicillin involve digestive tract upset. Nausea, vomiting, and diarrhea can be troublesome for some people. Less common but possibly more serious side effects include liver enzyme elevations, anemia, blood disorders, and psychological reactions. Report any unusual symptoms to your physician promptly. Long-term treatment with penicillin-type antibiotics requires periodic monitoring by a health professional.

Anaprox

naproxen sodium

Overview: **Anaprox** is a pain reliever used for arthritis, menstrual cramps, headaches, dental surgery, bursitis, tendinitis, sprains, strains, and other painful conditions. It belongs to a class of medications commonly called NSAIDs or nonsteroidal anti-inflammatory drugs.

Special Precautions: **Anaprox** is virtually identical to **Naprosyn**, a popular arthritis medicine, so these two drugs should never be taken together. The over-the-counter pain reliever **Aleve** is another guise naproxen may take and should not be mixed with **Anaprox**. People who are allergic to aspirin or other anti-inflammatory agents should avoid **Anaprox**. Signs of allergy include breathing difficulties, rash, fever, or a sudden drop in blood pressure, and require immediate medical attention.

Taking the Medicine: Because **Anaprox** and **Anaprox DS** can be hard on the digestive tract, the pills may be taken with food to reduce stomach trouble. This does not guarantee that the drug will be safe for the stomach.

Side Effects and Interactions: No matter how you swallow this medicine, the most common side effects involve the gastrointestinal tract. They include nausea, indigestion, heartburn, cramps, gas, constipation, and diarrhea.

Some people even develop ulcers and intestinal bleeding while taking **Anaprox**. These problems occasionally occur without obvious preliminary symptoms, leading to a sudden life-threatening crisis due to perforation of the stomach lining. Older people appear to be more susceptible to this problem and should be monitored carefully. Warning signs may include weight loss, persistent indigestion, a feeling of fullness after moderate meals, dark or tarry stools, anemia, and unusual fatigue. Home stool tests such as **Hemoccult** or **Fleet Detecatest** may provide an early indication of bleeding.

Other side effects to be alert for include headache, ringing in the ears, rash, itching, difficulty breathing, and fluid retention. Drowsiness, dizziness, light-headedness, difficulty concentrating, and confusion are possible; do not drive if you become impaired. Less commonly, **Anaprox** may produce jitteriness, insomnia, heart palpitations, hair loss, depression, tremor, tiredness, visual disturbances, and sores in the mouth. Some people become sensitive to sunlight while on **Anaprox**, so use an effective sunscreen, stay covered, or avoid the sun. Report any symptoms to your physician promptly. **Anaprox** can affect both the kidney and liver, so periodic blood tests to monitor the function of these organs is important.

This medication can adversely interact with many other drugs, including aspirin, alcohol, beta-blocker heart or blood pressure medicine, blood thinners, **Lasix**, lithium, and methotrexate. Over-the-counter pain relievers such as **Aleve** (which contains the same ingredient as **Anaprox**) or others containing ibuprofen or aspirin should not be combined with **Anaprox**. Check with your pharmacist and physician to make sure **Anaprox** is safe in combination with any other drugs you take.

Ansaid

flurbiprofen

Overview: **Ansaid** is a nonsteroidal anti-inflammatory drug, or NSAID. Medications in this class are used to relieve pain associated with arthritis, menstrual cramps, headaches, minor surgery, bursitis, tendinitis, sprains, strains, and other painful conditions. **Ansaid** is prescribed primarily for rheumatoid arthritis and osteoarthritis.

Special Precautions: People who are allergic to aspirin or other anti-inflammatory agents should avoid **Ansaid** because of the possibility of allergy. Symptoms include breathing difficulties, rash, fever, or a sudden drop in blood pressure, and require immediate medical attention.

Taking the Medicine: Because **Ansaid** can be hard on the digestive tract, the pills may be taken with food to reduce discomfort. Taking **Ansaid** with food will slow but not reduce its effects. There are no guarantees that the drug will be safe for the stomach, however.

Side Effects and Interactions: Without question, the most common side effects of arthritis drugs such as **Ansaid** involve the gastrointestinal tract. They include nausea, indigestion, heartburn, cramps, gas, constipation, and diarrhea. Even ulcers and intestinal bleeding are a possibility. These problems occasionally occur without obvious preliminary symptoms, leading to a sudden life-threatening crisis due to perforation of the stomach lining. Older people appear to be more susceptible to this problem and should be monitored carefully. Warning signs may include weight loss, persistent indigestion, a feeling of fullness after moderate meals, dark or tarry stools, anemia, and unusual fatigue. Home stool tests such as **Hemoccult** or **Fleet Detecatest** may provide an early indication of bleeding.

Other side effects to be alert for include headache, ringing in the ears, rash, itching, difficulty breathing, and fluid retention. Drowsiness, dizziness, lightheadedness, difficulty concentrating, and confusion are possible; do not drive if you become impaired. Less commonly, **Ansaid** may produce jitteriness, insomnia, heart palpitations, hair loss, depression, tremor, tiredness, visual disturbances, and sores in the mouth. Some people become sensitive to sunlight while on **Ansaid**, so use an effective sunscreen, stay covered, or avoid the sun. Report any symptoms to your physician promptly. **Ansaid** can affect both the kidney and liver, so periodic blood tests to monitor the function of these organs is important.

This medication may adversely interact with alcohol and many other drugs, including aspirin, beta-blocker heart or blood pressure medicine, blood thinners, **Lasix** and similar diuretics, lithium, and methotrexate. Over-the-counter pain medicines such as **Motrin IB** or **Aleve** should be avoided while you are on **Ansaid**. Check with your pharmacist and physician to make sure **Ansaid** is safe in combination with any other drugs you take.

Ativan

lorazepam

Overview: **Ativan** is an antianxiety agent, similar in many respects to **Valium.** Once called minor tranquilizers or sedatives, such drugs are prescribed to calm jittery nerves and relieve excessive tension. They belong to a class of medications called benzodiazepines. **Ativan** is a little more rapid in action than many other such drugs, and its calming effect lasts for a relatively short period of time.

Special Precautions: Regular reliance on **Ativan** for many months may lead to dependence. Sudden discontinuation of the drug could trigger withdrawal symptoms including nervousness, agitation, difficulty concentrating, insomnia, fatigue, headache, and nerve twitching. Never stop taking **Ativan** without medical supervision. This medication may have to be phased out gradually over a period of weeks or months.

Ativan, like several other short-acting benzodiazepines, may cause problems with memory for events that happen the day after the medicine is taken. People may appear normal to friends and family, but later be unable to recall some of the things they did or observed during that time.

Taking the Medicine: **Ativan** can be taken with food, especially if it upsets your stomach. Do not drink alcohol or use any other sedative while on this drug, because the combination may lead to dizziness, drowsiness, lack of coordination, or confusion.

Side Effects and Interactions: Side effects associated with **Ativan** include sedation, dizziness, unsteadiness, and confusion. These may fade after a few days or weeks. Do not drive, operate machinery, or undertake any activity that requires close attention. **Ativan** may make narrow-angle glaucoma worse and should not be taken by people diagnosed with this condition.

Other possible reactions include nausea, dry mouth, visual problems, depression, rash, itching, change in appetite, constipation, altered sex drive, urinary difficulties, and reduced blood pressure. Report any such symptoms to your physician promptly.

Many drugs, including erythromycin-type antibiotics, digitalis-type heart drugs, and the schizophrenia drug loxapine can interact with **Ativan**. Check with your pharmacist and physician to make sure **Ativan** is safe in combination with any other medicines you take.

Atrovent

ipratropium bromide

Overview: **Atrovent** is an inhaled medication used to open the airways in chronic conditions such as asthma, emphysema, and chronic bronchitis. It is generally used as preventive or maintenance therapy, rather than in an acute emergency, where it is less effective.

Special Precautions: People who are hypersensitive to atropine or related compounds must not take **Atrovent**, because a serious reaction could result. Let the prescribing doctor know if you have an enlarged prostate, urinary difficulties (due to obstruction of the neck of the bladder), or narrow-angle glaucoma, because the medication could aggravate these conditions.

Taking the Medicine: **Atrovent** comes in an aerosol inhaler. The usual dose is two puffs (36 micrograms) four times a day. The total dose should not exceed 12 inhalations in 24 hours. The medication should be stored at room temperature away from high humidity.

Side Effects and Interactions: Often **Atrovent** does not cause side effects, because it is not easily absorbed into the bloodstream. Possible side effects include dry mouth and irritation of the mouth or throat, cough, nausea, blurred vision, headache, nervousness, rash, or rapid heart rate. **Atrovent** is frequently used in combination with other asthma drugs, and does not seem to interact dangerously with compounds such as **Intal, Beclovent** or other inhaled steroids, and theophylline.

Augmentin

amoxicillin plus clavulanic acid

Overview: Amoxicillin is the most commonly prescribed antibiotic in the United States. Unfortunately, the widespread use of this penicillin-like drug has led many bacteria to develop resistance to it. By adding clavulanic acid to the formulation, scientists created a medication, **Augmentin**, that is effective against many bacteria that are not susceptible to amoxicillin alone.

This broad-spectrum antibiotic is effective in fighting infections in many parts of the body including the urinary tract, skin, sinuses, lungs, ears, throat, and genital tract.

Special Precautions: Because amoxicillin is related to penicillin, anyone who is allergic to this class of antibiotics must generally avoid such drugs like the plague. Symptoms such as breathing difficulty, wheezing, sneezing, hives, itching, and skin rash require immediate emergency treatment. Life-threatening anaphylactic shock may produce an inability to breathe and cardiovascular collapse, and can occur within minutes of exposure. If you experience a serious reaction and you ever have to go into the hospital, make sure a sign is placed over the bed alerting hospital personnel to penicillin allergy.

Taking the Medicine: **Augmentin** can be taken with meals or on an empty stomach. It is generally best swallowed with a full eight-ounce glass of water. To maintain adequate levels of the medicine in your body, it is usually recommended that doses be given every eight hours. Check with your pharmacist to see how you should adjust your schedule to get the third dose in on time.

Side Effects and Interactions: The most common side effects of **Augmentin** involve digestive tract upset. Nausea, vomiting, and diarrhea can be troublesome for some people. Other adverse reactions to be aware of include skin rash, itching, vaginal infections, stomachache, gas, headache, and vomiting. Less common but possibly more serious side effects include liver enzyme elevations, anemia, blood disorders, and psychological reactions. Report any symptoms to your physician promptly. Long-term treatment with penicillin-type antibiotics requires periodic monitoring by a health professional.

Augmentin may interfere with some urine tests for diabetes and produce false-positive results. **Augmentin** should not be taken with tetracycline or some other antibiotics. Notify your doctor if you are on such a drug for a different condition.

Axid

nizatidine

Overview: **Axid** is a popular treatment for ulcers that helps them clear up rapidly. It works in part by suppressing the secretion of stomach acid by blocking histamine receptors in the digestive tract (H_2 receptors). It is also used to treat the severe heartburn called reflux esophagitis, and may be prescribed as maintenance therapy to keep ulcers from coming back.

Special Precautions: Patients taking H_2 blockers such as **Axid** or **Zantac** have higher levels of certain microorganisms in their stomachs than would normally survive there. Scientists do not yet know whether these bacteria have negative long-term consequences, but it appears that vitamins C and E might provide some measure of protection.

Axid is eliminated almost completely by the kidneys. People with kidney problems may need the doctor to adjust the dose downward.

Taking the Medicine: **Axid** is usually taken once a day at bedtime. Absorption is slightly lower when this capsule is taken with food, and antacids also reduce absorption slightly.

Axid tablets should be kept away from heat, cold, light, and moisture. The container should be capped very tightly.

Side Effects and Interactions: Side effects associated with **Axid** are uncommon. Some people experience rash or anemia. Other reactions reported occasionally include diarrhea, headache, dizziness, muscle aches, and weakness. Report any symptoms to your physician promptly.

Axid appears to interact with very few other medications compared to its predecessor **Tagamet**. People who take high doses of aspirin may find blood levels of this salicylate increase if they start taking **Axid** as well. Check with your pharmacist and physician before taking other medicines in combination with **Axid**.

Biaxin

clarithromycin

Overview: **Biaxin** is a broad-spectrum antibiotic, a macrolide related to erythromycin. It is prescribed to fight respiratory tract infections including pneumonia and infections of the skin.

Special Precautions: Because **Biaxin**, like erythromycin, is eliminated from the body by the liver, this drug should be used very cautiously, if at all, by people with liver problems. Anyone with a history of allergy to macrolide (erythromycin-type) antibiotics should probably avoid **Biaxin**. Symptoms of an allergic reaction include hives, rash, and itching. In rare instances allergy may trigger life-threatening anaphylactic shock.

Pregnant women should avoid **Biaxin** unless the doctor finds no other appropriate therapy. This medication has caused birth defects in animal tests.

Taking the Medicine: **Biaxin** may be taken with or without food. Doses are usually spaced evenly throughout the day. Check with your physician or pharmacist for specific instructions, and be sure to complete the full course of medication unless directed otherwise.

Side Effects and Interactions: The most frequent side effects involve digestive tract upset. People taking **Biaxin** report fewer side effects than those on erythromycin, but diarrhea, nausea, abnormal taste, stomachache, and upset stomach are potential reactions. Headache has also been reported. Let your doctor know promptly of any symptoms you experience.

Biaxin interacts with a few other medicines. It may boost blood levels of the antiseizure medication **Tegretol** by 60 percent or more, leading to increased toxicity. The asthma drug theophylline, the blood thinner **Coumadin** (warfarin), and the anti-AIDS drug **Retrovir** (AZT) appear to interact with **Biaxin**. It should not be taken by people who are also taking the antihistamines **Seldane** or **Hismanal** because it could lead to a dangerous buildup of these drugs in the body. Check with your pharmacist and physician to make sure **Biaxin** is safe in combination with any other drugs you take.

Calan SR

verapamil (sustained release)

Overview: **Calan** belongs to a class of medicines called calcium channel blockers. Because of their safety and effectiveness, these drugs have helped revolutionize the treatment of high blood pressure. Other uses of calcium channel blockers include treatment of irregular heart rhythms and angina.

There is even some preliminary research that suggests some of these compounds may be able to prevent migraine headaches, ease nighttime leg cramps, asthma, and Raynaud's disease, and perhaps reduce atherosclerosis. Despite these future possibilities, **Calan SR** has been approved *only* for the treatment of hypertension.

Special Precautions: Although **Calan** may be prescribed for a variety of cardiac indications, there are some serious heart conditions that may be worsened by this drug. Your doctor should be fully informed about any heart problem, kidney disease, liver disease, low blood pressure, and muscular dystrophy. Careful monitoring is called for in any of these cases due to an increased risk of toxicity. In addition, older people may be more sensitive to the blood-pressure-lowering effects of **Calan SR**.

Taking the Medicine: The manufacturer recommends that this sustained-release formulation should be taken with food, preferably in the morning with breakfast. If a second dose is needed it should be swallowed approximately 12 hours later.

Do not stop taking **Calan SR** suddenly, because this could lead to complications. Your doctor will tell you how to taper off gradually if you no longer need this medication.

Side Effects and Interactions: One of the most common side effects of **Calan** is constipation. Although bothersome, this can often be controlled with fluid and fiber or a bulk-forming laxative such as psyllium. Another reaction to be alert for is low blood pressure, which may show up as light-headedness and dizziness.

Although uncommon, other adverse reactions include headache, fluid retention leading to swelling of arms and legs, nausea, tiredness, rash, and slowed heart rate. Report any symptoms or suspected side effects to your physician promptly.

Calan can interact with a number of other drugs, including several that are used to treat high blood pressure or heart conditions, the asthma medicine theophylline, the anticonvulsant **Tegretol** (carbamazepine), the transplant medication **Sandimmune** (cyclosporine), and the antituberculosis agent rifampin. The popular antidepressant **Prozac** (fluoxetine) may increase the likelihood of side effects from **Calan**.

Over-the-counter calcium supplements can reduce the effectiveness of **Calan**. Check with your doctor and pharmacist to make sure **Calan** is safe in combination with any other drugs you take.

Capoten

captopril

Overview: **Capoten** was the first of a new class of blood pressure medicines called ACE (for angiotensin-converting enzyme) inhibitors. The development of this unique drug reads almost like a medical mystery. It all started with the venom of a poisonous Brazilian snake, the deadly jararaca, whose bite causes severe hemorrhaging. An extract from the venom was found to affect the kidney and ultimately blood pressure regulation. This led to the creation of enzyme blockers, such as **Capoten** and **Vasotec**, that are radically altering the treatment of hypertension and congestive heart failure.

Special Precautions: The very first dose of **Capoten** may cause dizziness, especially for older people, Be especially careful until your body adjusts.

When you first start taking **Capoten**, be alert for a rare but serious reaction. Some people have experienced swelling of the face, lips, tongue, and throat, which can make breathing difficult if not impossible. This requires immediate emergency treatment.

Another uncommon but dangerous reaction is a drop in infection-fighting white blood cells. If you develop chills, fever, sore throat, and mouth sores, contact your physician promptly. Blood tests are required to detect this problem. This risk is greater for patients with certain predisposing conditions such as lupus, scleroderma, or kidney problems.

Capoten should not be taken by pregnant women in their second or third trimester unless there is no alternative. It may damage the fetus.

Taking the Medicine: The manufacturer recommends that **Capoten** be taken one hour before meals. Food can interfere with the absorption of this medicine, reducing the amount that gets into the bloodstream by up to 40 percent.

Do not stop taking **Capoten** suddenly, because this could lead to complications. If you must discontinue the drug, your physician will instruct you in tapering off gradually.

Side Effects and Interactions: **Capoten** can cause a number of uncomfortable side effects. Be alert for skin rash, itching, an annoying dry cough, fast or irregular heartbeats, chest pain, nausea, diarrhea, vomiting, insomnia, fatigue, dizziness, and headache. The skin may be more vulnerable to sunburn. An unusual adverse effect of **Capoten** may be loss of taste. Fortunately, this sense may return to normal after a few months. Report any symptoms or suspected side effects without delay.

People with kidney problems must be monitored extremely carefully, because **Capoten** can make kidney function worse. Even normal people should have their kidneys checked periodically.

A number of compounds can interact with **Capoten**, especially potassium and potassium-sparing diuretics. It is usually best to avoid potassium supplements, including low-sodium salt substitutes. Diuretics such as **Dyazide, Aldactazide,** and **Moduretic,** which preserve potassium, can also cause dangerous elevations in potassium.

Other drugs that can interact with **Capoten** include aspirin and the arthritis medicine **Indocin,** the gout medicine **Zyloprim,** and lithium for bipolar disorder. Check with your doctor and pharmacist to make sure **Capoten** is safe in combination with any other drugs you take.

Carafate

sucralfate

Overview: **Carafate** is a unique antiulcer medication that appears to work in part by forming a protective layer over stomach sores and speeding healing. It may also reduce some of the damage caused by irritating medicines such as aspirin and other anti-inflammatory arthritis drugs. **Carafate** can also be helpful in cases of severe heartburn called reflux esophagitis.

Special Precautions: Because aluminum makes up almost 20 percent of this compound, people with kidney disease or those who must rely on dialysis should be very cautious when taking **Carafate**. Kidney problems predispose people to aluminum toxicity, so such patients should use this ulcer medicine or any aluminum-containing antacid judiciously and only under careful medical supervision.

Taking the Medicine: The manufacturer recommends that **Carafate** be taken on an empty stomach. That usually means at least an hour before meals or two hours after eating. Antacids should not be taken at the same time you swallow **Carafate**. If such additional products become necessary, wait at least 30 minutes after swallowing **Carafate** before taking the antacid.

Side Effects and Interactions: Side effects associated with **Carafate** are uncommon. Some people have reported constipation, nausea, stomach upset, diarrhea, flatulence, and dry mouth. Other potential adverse reactions include rash, itching, dizziness, sleepiness or insomnia, headache, and back pain. Report any symptoms to your physician promptly.

Carafate is capable of interacting with a number of other medications. It may reduce the absorption of antibiotics like **Cipro, Floxin, Noroxin, Penetrex,** and tetracycline. **Carafate** may also affect such drugs as **Dilantin, Coumadin, Lanoxin, Tagamet,** and **Cuprimine**. Check with your pharmacist and physician for special instructions and precautions before taking any other medication.

Cardizem

diltiazem

Overview: **Cardizem** belongs to a class of medicines called calcium channel blockers. Because of their safety and effectiveness, these drugs have helped revolutionize the treatment of angina and high blood pressure.

Unlike certain other drugs in this class, **Cardizem** is not approved for treating irregular heart rhythms, but it is frequently prescribed to treat certain forms of angina and is a useful blood pressure drug.

Preliminary research suggests some calcium channel blockers may be able to prevent migraine headaches, ease nighttime leg cramps, relieve asthma brought on by exercise, and perhaps reduce atherosclerosis. **Cardizem** is being studied for its usefulness against tardive dyskinesia and Raynaud's disease.

Special Precautions: People with liver or kidney disease should use **Cardizem** only under close medical supervision. Careful monitoring is essential in such cases due to an increased risk of toxicity. Low blood pressure or a recent heart attack also signal serious problems.

Taking the Medicine: The manufacturer recommends that **Cardizem** be taken before meals and at bedtime. This usually means at least one hour before meals or two hours after eating.

A long-acting formulation, **Cardizem SR**, needs to be taken only twice daily.

Cardizem CD is a once-a-day formulation. The company does not provide guidelines on how these long-lasting pills should be swallowed with regard to meals. Check with your pharmacist for specific instructions. **Cardizem SR** has been approved only for treatment of high blood pressure, while **Cardizem CD** is also prescribed for angina.

Do not stop taking **Cardizem** suddenly, because this could lead to complications. Your doctor will tell you how to taper off gradually if you no longer need this medication.

Side Effects and Interactions: **Cardizem** is usually well tolerated with few side effects, but some people react to this drug with fluid retention, leading to swelling of the legs, feet, or hands. Another reaction to be alert for is low blood pressure, which may show up as light-headedness and dizziness. Headache, dizziness, loss of strength, slowed heart rate, or flushing may also occur. Although quite uncommon, other side effects include nausea, constipation, rash, heart problems, and changes in gait. The skin may be especially sensitive to sunburn, and precautions should be taken to avoid ultraviolet exposure. Report any symptoms or suspected side effects to your physician promptly.

Cardizem can interact with a number of other drugs, including several that are used to treat high blood pressure or heart conditions, the anticonvulsant **Tegretol**, the asthma medicine theophylline, tuberculosis medicines containing rifampin, and the transplant drug **Sandimmune**. Check with your doctor and pharmacist to make sure **Cardizem** is safe in combination with any other drugs you take.

Ceclor

cefaclor

Overview: **Ceclor** is one of the most commonly prescribed antibiotics in the United States. Its popularity is due largely to the drug's broad-spectrum activity against a wide range of bacteria. It is highly effective against many germs that cause skin and ear infections, pneumonia, bronchitis, sinusitis, and urinary tract infections.

Ceclor belongs to a class of medicines referred to as cephalosporins. These medicines were originally discovered in one of the world's most unlikely locations. A fungus found close to a sewer outlet along the coast of Sardinia turned out to cure a number of nasty infections. From this chance observation many extraordinary antibiotics have been developed.

Special Precautions: If you are allergic to penicillin-type antibiotics, alert your physician immediately. Some people who are sensitive to penicillin may also react to **Ceclor.** Symptoms such as breathing difficulty, wheezing, sneezing, hives, itching, and skin rash require immediate emergency treatment. Life-threatening anaphylactic shock may produce an inability to breathe, and cardiovascular collapse can occur within minutes of exposure.

People with kidney disease should take **Ceclor** only under careful medical supervision. Special dosage modifications will have to be made. This medicine may also cause a false-positive test for sugar in the urine with **Clinitest** tablets or similar products.

Prolonged use of an antibiotic like **Ceclor** sometimes leads to an overgrowth of fungus or resistant bacteria known as superinfection. If this occurs, the doctor may need to have you discontinue **Ceclor** and take a different medication.

Taking the Medicine: Although this antibiotic is absorbed more efficiently when it is taken on an empty stomach, the pills may be swallowed with food, especially if they upset your stomach. Be sure to finish the entire prescription unless your doctor directs you to stop.

Side Effects and Interactions: Side effects from cephalosporin antibiotics are generally mild. Nevertheless, be alert for skin rash, itching, arthritis or joint pain, fever, fluid retention, swollen glands, diarrhea, nausea, stomach upset, or vaginitis. Headache, dizziness, or confusion are unlikely, but have been reported.

If this medicine has to be taken for long periods of time, your physician will probably want to order periodic blood tests. Remember to report any symptoms or suspected side effects to your physician promptly.

Oral blood-thinners such as **Coumadin** interact with medications related to **Ceclor**. Prudence suggests careful monitoring of bleeding time if these drugs must be taken together.

Ceftin

cefuroxime axetil

Overview: **Ceftin** is a highly effective, broad-spectrum antibiotic that works against bacteria that cause a wide range of common problems. This drug is especially beneficial for skin, ear, and lung infections. It can help cure pneumonia, bronchitis, sinusitis, and cystitis.

Ceftin belongs to a class of medicines called cephalosporins, which were originally discovered in one of the world's most unlikely locations. A fungus found close to a sewer outlet along the coast of Sardinia turned out to cure a number of nasty infections. From this chance observation many extraordinary antibiotics have been developed.

Special Precautions: If you are allergic to penicillin-type antibiotics, alert your physician immediately. Some people who are sensitive to penicillin may also react to **Ceftin**. Symptoms such as breathing difficulty, wheezing, sneezing, hives, itching, and skin rash require immediate emergency treatment. Life-threatening anaphylactic shock may produce an inability to breathe and cardiovascular collapse, and can occur within minutes of exposure.

People with kidney or liver disease may need special medical supervision when they take **Ceftin**. This medicine may also cause a false positive test for sugar in the urine with **Clinitest** tablets or similar products.

Prolonged use of an antibiotic such as **Ceftin** sometimes leads to an overgrowth of fungus or resistant bacteria known as superinfection. If this occurs, the doctor may need to have you discontinue **Ceftin** and take a different medication.

Taking the Medicine: Unlike many antibiotics, this medicine gets into the bloodstream more efficiently when it is taken with food. Although it can be swallowed on an empty stomach, we recommend taking **Ceftin** at mealtime to reduce stomach upset and enhance drug absorption. Be sure to finish the entire prescription unless your doctor directs you to stop.

Side Effects and Interactions: Side effects from cephalosporin antibiotics are generally mild. Nevertheless, diarrhea can be troubling for some people and in rare instances may develop into colitis. Other reactions that have occasionally been reported with **Ceftin** include nausea, vomiting, vaginitis, itching, rash, stomachache, dizziness, and headache.

If this medicine has to be taken for long periods of time, your physician will probably want to order periodic blood tests. Remember to report any symptoms or suspected side effects of **Ceftin** to your physician promptly.

Oral blood-thinners such as **Coumadin** interact with medications related to **Ceftin**. Prudence suggests careful monitoring of bleeding time if these drugs must be taken together.

Cipro

ciprofloxacin

Overview: **Cipro** belongs to a class of potent antibiotics called quinolones. These drugs have become quite popular in recent years because they can help cure a wide variety of infections. Side effects are uncommon and bacteria appear slower to develop resistance to such medications. **Cipro** is especially useful against hard-to-treat infections that affect the lungs, urinary tract, skin, bones, and joints. This antibiotic also works against traveler's diarrhea and other bugs that invade the digestive tract.

Special Precautions: Pregnant women and children should not take **Cipro**. Others may be allergic to this medication. If you experience symptoms such as breathing difficulty, wheezing, sneezing, hives, or itching, obtain emergency medical attention. Life-threatening anaphylactic shock is rare, but it demands instant treatment.

People with kidney disease should take **Cipro** only under careful medical supervision, because special dosage modifications may have to be made. Liver enzyme elevations have also been noted, so periodic blood tests will be necessary if you have to take this medicine for any length of time.

Taking the Medicine: **Cipro** is absorbed more efficiently when it is taken on an empty stomach. The manufacturer recommends that it be swallowed two hours after a meal. If this medicine upsets your stomach, though, it may be swallowed with food without losing potency.

Side Effects and Interactions: **Cipro** may cause light-headedness. Do not drive or attempt any activity that requires coordination and judgment if you become impaired. Some people report restlessness, insomnia, nightmares, dizziness, tremor, headache, or irritability while taking this medicine. Such symptoms can be made worse by coffee or the asthma medicine theophylline. **Cipro** affects the liver and may allow caffeine and theophylline to build up to toxic levels in the body.

Because **Cipro** may cause digestive tract upset, nausea, pain, or diarrhea, you may be tempted to use an antacid. That could be a big mistake. Aluminum- or calcium-based products, including **Di-Gel, Gaviscon, Maalox, Mylanta**, and **Tums**, can dramatically interfere with the absorption of **Cipro**. Wait at least two hours after taking **Cipro** before swallowing an antacid. Vitamin and mineral formulas can also cause problems, so they should not be taken at the same time either.

Other side effects are rare, but be alert for changes in vision, rash, sores in the mouth, joint pain or stiffness, chest pain or heart palpitations, urinary changes, or breathing difficulty. Report any symptoms or suspected side effects to your physician promptly.

Claritin

loratidine

Overview: **Claritin** is the third of a new generation of allergy medicines called histamine H_1 receptor antagonists. These nonsedating antihistamines are changing the way doctors control allergy symptoms. Until these drugs became available, virtually all oral allergy medicines caused some degree of sedation. This made driving or operating machinery dangerous.

Nonsedating antihistamines such as **Claritin** now provide many people management of symptoms such as sneezing or hives without reducing alertness or coordination. And unlike other allergy medicine, **Claritin** does not appear to interact with sedatives.

Special Precautions: Antihistamines should be avoided for several days before allergy skin testing, because they could interfere with the results. People with liver problems should get a reduced dose of **Claritin**, as they process it less efficiently.

Recent animal research suggests that **Claritin** and other antihistamines may promote tumor growth. We hope that further research will clarify this risk. People with cancer or at high risk of cancer should discuss this animal data with their physicians.

Taking the Medicine: **Claritin** is a long-acting antihistamine. One tablet daily will provide 24-hour coverage. **Claritin** should be taken on an empty stomach—that means at least one hour before or two hours after eating a meal.

Side Effects and Interactions: Side effects with **Claritin** are not common, but people have reported headache, fatigue, drowsiness, and dry mouth. Other potential reactions include weight gain, blurred vision, weakness, dizziness, nausea, anxiety, depression, impotence, and menstrual changes. Report any symptoms to your doctor.

Certain drugs can interact with **Claritin** to raise blood levels of the antihistamine. **Nizoral** is known to boost blood levels of **Claritin**, but no changes in heart rhythm or electrocardiogram (ECG) were noted as a result. In general, it would be wise to check with your doctor or pharmacist if you must take **Claritin** in combination with a medicine known to interact with the similar drugs **Hismanal** and **Seldane**. These include erythromycin (**E.E.S.**, **E-Mycin, ERYC, Ery-Tab, Erythrocin Stearate**, etc.), **Biaxin**, and **Sporanox**. The manufacturer cannot rule out potential interactions with **Tagamet**, theophylline, or **Zantac**. Check with your pharmacist and physician to make sure **Claritin** is safe in combination with any other drugs you take.

Cognex

tacrine

Overview: Although **Cognex** is by no means a brand-new drug, it has only recently been approved for the treatment of Alzheimer's disease. This medication is not a cure, and not all patients respond well. For some, however, **Cognex** can slow the mental deterioration associated with this dread disease. A smaller proportion, perhaps 5 or 10 percent, may experience dramatic improvement. These individuals may regain the ability to recognize family members or to participate in the daily life of the family—feeding and dressing themselves, for example. Such improvements, while not permanent, are usually welcome.

Special Precautions: Response to **Cognex** seems to improve as the dose increases. Some individuals cannot tolerate **Cognex**, however, especially at higher doses. Reversible liver enzyme elevations have occurred. Patients on **Cognex** should have liver function monitored on a regular basis. People with liver problems may require closer supervision.

Taking the Medicine: Because food reduces the absorption of **Cognex,** the medicine should be taken on an empty stomach (one hour before meals or two hours after). It is best taken at the same time each day to maintain consistent blood levels. Discontinuing this medicine abruptly may worsen the patient's condition noticeably, so if the medicine must be stopped, check with the doctor about how to withdraw gradually.

Side Effects and Interactions: **Cognex** can cause a number of side effects, which are more common at higher doses. The most common include elevated liver enzymes, nausea and vomiting, diarrhea, muscle aches, loss of appetite, and trouble walking. Chills, fever, nervousness, fainting, headache, dizziness, swelling of the feet and legs, excessive sweating, and increased urination have also been reported. Slower heart rate, increased stomach acid, breathing difficulties, and convulsions could cause special problems in people with preexisting conditions such as heart disease, ulcers, asthma, or epilepsy.

Notify the doctor immediately if the patient develops a rash, yellow eyes or skin, or very pale or black tarry stools, or if he or she begins vomiting material resembling coffee grounds. These could indicate a serious adverse reaction.

If a person on **Cognex** needs an operation, be sure to tell the surgeon about the medication, because it could alter the response to drugs used in surgery. **Cognex** slows the body's elimination of the asthma drug theophylline and blood levels can double. If both drugs are needed, the doctor should monitor theophylline blood levels and adjust the dose if necessary.

Any gastrointestinal side effects should be treated cautiously, because some common stomach medicines, such as **Pro-Banthine**, are likely to interact with **Cognex**. In addition, **Tagamet** can increase the amount of **Cognex** circulating in the body. Because **Cognex** has not been widely prescribed for very long, there may be other drug interactions that have not yet been identified. Ask your doctor and pharmacist to check whether any other drug that must be taken is safe in combination with **Cognex**.

Corgard

nadolol

Overview: **Corgard** is known as a beta-blocker. That means the drug works in part by blunting the action of adrenaline, the body's natural fight-or-flight chemical. People normally respond to stressful situations with a rapid pulse, a pounding heart and an increase in blood pressure. **Corgard** helps block such reactions.

This medicine is normally prescribed for hypertension or chest pain caused by angina. Although the FDA has not specifically approved its use for other purposes, doctors have prescribed **Corgard** to treat glaucoma, irregular heart rhythms, tremor, bleeding from the esophagus, and performance anxiety such as stage fright. It has also been used to help prevent migraine headaches. The dose will vary depending upon the condition being treated.

Special Precautions: Some people should rarely, if ever, take beta-blockers such as **Corgard**. Asthmatics and patients with other respiratory problems are especially vulnerable, because these drugs can make breathing worse. People with heart failure must also be extremely cautious if prescribed beta-blockers because the medicine could lead to cardiac complications.

Never stop taking any beta-blocker medication abruptly unless you are under very close medical supervision. Angina or a heart attack could occur. These drugs may also make treatment of diabetes and thyroid disorders more complicated. Your doctor can tell you what additional tests and precautions you will need in managing these conditions.

Taking the Medicine: **Corgard** can be taken at mealtime or on an empty stomach. If you find this medicine causes digestive tract upset, it may be better tolerated when taken with food. Because of its long duration of action in the body, **Corgard** offers the convenience of once-daily dosing.

Side Effects and Interactions: **Corgard** can cause a number of side effects, including slow heart rate, cold hands and feet, insomnia, nightmares, blurred vision, and sexual difficulties. Symptoms of nerve tingling, dizziness, nausea, stomachache, gas, diarrhea, indigestion, rash, arthritis, and muscle pain trouble some people. This medicine may also have a negative effect on cholesterol and other blood fats, so a lipid test before treatment and periodically thereafter would be prudent.

Although **Corgard** is a little less likely to affect the nervous system than certain other drugs in this class, be alert for the beta-blocker blahs. Symptoms of psychological depression, fatigue, decreased concentration, memory loss, and mood swings may come on slowly and insidiously. Notify your physician promptly of any adverse reactions, especially breathing difficulties, fluid retention in the legs, or a night cough.

Corgard can interact with a number of other compounds, including several that are used to treat asthma, colds, allergies, diabetes, migraines, and heart problems. **Corgard** and the blood pressure medicine **Catapres** may not mix well, but neither one should be stopped suddenly. An allergic reaction to penicillin or ampicillin may be more severe in an individual taking **Corgard**. Arthritis medicine and aspirin may reduce its effectiveness. A barbiturate such as **Fiorinal** or a tuberculosis medicine such as **Rifadin** could also interfere with **Corgard**'s effectiveness. Check with your doctor and pharmacist to make sure **Corgard** is safe in combination with any other drugs you may take.

Coumadin

warfarin

Overview: **Coumadin** is known as a blood thinner or anticoagulant. That means it is prescribed to prevent the formation or recurrence of blood clots. People who experience a pulmonary embolism or thrombophlebitis in their legs often receive **Coumadin** to reduce the risk of more serious complications. When clots are feared, this medicine may lower the likelihood of a heart attack or stroke.

Coumadin works by blocking key factors necessary for normal blood coagulation. Getting the right dose can be a very tricky process. Too little **Coumadin** may not allow for adequate clot protection, but too much could lead to life-threatening hemorrhage. Like Goldilocks and the porridge, it may take some experimentation to get things just right. That requires frequent blood tests for prothrombin (clotting) time, especially in the early phase of treatment.

Special Precautions: Anyone taking **Coumadin** must monitor his body carefully. Be alert for any early warning signs of bleeding. Symptoms to watch for include bruising or red spots under the skin, red or dark urine, red, black, or tarry stools, nosebleeds, or bleeding around the gums after gentle toothbrushing. Internal hemorrhaging may manifest itself in a variety of ways including pain in joints, chest, stomach, or head. Shortness of breath, difficulty breathing, or unexplained swelling could indicate bleeding. Alert your physician immediately if you notice any unusual symptoms or signs of spontaneous bleeding.

Taking the Medicine: Although the absorption of **Coumadin** may be slightly slowed by food, the medicine may be taken at mealtime, especially if it upsets your stomach. There are, however, certain foods that may reduce the effectiveness of this drug. Because vitamin K can counteract **Coumadin**'s action, be careful not to overdo on foods that are rich in this nutrient. These include broccoli, cabbage, spinach, collard greens, kale, brussels sprouts, and lettuce. This doesn't mean that you must avoid such healthy vegetables, but don't suddenly increase your intake without careful monitoring of prothrombin time. The same warning would hold if you suddenly eliminated one of these foods from your diet.

Side Effects and Interactions: Side effects of **Coumadin** therapy are uncommon if the dose is appropriate and the blood is carefully monitored. Some people have occasionally reported hair loss, skin rash, itching, nausea, fever, digestive upset, diarrhea, hepatitis, purple toes, red-orange urine, prolonged, painful erections, and mouth ulcers. Report any symptoms to your physician promptly.

A large number of over-the-counter and prescription medications may interact with **Coumadin** in a dangerous way. Some drugs, including barbiturates and the anticonvulsant **Tegretol** (carbamazepine), can reduce the effectiveness of **Coumadin** and increase the risk of blood clots. Others, such as the antibiotics metronidazole (**Flagyl**) or co-trimoxazole (**Bactrim, Septra**, etc.), can increase the blood-thinning potential of **Coumadin** and thereby raise the risk of dangerous bleeding. The drugs **Nolvadex** (tamoxifen) and **Danocrine** (danazol) can also increase susceptibility to hemorrhage when a woman is taking **Coumadin**. Because aspirin also acts as an anticoagulant, though it works differently from **Coumadin**, it should be avoided unless your doctor specifically prescribes it and monitors clotting time.

The heart drug **Cordarone** (amiodarone), the ulcer drug **Tagamet** (cimetidine), anabolic steroids such as **Anadrol-50** (oxymetholone), and antibiotics such as **Biaxin** (clarithromycin), erythromycin, or tetracycline can also make bleeding more hazardous for people on **Coumadin**. Some individuals may also be vulnerable to increased bleeding when they take the new antidepressants **Paxil** (paroxetine), **Prozac** (fluoxetine) or **Zoloft** (sertraline). Also beware of quinine derivatives, including heart medicines.

Patients should also be wary of taking thyroid drugs, cholesterol medications, and tuberculosis medicines in combination with **Coumadin**. Vitamins E and K could also be problematic. As a general rule, do not take any other medication without first checking with your physician and pharmacist.

Darvocet-N 100

propoxyphene napsylate plus acetaminophen

Overview: **Darvocet-N 100** is a popular pain reliever containing propoxyphene and acetaminophen. Propoxyphene, a mild synthetic analgesic, is almost as effective as codeine. In combination with acetaminophen, it offers relief for mild to moderate pain, such as that caused by a bad toothache or the aftermath of minor surgery.

Special Precautions: Like any narcotic, propoxyphene may make you drowsy. Do not drive or attempt any activity that requires coordination and judgment. Older people may be more susceptible to this reaction. Light-headedness or dizziness could make walking dangerous. Standing up suddenly could make you feel faint.

Taking the Medicine: Some people react to **Darvocet-N 100** with nausea or vomiting. Taking it with food may reduce stomach upset. Nausea, dizziness, and other common reactions may be less troublesome if you lie down for a while.

Side Effects and Interactions: Other side effects to be aware of include headache, euphoria, abdominal pain, sweating, and constipation. Some people experience shortness of breath, especially if they have asthma. Other less common reactions include skin rash, disorientation, dry mouth, visual problems, and urinary difficulties. Report any such symptoms to your physician promptly.

Long-term use of **Darvocet-N 100** has drawbacks. Like any narcotic, it may be habit-forming if you take it regularly in large doses. Do not increase the dose on your own in a quest to achieve greater pain relief. But don't play the hero by skipping doses during an acute crisis. Pain is more easily managed if it can be nipped in the bud instead of trying to play catch-up when it has gotten out of control.

Acetaminophen and propoxyphene may both cause liver problems in large doses or over long periods, so liver function should be monitored. As kidney damage is also a potential risk, your physician should evaluate your need for this combination pain reliever periodically.

If you are taking any other medicines, check with a physician or pharmacist. Alcohol as well as certain over-the-counter and prescription drugs can add to the sedative effect of this analgesic. Antihistamines, antianxiety agents, antidepressants, and sleeping pills can all cause drowsiness and might make this effect worse. An anticonvulsant such as **Dilantin** (phenytoin) could increase the risk of liver trouble for patients on **Darvocet-N 100.**

DiaBeta

glyburide

Overview: **DiaBeta** is used together with diet and exercise to control non–insulin-dependent, or Type II, diabetes. This condition, formerly called "adult-onset" diabetes, seems to result when the body does not respond adequately to insulin made by the pancreas. This pill seems to stimulate the pancreas to make more insulin and encourages greater sensitivity to insulin in the body.

Special Precautions: **DiaBeta** must not be taken by people who are allergic to sulfa drugs. Your doctor will need frequent blood tests to adjust the dose of **DiaBeta** when you begin taking it. Illness or a change in your exercise program may also make it necessary to adjust the dose later on.

Taking the Medicine: **DiaBeta** may be taken with food, especially if it upsets your stomach. The manufacturer suggests that it be taken with breakfast or the first meal of the day.

Side Effects and Interactions: Episodes of dangerously low blood sugar, or hypoglycemia, are a hazard with **DiaBeta** as with any oral diabetes drug. Be alert for symptoms of fatigue, shakiness, headache, cold sweat, or confusion, because they could signal this hazardous reaction. Be sure to discuss the symptoms and treatment of hypoglycemia with your health care provider.

Other possible side effects of this medication include nausea, heartburn, skin rash, changes in liver enzymes, susceptibility to sunburn, ringing in the ears, and blood changes. Fever, sore throat, and bruising or bleeding could signal a rare but serious reaction that requires immediate attention. Report any symptoms or suspected side effects without delay.

A number of compounds may interact with **DiaBeta**. Alcohol should be avoided if you are on this drug, because it could cause low blood sugar. Other drugs that might lead to drops in blood sugar include large doses of aspirin, the ulcer drugs **Tagamet** and **Zantac**, the cholesterol medicine **Lopid,** and the MAO-inhibitor antidepressant **Nardil**. Be aware that a magnesium-based antacid such as **Maalox** or a laxative such as milk of magnesia could boost the power of **DiaBeta** and lead to unexpectedly low blood sugar levels.

Many blood pressure pills and heart medicines may also interact with **DiaBeta**. Of special concern are the beta-blockers such as **Corgard, Inderal,** or **Tenormin**, because they may mask the warning symptoms of hypoglycemia. Thiazide diuretics such as **HydroDIURIL** or **Lozol** can raise blood sugar and may interfere with **DiaBeta**'s effects. Check with your doctor and pharmacist to make sure **DiaBeta** is safe in combination with any other drugs you take.

Dilantin

phenytoin

Overview: Dilantin is one of the oldest and best-studied antiseizure medications on the market. Although it was first developed in 1908, the drug's ability to prevent epilepsy wasn't discovered until 1938.

Dilantin works in part by stabilizing nerve cells and making them less excitable. It also exerts a similar action in the heart and is sometimes prescribed for irregular rhythms or a painful nerve condition that affects the face called trigeminal neuralgia.

Special Precautions: Determining the proper dose of **Dilantin** is not always easy. Some individuals metabolize this medicine more rapidly than normal and may need higher amounts. Others, especially older people or those with liver problems, may need lower doses or a different antiseizure medication to avoid toxicity. Periodic blood tests can help determine if the dose is appropriate.

Diabetics will need to be even more careful than usual in monitoring blood sugar. **Dilantin** may interfere with normal control.

Taking the Medicine: **Dilantin** is best taken at mealtime to increase absorption and reduce the risk of stomach upset. Do not swallow your pill with milk, however, or take it at the same time you eat foods high in calcium, because this mineral may reduce the effectiveness of your medicine.

Side Effects and Interactions: **Dilantin** can cause a number of side effects, which are more common at higher doses. Symptoms to be alert for include slurred speech, confusion, clumsiness, tremor, poor coordination, dizziness, drowsiness, uncontrollable eye movements, blurred vision, muscle twitching, insomnia, headaches, nervousness, and hyperactivity. If these adverse reactions do not disappear within a few weeks of starting therapy, contact your physician promptly and request a blood test.

If you develop a skin rash call your doctor immediately. This side effect usually calls for the discontinuation of the medicine, though this may require a gradual tapering of the dose and the substitution of another drug. Other less common side effects include chest pain, nausea, diarrhea or constipation, water retention, numbness or tingling of hands and feet, hair loss, fever, blood changes, weight gain, and liver problems. Some women note unwanted hair growth on their faces or bodies. Report any symptoms to your physician promptly.

Many people who take **Dilantin** for long periods of time experience overgrowth of the gums (called gingival hyperplasia). In this case practicing good dental hygiene is especially important. Frequent dental visits are advisable.

A large number of over-the-counter and prescription medications may interact with **Dilantin** in a dangerous way. This anticonvulsant can interfere with the transplant drug **Sandimmune**, increasing the risk of rejection. Certain other anticonvulsants may increase **Dilantin**'s toxicity, as may **Prozac** or related antidepressants. Some drugs, such as theophylline or tuberculosis drugs, can reduce the effectiveness of **Dilantin** and make people more vulnerable to seizures. In addition, **Dilantin** can interfere with the effectiveness of many other medications, including doxycycline, birth control pills, and the heart medicine **Cordarone**.

Other drugs that interact with **Dilantin** include alcohol, calcium-based antacids, pain relievers containing acetaminophen, folic acid, quinidine heart drugs, the blood thinner **Coumadin**, certain antidepressants, and the ulcer medicines **Tagamet** and **Prilosec**. Do not take any other medication without first checking with your physician and pharmacist.

Duricef

cefadroxil

Overview: **Duricef** belongs to a class of potent antibiotics called cephalosporins. It may also be prescribed as **Ultracef**. This drug works against a wide variety of germs, including staphylococcus and Group A beta-hemolytic streptococcus. It is used to treat infections of the urinary tract, skin, throat, and tonsils.

Cephalosporins are broad-spectrum medicines that were originally discovered in one of the world's most unlikely locations. A fungus found close to a sewer outlet along the coast of Sardinia turned out to cure a number of nasty infections. From this chance observation many extraordinary antibiotics have been developed.

Special Precautions: If you are allergic to penicillin-type antibiotics, alert your physician immediately. Some people who are sensitive to penicillin may also react to cephalosporins such as **Duricef**. Symptoms such as breathing difficulty, wheezing, sneezing, hives, itching, and skin rash require immediate emergency treatment. Life-threatening anaphylactic shock may produce an inability to breathe, and cardiovascular collapse can occur within minutes of exposure. If you have reacted to another cephalosporin, such as **Keflex**, you should avoid **Duricef**.

People with kidney problems should receive **Duricef** only under careful medical supervision, because the dosage will most likely have to be modified to prevent toxicity.

Taking the Medicine: **Duricef** may be taken with or without food. It may cause less stomach upset if taken with meals.

Side Effects and Interactions: Side effects from cephalosporin-type antibiotics are generally mild. Nevertheless, **Duricef** can cause digestive-tract discomfort, with diarrhea, nausea, or vomiting. If you develop diarrhea, contact your physician, because it may be a warning of drug-induced colitis.

Other infrequent reactions to be aware of include rash, itching, swelling of the face and throat, vaginitis, and yeast infections. **Duricef** may affect laboratory test results. Liver enzymes may become elevated and false-positive results may show up on a blood test for certain anemias or lupus. Make sure that the laboratory personnel are aware you are taking **Duricef** if you have blood drawn. And remember to report any symptoms or suspected side effects of cefadroxil to your physician promptly.

Dyazide

hydrochlorothiazide plus triamterene

Overview: **Dyazide** is a diuretic, or water pill, that has long been a staple of treatment for high blood pressure. This medication has been available about 30 years. **Dyazide** has maintained its popularity because of its ability to keep potassium in the system. Many other diuretics deplete the body of this essential mineral.

Special Precautions: Because diuretics may increase cholesterol levels, it is wise to have a blood test before starting on this medicine and at periodic intervals to make sure this drug is not having an adverse effect upon blood fats.

Taking the Medicine: **Dyazide** is absorbed more effectively when it is taken with meals, especially if the food is a little high in fat. Because of its potassium-sparing effects, avoid using a potassium-based salt substitute on your food. This could lead to a dangerous overload of the mineral. Likewise, potassium supplements should be avoided unless specifically recommended by your physician. Periodic blood tests are crucial to monitor potassium levels in the body.

Side Effects and Interactions: Diuretics such as **Dyazide** are generally well tolerated. Although side effects are relatively rare, be alert for symptoms such as upset stomach, cramps, loss of appetite, and diarrhea. Increased frequency of urination is common but may be less bothersome if you take your medicine at breakfast rather than at night.

Infrequent adverse reactions include sensitivity to sunlight leading to sunburn, dizziness or faintness if you stand up suddenly, rash, unexplained sore throat with fever, bruising, blurred vision, sexual difficulties, increases in blood sugar, headache, and gout. Report any symptoms to your physician promptly.

Dyazide can interact with a number of other medications. Potassium supplements such as **K-Lor, Slow-K, K-Lyte,** and **Micro-K** are generally inappropriate in combination with **Dyazide**. Cholesterol-lowering medications such as **Questran, Cholybar,** or **Colestid** decrease absorption of **Dyazide.** The stomach and antiulcer medicine **Tagamet** can increase blood levels of **Dyazide,** with a greater possibility of side effects. Some compounds may become more toxic when combined with **Dyazide; Indocin** and **Symmetrel** are among these.

Other blood pressure drugs such as **Accupril, Altace, Capoten, Vasotec, Prinivil,** or **Zestril** can lead to dangerously high potassium levels in combination with **Dyazide.** Check with your doctor and pharmacist to make sure this medicine is safe in combination with any other drugs you take.

E-Mycin

erythromycin

Overview: **E-Mycin** is a broad-spectrum antibiotic that is effective against a large number of bacteria. It helps fight infections in many places in the body including the urinary, genital and digestive tracts, lungs, heart, ears, throat, and skin.

Special Precautions: Because **E-Mycin**, like other erythromycins, is eliminated from the body by the liver, this drug should be used very cautiously, if at all, by people with liver problems. Anyone with a history of allergy to erythromycin-type antibiotics should probably avoid **E-Mycin**. Symptoms of an allergic reaction include hives, rash, and itching. In rare instances allergy may trigger life-threatening anaphylactic shock.

Taking the Medicine: **E-Mycin** is an enteric-coated tablet and may be taken with or without food. Doses are usually spaced evenly throughout the day. Check with your physician or pharmacist for specific instructions.

Side Effects and Interactions: The most frequent side effects of erythromycin-type antibiotics involve digestive tract upset. Stomach pain and cramping are not uncommon. Nausea, vomiting, loss of appetite, and diarrhea can be troublesome for some people. Less common adverse reactions include jaundice, pale stools, confusion, hairy tongue, itching of the anus or vagina, and hearing loss, especially in older people or individuals with kidney problems. Report any symptoms to your physician promptly.

E-Mycin can interact with several other medicines including the asthma drug theophylline, the antiseizure medication **Tegretol**, the blood thinner **Coumadin**, the sleeping pill **Halcion**, and the migraine medicine ergotamine. It should not be taken by people who are also taking the antihistamines **Seldane** or **Hismanal**, because it could lead to a dangerous buildup of these drugs in the body. Check with your pharmacist and physician to make sure **E-Mycin** is safe in combination with any other drugs you take.

Effexor

venlafaxine

Overview: **Effexor** is one of the new generation of antidepressants. This medication affects many systems of chemical messengers (the neurotransmitters serotonin, norepinephrine, and dopamine) in the brain. Studies indicate that it is an effective first-line treatment for depression, with improvement often appearing by the second week of treatment.

Special Precautions: Some depressed people experience anxiety and insomnia as part of the symptoms of their condition. **Effexor** may exacerbate these problems in some patients. The drug may also worsen the manic phase for some manic-depressive individuals and so may not be appropriate for continued treatment.

Any medicine affecting the brain may have the potential to slow reflexes or impair judgment. Such problems did not appear significant in clinical trials, but patients are best advised not to drive or use hazardous machinery until they can determine (preferably through an objective assessment) that they are not adversely affected by **Effexor**.

As of this writing, **Effexor** is a new drug with relatively little data available. Studies have not established that it is effective for long-term use of more than six weeks. It is advisable for doctor and patient to reevaluate this therapy periodically to make sure that it continues to be appropriate.

Taking the Medicine: **Effexor** should be taken with food. The dosage should be individually adjusted and will determine whether **Effexor** is taken two or three times daily. When going off **Effexor**, a person should ask the doctor for guidelines on gradual withdrawal.

Side Effects and Interactions: The side effects of **Effexor** are similar, in general, to those of **Prozac** or similar antidepressants. Nausea, headache, anxiety or agitation, insomnia, drowsiness, excessive sweating, and loss of appetite were reported during clinical trials. Appetite problems may result in weight loss, which could be serious for an underweight patient. Dry mouth, constipation, tremor, and blurred vision are other possible side effects. **Effexor** may lead to increased blood pressure in some people, so blood pressure should be monitored. As with other antidepressants, a small number of patients on **Effexor** have experienced seizures. Report any symptoms or suspected side effects without delay.

Because of the possibility of a life-threatening interaction, **Effexor** should not be taken by anyone also taking **Nardil** or **Parnate**. A person who has been taking one of these antidepressants (MAO-inhibitor type) should wait at least 14 days after stopping it before beginning to take **Effexor**; after stopping **Effexor**, a person should wait 7 days before starting on an MAO inhibitor. **Tagamet** can slow removal of **Effexor** from the body, and a person who must take both may need a dosage adjustment. This is most likely to affect individuals with high blood pressure or liver problems, and the elderly. Certain other medications, such as quinidine, may increase blood levels of **Effexor**, but there is limited data on interactions, and there may be other drug interactions that have not yet been identified. Ask your doctor and pharmacist to check whether any other drug that must be taken is safe in combination with **Effexor**.

ERYC

erythromycin

Overview: **ERYC** is a broad-spectrum antibiotic that is effective against a large number of bacteria. It helps fight infections in many places in the body including the urinary, genital, and digestive tracts, lungs, heart, ears, throat, and skin.

Special Precautions: Because **ERYC**, like other erythromycins, is eliminated from the body by the liver, this drug should be used very cautiously, if at all, by people with liver problems. Anyone with a history of allergy to erythromycin-type antibiotics should probably avoid **ERYC**. Symptoms of an allergic reaction include hives, rash, and itching. In rare instances allergy may trigger life-threatening anaphylactic shock.

Taking the Medicine: **ERYC** is best absorbed when taken on an empty stomach. That means at least one hour before meals or two hours after eating. Doses are usually spaced evenly throughout the day. Check with your physician or pharmacist for specific instructions.

Side Effects and Interactions: The most frequent side effects of erythromycin-type antibiotics involve digestive-tract upset. Stomach pain and cramping are not uncommon. Nausea, vomiting, loss of appetite, and diarrhea can be troublesome for some people. Less common adverse reactions include jaundice, pale stools, confusion, hairy tongue, itching of the anus or vagina, and hearing loss, especially in older people or individuals with kidney problems. Report any symptoms to your physician promptly.

ERYC can interact with certain other medicines including the asthma drug theophylline, the antiseizure medication **Tegretol**, the blood thinner **Coumadin**, the sleeping pill **Halcion**, the heart medicine **Lanoxin**, and the migraine medicine ergotamine. It should not be taken by people who are also taking the antihistamines **Seldane** or **Hismanal**, because it could lead to a dangerous buildup of these drugs in the body. Check with your pharmacist and physician to make sure **ERYC** is safe in combination with any other drugs you take.

Erythrocin Stearate

erythromycin stearate

Overview: **Erythrocin** is a broad-spectrum antibiotic that is effective against a large number of bacteria. It helps fight infections in many places in the body including the urinary, genital and digestive tracts, lungs, heart, ears, throat, and skin.

Special Precautions: Because erythromycin is eliminated from the body by the liver, this drug should be used very cautiously, if at all, by people with liver problems. Anyone with a history of allergy to erythromycin-type antibiotics should probably avoid **Erythrocin**. Symptoms of an allergic reaction include hives, rash, and itching. In rare instances allergy may trigger life-threatening anaphylactic shock.

Taking the Medicine: **Erythrocin** is best swallowed on an empty stomach.

That means it should be taken at least one hour before meals or two hours after eating.

Side Effects and Interactions: The most frequent side effects of erythromycin-type antibiotics involve digestive-tract upset. Stomach pain and cramping are not uncommon. Nausea, vomiting, loss of appetite, and diarrhea can be troublesome for some people. Less common adverse reactions include jaundice, pale stools, confusion, hairy tongue, itching of the anus or vagina, and hearing loss, especially in older people or individuals with kidney problems. Report any symptoms to your physician promptly.

Erythrocin can interact with certain other medicines including the asthma drug theophylline, the antiseizure medication **Tegretol**, the blood thinner **Coumadin**, the heart medicine **Lanoxin**, the sleeping pill **Halcion**, and the migraine medicine ergotamine. It should not be taken by people who are also taking the antihistamines **Seldane** or **Hismanal**, because it could lead to a dangerous buildup of these drugs in the body. Check with your pharmacist and physician to make sure **Erythrocin** is safe in combination with any other drugs you take.

Estraderm

estradiol transdermal system

Overview: This unique skin patch is designed to release estrogen through the skin and into the body. It provides a long-lasting steady level of this female hormone. Each patch is effective for roughly half a week.

Estraderm is prescribed primarily to relieve menopausal symptoms such as hot flashes and to prevent postmenopausal bone loss. It can also be helpful in various conditions when a woman does not produce enough natural estrogen.

Special Precautions: There are a number of situations in which estrogen may be inappropriate. Pregnant women should not use this medication because it could affect the fetus. Women with a history of breast cancer or other malignant disease susceptible to estrogen should also generally avoid this hormone. Blood-clotting disorders such as thrombophlebitis are also a reason to be wary of estrogen.

Prolonged use of postmenopausal estrogen has been controversial because of questions about cancer. Endometrial carcinoma or cancer of the uterine lining is more of a risk for women exposed to estrogen. This adverse reaction may be counteracted by simultaneous administration of progestins. Vaginal bleeding could be an early warning sign of cancer and requires immediate medical attention.

The risk of breast cancer is more uncertain. Studies have provided conflicting results, and more research is needed. Women with a strong family history of breast cancer will want to discuss this issue with their doctor.

Estrogen therapy can affect thyroid-function tests, so if you need one, be sure to tell the laboratory technicians you are using **Estraderm**.

Taking the Medicine: After removing the patch from its pouch, place it on a clean, dry area of the body. Belly and buttocks are fine, but do not place it on the breasts. It's best to avoid the waistline or other places where tight clothing might rub the patch off. Each application lasts half a week; then a new patch is applied to a different spot.

Side Effects and Interactions: Side effects of **Estraderm** include redness and itching where the patch is applied. In addition, some women experience break-through menstrual bleeding, breast tenderness, bloating, nausea, vomiting, stomach pain, headache, fluid retention, gallbladder problems, liver tumors, jaundice, and high blood pressure. Susceptible women may experience an increase in blood sugar and go on to develop diabetes.

Some kinds of vaginal infections could be more common in women using estrogen. Candida or yeast overgrowth may be a problem. Other adverse reactions include a change in weight, alteration in sex drive, hair loss, and change in the curvature of the cornea. This may make contact lenses inappropriate.

Estraderm may interact with several other medications, such as **Dilantin**, **Mesantoin**, cortisone and other steroids, and certain antidepressants. Blood thinners such as **Coumadin** may be less effective. Check with your doctor and pharmacist before taking any other medicine while wearing an **Estraderm** patch.

furosemide

Lasix

Overview: Furosemide, sometimes prescribed under the brand name **Lasix**, is a potent diuretic, or water pill. It is used to treat high blood pressure as well as a number of serious conditions in which fluid builds up in body tissues.

Special Precautions: Like many diuretics, furosemide depletes the body of potassium and other important minerals. People taking this medicine may need to include potassium-rich foods in their diet. Vegetables such as potatoes, beets, brussels sprouts, spinach, cabbage, broccoli, carrots, peppers, and squash are good sources of potassium. So are apricots, strawberries, bananas, oranges, peaches, and plums. Most fish also provide good quantities of this mineral.

Some people may not be able to maintain adequate potassium levels even with a diet rich in fish, fruits, and vegetables. Periodic blood tests are crucial to monitor potassium levels in the body. If such a test shows that potassium levels are low, your physician may recommend you cook with a potassium-based salt substitute or he may prescribe a potassium supplement.

Taking the Medicine: Furosemide is absorbed most completely when it is taken on an empty stomach. This medication may cause stomach upset, however, which tends to be less of a problem when it is taken with food or milk. Because the dose should be adjusted individually, with the help of blood tests, let your doctor know if you will change the way you take this drug.

Side Effects and Interactions: People on furosemide may feel dizzy or faint if they stand up rapidly. Older people especially may need to take care to avoid falling when they first get up. Increased frequency of urination is common but may be less bothersome if you take your medicine at breakfast rather than at night.

Other adverse reactions to be alert for include rash, itching, sensitivity to sunlight leading to sunburn, ringing in the ears, nausea, diarrhea or constipation, muscle cramps, hearing loss, unexplained sore throat with fever, bruising, blurred vision, loss of appetite, increases in blood sugar, headache, gout, and tingling or numbness in hands or feet. Report any symptoms to your physician promptly.

Furosemide can interact with a number of other medications. **Lanoxin** and other digitalis heart medicines may cause abnormal heart rhythms if potassium levels are decreased by diuretics. **Indocin, Clinoril,** ibuprofen, **Dilantin,** and activated charcoal may interfere with the effectiveness of furosemide. At high doses, furosemide can increase the activity of the blood thinner **Coumadin.** Adding furosemide to thiazide diuretics may deplete the body rapidly of fluid and minerals, and calls for careful monitoring. Check with your doctor and pharmacist to make sure furosemide is safe in combination with any other drugs you take.

Glucotrol

glipizide

Overview: **Glucotrol** is used together with diet and exercise to control non–insulin-dependent, or Type II, diabetes, which was once called "adult-onset diabetes." This pill seems to stimulate the pancreas to make more insulin in response to a meal.

Special Precautions: **Glucotrol** must not be taken by people who are allergic to sulfa drugs. Your doctor will need frequent blood tests to adjust the dose of the medicine when you begin taking it. Illness or a change in your exercise program may also make it necessary to adjust the dose later on.

Taking the Medicine: For greatest effectiveness, **Glucotrol** should be taken approximately half an hour before a meal. Your doctor will tell you if you should take it once or twice a day.

Side Effects and Interactions: Episodes of dangerously low blood sugar, or hypoglycemia, are a hazard with **Glucotrol** as with any oral diabetes drug. Be alert for symptoms of fatigue, shakiness, headache, cold sweat or confusion, as they could signal this hazardous reaction. Be sure to discuss the symptoms and treatment of hypoglycemia with your health care provider.

Other possible side effects of this medication include nausea, diarrhea, dizziness, skin rash, drowsiness, stomachache, changes in liver enzymes, constipation, and blood changes. Fever, sore throat, and bruising or bleeding could signal a rare but serious reaction that requires immediate attention. Report any symptoms or suspected side effects without delay.

A number of compounds may interact with **Glucotrol**. Alcohol should be avoided if you are on this drug, because it could cause low blood sugar or uncomfortable skin flushing and breathlessness. Other drugs that could lead to drops in blood sugar include nonsteroidal arthritis medicines like **Motrin**, aspirin and similar medicines, and antidepressants such as **Nardil**.

Many blood pressure pills and heart medicines also interact with **Glucotrol**, including beta-blockers such as **Tenormin** and **Corgard** as well as calcium channel blockers such as **Procardia** or **Cardizem**. So may estrogen or thyroid hormones, corticosteroids, niacin used to lower cholesterol, and the seizure medication **Dilantin**. Check with your doctor and pharmacist before starting or stopping any other medication.

hydrochlorothiazide

HydroDIURIL

Esidrix

Oretic

Overview: Hydrochlorothiazide is one of the most frequently prescribed medications in the world. It is commonly found in combination blood pressure medicines.

Special Precautions: Like many diuretics, hydrochlorothiazide depletes the body of potassium and other important minerals. People taking this drug may need to include potassium-rich foods in their diet. Vegetables such as potatoes, beets, brussels sprouts, spinach, cabbage, broccoli, carrots, peppers, and squash are good sources of potassium. So are apricots, strawberries, bananas, oranges, peaches, and plums. Most fish also provide good quantities of this mineral.

Some people may not be able to maintain adequate potassium levels even with a diet rich in fish, fruits and vegetables. Periodic blood tests are crucial to monitor potassium levels in the body. If such a test shows that potassium levels are low, your physician may recommend a potassium-based salt substitute for food or he may prescribe either a potassium supplement or a combination medicine with a potassium-sparing component.

Because diuretics may increase cholesterol levels, it is wise to have a blood test before starting on this medicine and at periodic intervals to make sure this drug is not having an adverse effect upon blood fats.

Taking the Medicine: There is some controversy about the best way to swallow hydrochlorothiazide. Some researchers have found that it is absorbed best when it is taken with food, while others report that it is best taken on an empty stomach. This medication may cause stomach upset. If it does, we suggest you take it with food or milk.

Side Effects and Interactions: Diuretics such as hydrochlorothiazide are generally well tolerated. Although side effects are relatively rare, be alert for symptoms such as upset stomach, cramps, loss of appetite and diarrhea. Increased frequency of urination is common but may be less bothersome if you take your medicine at breakfast rather than in the evening, so you won't have to get up as much at night.

Infrequent adverse reactions include rash, itching, sensitivity to sunlight leading to sunburn, dizziness or faintness if you stand up suddenly, muscle cramps, unexplained sore throat with fever, bruising, blurred vision, sexual difficulties, increases in blood sugar, headache, and gout. Report any symptoms to your physician promptly.

Hydrochlorothiazide can interact with a number of other medications. Cholesterol-lowering drugs such as **Questran, Cholybar**, or **Colestid** decrease absorption of hydrochlorothiazide. **Lanoxin** and other digitalis heart medicines may cause abnormal heart rhythms if potassium levels are decreased by diuretics. While it can make blood sugar rise, hydrochlorothiazide can also interfere with oral diabetes pills such as **DiaBeta, Diabinese, Glucotrol**, or **Micronase** and make them less effective.

Adding hydrochlorothiazide to other diuretics such as **Lasix** may deplete the body rapidly of fluid and minerals, and calls for careful monitoring. Some compounds may become more toxic when combined with hydrochlorothiazide. Lithium, allopurinol (**Zyloprim** or **Lopurin**), and amantadine (**Symmetrel** or **Symadine**) are among these. Check with your doctor and pharmacist to make sure hydrochlorothiazide is safe in combination with any other drugs you take.

Hismanal

astemizole

Overview: **Hismanal** is the second of a new generation of allergy medicines called histamine (H_1) receptor antagonists. These nonsedating antihistamines are changing the way doctors control allergy symptoms. Until these drugs became available, virtually all oral allergy medicines caused some degree of sedation. This made driving or operating machinery dangerous.

Nonsedating antihistamines such as **Hismanal** now provide many people management of symptoms such as sneezing or hives without reducing alertness or coordination. And unlike other allergy medicine, **Hismanal** does not appear to interact with sedatives.

Special Precautions: If **Hismanal** is taken in overdose, irregular heart rhythms could occur. They may be quite dangerous. Never exceed the dose recommended by your physician, and avoid the drugs that interact with **Hismanal.** If you feel faint or experience heart palpitations, contact your doctor immediately as this could be a sign of heart rhythm disturbance.

Taking the Medicine: **Hismanal** is a long-acting antihistamine. One tablet daily will provide 24-hour coverage. **Hismanal** should be taken on an empty stomach, as food substantially interferes with absorption. That means at least one hour before or two hours after eating a meal.

Side Effects and Interactions: Side effects with **Hismanal** are relatively rare, but people occasionally report fatigue, nervousness, dry mouth, headache, nausea, dizziness, nosebleeds, breathing difficulty, depression, and increased appetite.

Weight gain has been noted in roughly 4 percent of patients in early trials. If you suddenly start to gain weight, it may be associated with this antihistamine. Report this or any other symptoms or suspected side effects to your physician promptly.

Certain drugs can greatly increase the danger of heart rhythm changes. Erythromycin (**E.E.S., E-Mycin, ERYC, Ery-Tab, Erythrocin Stearate**, etc.), **Biaxin, Sporanox, Luvox,** and **Nizoral** should generally be avoided by people taking **Hismanal**. If you need one of these important infection-fighters, ask your doctor if you should stop the **Hismanal.**

All of these medications affect an important enzyme in the liver (cytochrome P450 3A4) that is needed to metabolize the antihistamine. Grapefruit juice also affects this enzyme. Although we haven't yet heard of anyone landing in the hospital from this combination, we suggest you avoid grapefruit and grapefruit juice while you are taking **Hismanal**.

Certain other medications that can affect heart rhythm might make a person more vulnerable to problems while on **Hismanal**. Be sure to discuss this situation with your doctor before adding the cholesterol medicine **Lorelco**, a heart medicine designed to control rhythm disturbances (for example, **Betapace, Norpace, Cardioquin,** or **Procan SR**), or a medicine that is supposed to control hallucinations (**Haldol** or **Mellaril**).

hydrocodone with acetaminophen

Anexsia	Vicodin
Lorcet	Zydone
Lortab	

Overview: Hydrocodone is a semisynthetic analgesic similar in most respects to codeine. In combination with acetaminophen, it offers excellent relief for moderate pain. It can ease the discomfort of a bad toothache or the aftermath of minor surgery.

Hydrocodone with acetaminophen is sold under a number of names, including **Anexsia 5/500, Anodynos-DHC, Bancap, Co-Gesic, Dolacet, Duradyne DHC, Hydrocet, Lortab, Norcet, T-Gesic,** and **Zydone. Vicodin** is the most popular brand name for this medication.

Special Precautions: Like any narcotic, hydrocodone may make you drowsy. Do not drive or attempt any activity that requires coordination and judgment.

Older people may be more susceptible to this reaction. Light-headedness or dizziness could make walking dangerous. Never stand up suddenly because this may make you feel faint.

Long-term use of hydrocodone and acetaminophen has drawbacks. Hydrocodone, like other narcotics, may be habit-forming if you take it regularly. Do not increase the dose on your own in a quest to achieve greater pain relief. But don't play the hero by skipping doses during an acute crisis. Pain is more easily managed if it can be dealt with immediately instead of after it has gotten out of control.

Taking the Medicine: Some people react to hydrocodone with nausea or vomiting. Taking it with food may reduce stomach upset. Nausea, dizziness, and other common reactions may be less troublesome if you lie down for a while.

Side Effects and Interactions: Possible side effects to be aware of include weakness, euphoria, loss of appetite, sweating, and constipation. Some people experience shortness of breath, especially if they have asthma. Other less common reactions include an allergic rash, disorientation, dry mouth, and urinary difficulties. Report any such symptoms to your physician promptly.

Acetaminophen may cause liver or kidney problems in large doses or over long periods. Your physician should evaluate your need for this combination pain reliever periodically.

If you are taking any other medicines, check with a physician or pharmacist. Alcohol as well as many over-the-counter and prescription drugs can add to the sedative effect of this analgesic. Antihistamines, antianxiety agents, antidepressants, and sleeping pills require extra caution. Both tricyclic and MAO-type antidepressants may interact with this analgesic to cause greater toxicity, and the anticonvulsant **Dilantin** may increase the risk of liver damage.

Hytrin

terazosin

Overview: **Hytrin** is a blood pressure medicine that relaxes the muscles lining the blood vessels. This reduces their resistance to blood flow. This same action, of smooth muscle relaxation, is often helpful in managing the urinary difficulties that may result from an enlarged prostate gland (benign prostatic hypertrophy).

Special Precautions: **Hytrin** can cause a potentially dangerous "first-dose effect" soon after you begin taking it. A person may feel faint or dizzy, especially when he or she stands up from sitting or lying down. This is apparently due to excessive lowering of the blood pressure at first. Your doctor will probably start you on a low dose of **Hytrin** and gradually increase it to reduce this problem. Remember that if you miss a few doses, starting again could produce this first-dose effect. Avoid driving and other dangerous activities for at least 12 hours after your first pill or after resuming medication. Don't stand up suddenly without holding on to something.

Taking the Medicine: **Hytrin** is started as a 1-mg pill given at bedtime. The dose will be increased gradually until the response is satisfactory. Your doctor will tell you if you should take it once or twice a day.

Side Effects and Interactions: The most common side effects of **Hytrin** are light-headedness or dizziness when standing up from sitting or lying down. Even after you have been taking **Hytrin** for some time, this effect is more likely within the first few hours after swallowing the pill. Palpitations and occasionally fainting may also occur.

Other side effects include a feeling of tiredness or weakness, headaches, nausea, fluid buildup in arms and legs, weight gain, drowsiness, nasal stuffiness, and blurred vision. Tell your doctor about any symptoms you experience.

Few interactions have been reported between **Hytrin** and other drugs. If other blood pressure drugs must be added, keep in mind that the first-dose effect may crop up, and exercise precautions against fainting and falling.

ibuprofen

Advil	**Motrin IB**
Children's Advil	**Nuprin**
Excedrin IB	**Pamprin-IB**
Ibu-Tab	**PediaProfen**
Midol 200	**Rufen**
Motrin	**Trendar**

Overview: Ibuprofen is a pain reliever used primarily for arthritis. It may also be prescribed for menstrual cramps, bursitis, tendinitis, sprains, strains, and other painful conditions. It belongs to a class of medications commonly called NSAIDs or nonsteroidal anti-inflammatory drugs. It is now available generically, but previously it was one of the most popular arthritis drugs on the market under the brand name **Motrin**.

Ibuprofen may be prescribed generically or by brand names such as **Children's Advil, Ibu-Tab, Motrin,** or **Rufen**. It is also available without prescription under such names as **Advil, Bayer Select Pain Relief, Medipren, Nuprin,** or **Motrin IB**, among others.

Special Precautions: People who are allergic to aspirin or other anti-inflammatory agents should avoid ibuprofen. Signs of allergy include breathing difficulties, rash, fever, or a sudden drop in blood pressure, and require immediate medical attention.

Taking the Medicine: Because ibuprofen can be hard on the digestive tract, it may be taken with food to reduce stomach trouble. This does not guarantee, however, that the drug will be safe for the stomach. Alcohol may contribute to indigestion, ulcers, and irritation and should be avoided.

Side Effects and Interactions: Unquestionably the most common side effects of ibuprofen involve the gastrointestinal tract. They include nausea, indigestion, heartburn, cramps, gas, constipation, and diarrhea.

Some people may develop ulcers and intestinal bleeding while taking ibuprofen. Occasionally these problems can occur without obvious symptoms and lead to a life-threatening crisis due to perforation of the stomach lining.

Older people appear to be more susceptible to this problem and should be monitored carefully. Warning signs include weight loss, persistent indigestion, a feeling of fullness after moderate meals, dark or tarry stools, anemia, and unusual fatigue. Home stool tests such as **Hemoccult** or **Fleet Detecatest** may provide an early indication of bleeding.

Other side effects to be alert for include headache, ringing in the ears, rash, itching, nervousness, fluid retention, and loss of appetite. Drowsiness, dizziness, light-headedness, and confusion are possible, so do not drive if you become impaired.

Less common adverse reactions include insomnia, heart palpitations, hair loss, depression, tiredness, anemia or other blood changes, fever, visual disturbances, meningitis, and sores in the mouth. Some people might become sensitive to sunlight while on ibuprofen, so use an effective sunscreen or stay well covered. Report any symptoms to your physician promptly. Ibuprofen can affect both the kidney and liver, so periodic blood tests to monitor the function of these organs are important for anyone on this drug long-term.

This medication can adversely interact with many other drugs. A person taking a blood thinner such as **Coumadin** may become far more vulnerable to a dangerous bleeding ulcer. Aspirin may reduce the effectiveness of ibuprofen for reducing inflammation. All the NSAIDs, including ibuprofen, can make methotrexate (**Folex, Mexate, Rheumatrex**) and lithium (**Eskalith, Lithobid**, etc.) far more toxic. Other potentially serious interactions may occur with ibuprofen reducing the effectiveness of ACE-inhibitor blood pressure medicines such as **Altace, Lotensin,** or **Vasotec;** beta-blocker blood pressure drugs such as **Corgard, Inderal,** or **Tenormin**; and diuretics such as **Bumex, Dyazide, Lasix,** or **Maxzide.** Check with your pharmacist and physician to make sure ibuprofen is safe in combination with any other drugs you take.

Imitrex

sumatriptan

Overview: **Imitrex** is an injection administered either by the physician or by the patient him- or herself. It works through serotonin receptors to cause constriction of blood vessels to the brain. This in turn stops a migraine in progress.

This subcutaneous injection is extremely effective in relieving the symptoms of migraine. Two hours after the injection, over 80 percent of patients receiving **Imitrex** have substantial pain relief, compared to only 30 to 40 percent of those receiving a placebo injection. The autoinjector device used by patients is apparently easy to master.

This medication is also available in an oral formulation.

Special Precautions: **Imitrex** should not be injected in people with heart disease, whether they have had angina or a heart attack, or have been told they have silent ischemia. Because it could cause coronary blood-vessel spasm, a life-threatening condition, it should never be injected intravenously. **Imitrex** may also raise blood pressure and should not be given to anyone with uncontrolled hypertension. There is some controversy about how well it can be determined who has heart disease and therefore should not get **Imitrex**. (See page 187.)

The diagnosis of migraine should be confirmed with care before **Imitrex** is administered, because it can be dangerous if given to people with other neurological problems. **Imitrex** is inappropriate for basilar or hemiplegic migraine.

Taking the Medicine: **Imitrex** is injected just below the skin, preferably as soon as the symptoms of a migraine are recognized. If necessary, a second injection may be administered at least one hour later. Do not exceed more than two 6-mg injections in a 24-hour day. **Imitrex** should be stored between 36 and 86 degrees Fahrenheit away from light.

Side Effects and Interactions: **Imitrex** may produce a number of side effects, including most commonly a reaction at the injection site. Chest, jaw, or neck tightness; a sensation of tingling; a warm, hot, or burning sensation; sensations of pressure, heaviness, or tightness; flushing, fatigue, dizziness, and drowsiness are not uncommon. Other reported reactions include numbness, a tight feeling in the head, a cold sensation, and discomfort of the throat, mouth, nose, or sinuses. There are rare cases abroad of serious changes in heart rhythm or of episodes of angina. Report any symptoms to your physician.

Few interactions with **Imitrex** have been noted. It should not be given at the same time as ergot-containing migraine medicine such as **Cafergot, Ergostat**, or **Wigraine**. Avoid **Imitrex** if you are taking any drug that is an MAO-type antidepressant such as **Nardil** or **Parnate**. As doctors and patients acquire more experience with **Imitrex**, more interactions may become apparent. Check with your doctor and pharmacist to make sure **Imitrex** is safe in combination with any other drugs you take.

Inderal LA

propranolol

Overview: **Inderal LA** is a special long-acting formulation of a propranolol, the preeminent member of a class of medicines called beta-blockers. That means these drugs work in part by blunting the action of adrenaline, the body's natural fight-or-flight chemical. People normally respond to stressful situations with a rapid pulse, a pounding heart and an increase in blood pressure. **Inderal LA** helps block such reactions.

Inderal LA is prescribed for a wide range of health conditions including irregular heart rhythms, angina, high blood pressure, prevention of migraine headaches or a second heart attack and tremor. Although the FDA has not specifically approved its use for other purposes, doctors have employed **Inderal LA** to relieve involuntary movements caused by major tranquilizers, stage fright and panic disorders. The dose will vary depending upon the condition being treated.

Special Precautions: Some people should rarely, if ever, take beta-blockers such as **Inderal**. Asthmatics and patients with other respiratory problems are especially vulnerable, because these drugs can make breathing worse. People with heart failure must also be extremely cautious if prescribed beta-blockers because the medicine could lead to cardiac complications.

Never stop taking any beta-blocker medication abruptly unless you are under very close medical supervision. Angina or a heart attack could occur. These drugs may also make treatment of diabetes and thyroid disorders more complicated. Your doctor can tell you what additional tests and precautions you will need in managing these conditions.

Taking the Medicine: **Inderal LA** is more convenient than regular **Inderal** because its sustained release formulation provides blood levels that last substantially longer in the body. This means that most people only need to take one capsule a day. To maintain a constant level of the medicine in your system, try to maintain a regular regimen, taking **Inderal LA** at roughly the same time each day.

Side Effects and Interactions: **Inderal LA** can cause a number of side effects. They include slow heart rate, cold hands and feet, insomnia, nightmares, blurred vision, sexual difficulties, nerve tingling, dizziness, nausea, stomachache, gas, diarrhea, indigestion, rash, arthritis, and muscle pain. This medicine may also have a negative effect on cholesterol and other blood fats so a lipid test before treatment and periodically thereafter would be prudent.

Inderal LA is a little more likely to affect the nervous system than certain other drugs in this class. Be alert for the beta-blocker blues. Symptoms of psychological depression, fatigue, decreased concentration, memory loss and mood swings may come on slowly and insidiously. Notify your physician promptly of any adverse reactions, especially breathing difficulties, fluid retention in the legs, or a night cough.

Inderal LA can interact with a number of other compounds, including several that are used to treat asthma, colds, allergies, diabetes, and heart problems. Arthritis medicine and aspirin may also reduce the effectiveness of some beta-blockers. Check with your doctor and pharmacist to make sure **Inderal LA** is safe in combination with any other drugs you may take.

Keflex

cephalexin

Overview: **Keflex** belongs to a class of potent antibiotics called cephalosporins. It is one of the first of these to become available generically and is now often prescribed as cephalexin. This drug works against a wide variety of germs, including those that cause infections of the skin, lungs, throat, prostate, urinary tract, bones, and ears.

Cephalosporins are broad-spectrum medicines that were originally discovered in one of the world's most unlikely locations. A fungus found close to a sewer outlet along the coast of Sardinia turned out to cure a number of nasty infections. From this chance observation many extraordinary antibiotics have been developed.

Special Precautions: If you are allergic to penicillin-type antibiotics, alert your physician immediately. Some people who are sensitive to penicillin may also react to cephalexin. Symptoms such as breathing difficulty, wheezing, sneezing, hives, itching, and skin rash require immediate emergency treatment. Life-threatening anaphylactic shock may produce an inability to breathe, and cardiovascular collapse can occur within minutes of exposure.

People with kidney problems should receive cephalexin only under careful medical supervision because the dosage will most likely have to be modified to prevent toxicity.

Taking the Medicine: Although this antibiotic is absorbed more efficiently when it is taken on an empty stomach, the pills may be swallowed with food, especially if they upset your stomach.

Side Effects and Interactions: Side effects from cephalosporin-type antibiotics are generally mild. Nevertheless, cephalexin can cause a range of digestive tract disorders. Indigestion, stomach pain, nausea, vomiting, and diarrhea have been reported. If diarrhea becomes severe, contact your physician, since it may be a warning of drug-induced colitis.

Other infrequent reactions to be aware of include rash, itching, vaginitis, headache, confusion, joint pain, fatigue, and dizziness. Cephalexin may affect laboratory test results. Liver enzymes may become elevated and false-positive results may show up during certain diabetes tests. Make sure that the laboratory personnel are aware you are taking cephalexin if you have blood drawn. And remember to report any symptoms or suspected side effects of cephalexin to your physician promptly.

Lanoxin

digoxin

Overview: **Lanoxin** is among the most frequently prescribed drugs in this country. It is a digitalis heart medicine that to this day is derived from the leaves of a plant related to foxglove. Digitalis has been used medically for more than 200 years.

Lanoxin is prescribed for congestive heart failure and certain irregular heart rhythms, or arrhythmias. People with heart failure often experience fluid retention, sensitivity to cold, fatigue and difficulty breathing after mild exercise, and a nighttime cough, especially when they lie down. **Lanoxin** works partly by increasing the pumping power of the heart. It can also help slow an abnormal heart when atrial rhythms get out of control. But **Lanoxin** is complex to manage, especially in older people. This medication requires careful monitoring to prevent an overdose, as the therapeutic level is very close to the toxic dose. Periodic blood tests are crucial.

Special Precautions: People with reduced kidney function generally require less **Lanoxin**. As people age, their kidneys may no longer process this medicine as efficiently. This is another reason why periodic blood tests for digoxin levels are essential. It is also crucial to monitor both potassium and magnesium levels. If these essential minerals become depleted because of diuretic therapy, **Lanoxin** can become extremely dangerous. Blood tests are the only way to determine electrolyte levels.

Taking the Medicine: It is usually recommended that **Lanoxin** be taken at the same time and in the same way each day. For many people the most convenient time is with breakfast. However, food high in fiber may reduce the absorption of this drug. If your breakfast tends to be high in such foods, you might want to schedule your **Lanoxin** for another time of day.

Side Effects and Interactions: Signs of digitalis toxicity include loss of appetite, nausea, diarrhea, vomiting, stomach pain, blurred or disturbed color vision, headache, drowsiness, fatigue, and muscle weakness. If any of these symptoms occur, contact your physician immediately. Other adverse reactions may include personality change, depression, confusion, disorientation, apathy, bad dreams, and hallucinations. Any side effects should be brought to a doctor's attention promptly.

Lanoxin can interact with a wide range of over-the-counter and prescription medications. Antacids, for example, may diminish the proper absorption of digoxin. So can certain diarrhea medicines and drugs to control cholesterol such as **Questran** or **Colestid**. A number of other medications, such as **Cordarone, Rythmol,** and quinidine drugs, may make **Lanoxin** more toxic. So can **Sandimmune**, used to prevent transplant rejection. Calcium-blocking blood pressure medicines such as **Procardia, Cardizem,** or **Calan** may also increase digoxin levels dangerously.

Diuretics such as **Lasix** are often prescribed in conjunction with **Lanoxin**. A patient taking both medicines should be monitored carefully, however, because the diuretic may make the body lose too much potassium or magnesium. This could lead to serious changes in heart rhythm. Potassium-sparing diuretics such as **Aldactazide** or **Moduretic** could make monitoring and interpreting tests far more complicated.

One of the trickiest interactions is that of **Lanoxin** with erythromycin and tetracycline. For reasons that are not well understood, about one person in ten harbors bacteria in the gut that metabolizes digoxin. If this intestinal flora is wiped out with an antibiotic, the person may suddenly be exposed to much more **Lanoxin** than usual, even though he or she may still be swallowing the exact same dose. Because of these possible complications, never add any other prescription or over-the-counter medication to **Lanoxin** without first checking with your pharmacist and physician.

Never stop taking **Lanoxin** or switch to another brand of digoxin unless your physician is monitoring you closely. Because the effective dose is so close to the toxic dose, this might be dangerous.

Lasix

furosemide

Overview: **Lasix** is a potent diuretic, or water pill. It is used to treat high blood pressure and congestive heart failure as well as a number of other serious conditions in which fluid builds up in body tissues.

Special Precautions: Like many diuretics, **Lasix** depletes the body of potassium and other important minerals. People taking this medicine may need to include potassium-rich foods in their diet. Vegetables such as potatoes, beets, brussels sprouts, spinach, cabbage, broccoli, carrots, peppers, and squash are good sources of potassium. So are apricots, strawberries, bananas, oranges, peaches, and plums. Most fish also provide good quantities of this mineral.

Some people may not be able to maintain adequate potassium levels even with a diet rich in fish, fruits, and vegetables. Periodic blood tests are crucial to monitor potassium levels in the body. If such a test shows that potassium levels are low, your physician may recommend a potassium-based salt substitute or he may prescribe a potassium supplement.

Taking the Medicine: **Lasix** is absorbed most completely when it is taken on an empty stomach. This medication may cause stomach upset, however, which tends to be less of a problem when it is taken with food or milk. Because the dose should be adjusted individually, with the help of blood tests, let your doctor know if you will change the way you take this drug.

Side Effects and Interactions: People on **Lasix** may feel dizzy or faint if they stand up rapidly. Older people especially may need to take care to avoid falling when they first get up. Increased frequency of urination is common but may be less bothersome if you take your medicine at breakfast rather than at night.

Other adverse reactions to be alert for include rash, itching, sensitivity to sunlight leading to sunburn, ringing in the ears, nausea, diarrhea or constipation, muscle cramps, hearing loss, unexplained sore throat with fever, bruising, blurred vision, loss of appetite, increases in blood sugar, headache, gout, and tingling or numbness in hands or feet. Report any symptoms to your physician promptly.

Lasix can interact with a number of other medications. **Lanoxin** and other digitalis heart medicines may cause abnormal heart rhythms if potassium levels are decreased by diuretics. Other blood pressure medicines such as **Accupril, Lotensin,** or **Vasotec** could cause serious kidney problems in combination with **Lasix**, while diuretics such as **HydroDIURIL** or **Esidrix** may combine with **Lasix** to cause an excessive loss of water and minerals.

Lasix may increase blood levels of the blood thinner **Coumadin** and the manic-depressive drug lithium. On the other hand, **Indocin, Clinoril**, ibuprofen, **Dilantin**, and activated charcoal may interfere with the effectiveness of **Lasix**. Check with your doctor and pharmacist to make sure **Lasix** is safe in combination with any other drugs you take.

Lodine

etodolac

Overview: **Lodine** belongs to a class of medications commonly called NSAIDs or nonsteroidal anti-inflammatory drugs. It is prescribed for the management of pain and is also used both for short-term and long-term treatment of arthritis.

Pain relief begins within 30 minutes of taking **Lodine** and lasts 4 hours or more (up to 12 hours in a few patients).

Special Precautions: People who are allergic to aspirin, ibuprofen, or other anti-inflammatory agents should avoid **Lodine**. Signs of allergy include breathing difficulties, rash, fever, or a sudden drop in blood pressure, and require immediate medical attention.

Taking the Medicine: Taking **Lodine** with an antacid or a meal may help reduce possible stomach irritation. This will, however, decrease the peak concentration of **Lodine** in the body and may delay the onset of pain relief. Taking an NSAID with food does not guarantee that the drug will be safe for the stomach.

Side Effects and Interactions: Unquestionably the most common side effects of **Lodine** involve the gastrointestinal tract. They include indigestion, cramps, diarrhea, gas, nausea, and constipation. Some people may develop ulcers and intestinal bleeding while taking **Lodine**. Occasionally these problems can occur without obvious symptoms and lead to a life-threatening crisis due to perforation of the stomach lining.

Older people appear to be more susceptible to this problem and should be monitored carefully. Warning signs include weight loss, persistent indigestion, a feeling of fullness after moderate meals, dark or tarry stools, anemia, and unusual fatigue. Home stool tests such as **Hemoccult** or **Fleet Detecatest** may provide an early indication of bleeding.

Other side effects to be alert for include fatigue, dizziness, nervousness, ringing in the ears, blurred vision, rash, itching, fluid retention, frequent urination, sensitivity to sunlight leading to sunburn, and chills or fever. Drowsiness or insomnia is possible, so do not drive if you become impaired. Report any symptoms to your physician promptly.

Lodine can affect both the kidney and liver, so periodic blood tests to monitor the function of these organs are important for anyone on this drug long-term.

This medication may interact adversely with certain other drugs. A person taking a blood thinner such as **Coumadin** may become more vulnerable to a dangerous bleeding ulcer. Aspirin may interfere with **Lodine**'s effectiveness for reducing inflammation, although data on this point are not clear. All the NSAIDs, including **Lodine**, can make methotrexate (**Folex, Mexate, Rheumatrex**), lithium (**Eskalith, Lithobid,** etc.) and **Lanoxin** far more toxic. When **Lodine** is combined with the immunosuppressant cyclosporine (**Sandimmune**) the risk of kidney damage is increased. **Lodine** is still a relatively new drug and more interactions may become apparent as clinical experience accumulates. Ask your doctor and pharmacist to check whether **Lodine** interacts with any other drugs you take.

Lopid

gemfibrozil

Overview: **Lopid** is prescribed primarily to lower cholesterol and triglycerides. Heart specialists recognize that coronary artery disease is associated with certain risk factors, including high serum cholesterol, bad LDL cholesterol, elevated triglycerides, and reduced levels of protective HDL cholesterol.

Diet, exercise, and weight control are usually considered important first-line preventive approaches. When they are insufficient, drugs such as **Lopid** may be important in reducing the risk of heart disease. It increases HDL cholesterol while lowering triglycerides and certain other negative blood fats. A well-controlled study from Helsinki, Finland, revealed that this medication appears to lower the risk of heart attacks by about one third.

Special Precautions: Anyone with kidney or liver problems should probably not take **Lopid**. This medicine must also be used with great caution by anyone with gallstones or gallbladder disease, as **Lopid** may precipitate or aggravate problems. Tests for liver function and blood sugar should be carried out periodically.

Women who are pregnant should also avoid **Lopid** because animal studies have shown an increased risk of damage to the fetus. Research on animals has also linked **Lopid** to liver and testicular tumors, but only at relatively high doses. Whether there is a risk for humans remains to be determined.

Taking the Medicine: The manufacturer recommends that people take **Lopid** half an hour before breakfast and your evening meal. If you feel dizzy or your vision becomes blurred, do not drive.

Side Effects and Interactions: The most common side effects of **Lopid** are digestive tract problems: heartburn, stomach pain, diarrhea, nausea, vomiting, and flatulence. Other possible adverse reactions include skin rash, itching, dizziness, headache, blurred vision, muscle or joint pain, or unusual sore throat and fever. Notify your physician promptly of any symptoms.

Lopid can interact dangerously with cholesterol-lowering drugs such as **Mevacor, Pravachol,** or **Zocor**. Such a combination of cholesterol-lowering drugs could trigger destruction of muscle tissue, resulting in muscle pain, weakness, and ultimately kidney damage. If your doctor decides both drugs are necessary, close monitoring of kidney function is essential.

Lopressor

metoprolol

Overview: **Lopressor** belongs to the group of drugs known as beta-blockers. That means it works partly by blunting the action of adrenaline, the body's natural fight-or-flight chemical. People normally respond to stressful situations with a rapid pulse, a pounding heart, and an increase in blood pressure. **Lopressor** helps block such reactions.

This medicine is normally prescribed for hypertension, chest pain caused by angina, and prevention of a second heart attack. Although the FDA has not specifically approved its use for other purposes, doctors have prescribed **Lopressor** to treat irregular heart rhythms, tremor, and aggressive behavior, and to prevent migraine headaches. The dose will vary depending upon the condition being treated.

Special Precautions: Some people must be very careful if they take beta blockers. Asthmatics and patients with other respiratory problems are especially vulnerable, because these drugs can make breathing more difficult. **Lopressor** is a little better than other beta-blockers in this regard, but monitor your breathing carefully. People with heart failure must also be extremely cautious if prescribed beta-blockers because the medicine could lead to cardiac complications.

Taking the Medicine: **Lopressor** can be taken on an empty stomach, though it is best absorbed when swallowed at mealtime. Food may also reduce the risk of digestive tract upset. To maintain a constant level of the medicine in your bloodstream, try to maintain a regular regimen, taking **Lopressor** at roughly the same times each day.

Side Effects and Interactions: **Lopressor** can cause a number of side effects. These include slow heart rate, cold hands and feet, insomnia, nightmares, blurred vision, sexual difficulties, nerve tingling, dizziness, nausea, stomachache, gas, diarrhea, indigestion, rash, arthritis, and muscle pain. This medicine may also have a negative effect on cholesterol and other blood fats, so a lipid test before treatment and periodically thereafter would be prudent.

Lopressor is a little more likely to affect the nervous system than certain other drugs in this class. Be alert for the beta-blocker blues. Symptoms of psychological depression, fatigue, decreased concentration, memory loss, and mood swings may come on slowly and insidiously. Notify your physician promptly of any adverse reactions, especially breathing difficulties, fluid retention in the legs, or a night cough.

Never stop taking any beta-blocker medication abruptly unless you are under very close medical supervision. Angina or a heart attack could occur. These drugs may also make treatment of diabetes and thyroid disorders more complicated. Your physician will need to monitor such conditions closely.

Lopressor can interact with a number of other medicines. Antacids containing aluminum or calcium can reduce absorption and interfere with the effectiveness of **Lopressor**, as can many arthritis drugs and aspirin. Cholesterol-lowering medications such as **Questran** or **Colestid** and penicillin-type antibiotics might have the same effect on this beta-blocker. The ulcer medicines **Tagamet** and **Zantac** may increase the effects of **Lopressor**, however.

Other blood pressure medicines such as **Apresoline** or calcium channel blockers such as **Calan** or **Procardia** could interact with **Lopressor** so that the blood pressure–lowering power of each drug is enhanced. **Minipress** is more likely to cause fainting problems when combined with **Lopressor.** Be aware that over-the-counter asthma medicines containing epinephrine, the blood thinner **Coumadin,** or ergotamine-containing migraine drugs such as **Cafergot** could all interact badly with **Lopressor.** Check with your doctor and pharmacist before taking any other drugs to make sure you are aware of the risks the combination may carry.

Lotrisone Cream

betamethasone and clotrimazole

Overview: This antifungal cream is effective against skin problems such as athlete's foot, jock itch, ringworm, and other fungal infections. The steroid component can relieve itching and inflammation for symptomatic improvement.

Special Precautions: If you are suffering from a fungal infection in the groin area, such as jock itch, be stingy in your use of **Lotrisone**. Wear clothes that are loose and comfortable. If your condition does not clear up within two weeks, check back with your doctor.

Taking the Medicine: **Lotrisone** is usually applied to the affected skin twice daily. Unless your doctor tells you otherwise, do not cover this area with a bandage or tight dressing, because more of the medicine may be absorbed into your body than intended.

Side Effects and Interactions: Side effects associated with **Lotrisone** are uncommon. Some people report rash, itching, burning, stinging, blistering, swelling, redness, and skin irritation. Even more rare are symptoms such as loss of pigmentation of the skin, tingling or numbness, acne, and thinning of the skin. Report any symptoms to your physician promptly.

Lozol

indapamide

Overview: **Lozol** is a new kind of diuretic, or water pill. It is used to treat high blood pressure and congestive heart failure as well as certain other serious conditions in which fluid builds up in body tissues. Unlike many other diuretics, **Lozol** does not appear to raise cholesterol levels. This may be an important benefit for some people.

Special Precautions: Like many diuretics, **Lozol** depletes the body of potassium and other important minerals. People taking this medicine may need to include potassium-rich foods in their diet. Vegetables such as potatoes, beets, brussels sprouts, spinach, cabbage, broccoli, carrots, peppers, and squash are good sources of potassium. So are apricots, strawberries, bananas, oranges, peaches, and plums. Most fish also provide good quantities of this mineral.

Some people may not be able to maintain adequate potassium levels even with a diet rich in fish, fruits, and vegetables. Periodic blood tests are crucial to monitor potassium levels in the body. If such a test shows that potassium levels are low, your physician may recommend a potassium-based salt substitute you can cook with or he may prescribe a potassium supplement.

People who are allergic to sulfa drugs or who have kidney or liver disease will probably have to avoid **Lozol**.

Taking the Medicine: Because **Lozol** is likely to cause increased frequency of urination, the normal recommendation is to take one dose in the morning. This way the natural effect of the diuretic may be less bothersome.

Side Effects and Interactions: People on **Lozol** may feel dizzy or faint if they stand up rapidly. Older people especially may need to take care to avoid falling when they first get up.

Other adverse reactions to be alert for include headache, tiredness, weakness, muscle cramps, anxiety, rash, itching, insomnia, depression, nausea, diarrhea or constipation, unexplained sore throat with fever, bruising, blurred vision, loss of appetite, increases in blood sugar, gout, sexual difficulties, and tingling or numbness in hands or feet. Report any symptoms to your physician promptly.

Lozol can interact with a number of other medications. Lithium can become significantly more toxic if you combine it with **Lozol**. **Lanoxin** and other digitalis heart medicines may cause abnormal heart rhythms if potassium levels are decreased by diuretics such as **Lozol**. Careful monitoring of serum potassium is essential to prevent this serious complication.

Lozol is sometimes prescribed together with other drugs that lower blood pressure, and may increase their action. Close monitoring of blood pressure is extremely important while such a regimen is beginning. Certain diabetes medications, cholesterol-lowering drugs, and antibiotics may cause complications in combination with **Lozol**. Over-the-counter cold or allergy medicines could also pose problems. Check with your doctor and pharmacist to make sure this diuretic is safe with any other drugs you take.

Mevacor

lovastatin

Overview: **Mevacor** is prescribed primarily to lower cholesterol. Heart specialists recognize that coronary artery disease is associated with certain risk factors, including high serum cholesterol, bad LDL cholesterol, elevated triglycerides, and reduced levels of protective HDL cholesterol.

Diet, exercise, and weight control are usually considered important first-line preventive approaches. When they are insufficient, drugs such as **Mevacor** may be important in reducing the risk of heart disease. This medication has been found to increase good HDL cholesterol while lowering triglycerides and certain other negative blood fats.

Special Precautions: Anyone with liver problems should probably not take **Mevacor**. Liver enzyme changes have been reported in a small proportion of patients using this medicine, and may indicate serious problems. Liver function should be tested before anyone starts taking **Mevacor** and every month or so for the first year. Periodic tests are needed thereafter.

Because cholesterol is essential for the developing fetus, pregnant women should not take **Mevacor**.

Research on animals has also linked **Mevacor** to liver tumors, but only at relatively high doses. Whether there is a risk for humans remains to be determined.

It is important to see an ophthalmologist before starting on **Mevacor**. An eye test should also be performed annually to ensure there is no damage to the lens.

Taking the Medicine: The manufacturer recommends that **Mevacor** be taken with supper. If you need more than one dose daily, take them with meals.

Side Effects and Interactions: **Mevacor** has relatively few side effects and most people tolerate it well. Some adverse reactions that may occur include headache, skin rash, flatulence, constipation, diarrhea, nausea, and stomachache. Less common complications include muscle pain, blurred vision, dizziness, insomnia, and numbness or tingling of the hands or feet. Muscle aches or weakness could be a sign of a serious reaction called rhabdomyolysis or myopathy, and call for a test of kidney function. Kidney failure might be the outcome of untreated myopathy. Report any symptoms to your physician promptly.

The danger of rhabdomyolysis or myopathy is increased when **Mevacor** is combined with certain other drugs. Troleandomycin or erythromycin antibiotics such as **E.E.S., E-Mycin, Erythrocin,** or **PCE** have been involved in several cases. The new antibiotics **Biaxin** and **Zithromax** belong to the same class of drugs, but it is not clear if they have a potential for such an interaction. When **Mevacor** is combined with other cholesterol-lowering medicines such as **Lopid** or niacin, be alert for muscle pain, weakness, and kidney damage, because rhabdomyolysis is more common in this situation (affecting perhaps 3 or 4 percent of those on **Mevacor** and **Lopid**). The transplant drug **Sandimmune** increases the risk of this dangerous reaction dramatically, with some reports estimating that around 30 percent of patients on this immunosuppressant together with **Mevacor** experience myopathy. **Mevacor** may also increase the action of the blood thinner **Coumadin**, with prolonged prothrombin time. Check with your physician and pharmacist to make sure **Mevacor** is safe in combination with any other drug you may take.

Micro-K

potassium chloride (controlled release)

Overview: **Micro-K** is a specially formulated potassium supplement designed to slowly release potassium and chloride over 8 to 10 hours. By taking potassium this way, patients are not supposed to experience the unpleasant taste many liquid potassium supplements leave in the mouth, and it is hoped they will also have a lower risk of digestive tract irritation. Potassium is an essential mineral that plays an important role in every cell in the body. It is crucial for normal heart rhythms. Many medications can deplete the body of potassium, including diuretics and cortisone-type compounds. This can be extremely dangerous, especially for people taking digitalis heart medicine. Symptoms of potassium loss include weakness, palpitations, irregular heart rhythms, and fatigue. However the only way you can really tell if your body is low in potassium is to have a blood test.

Normally, doctors prefer that patients with mild to moderate potassium loss replace this mineral through the diet. Potassium-rich foods include vegetables such as potatoes, beets, brussels sprouts, spinach, cabbage, broccoli, carrots, peppers, and squash. Fish and fruits like apricots, strawberries, bananas, oranges, peaches, and plums are also good sources of potassium.

Some people may not be able to maintain adequate potassium levels even with a diet rich in such fruits and vegetables. Periodic blood tests are crucial to monitor potassium levels in the body. If such a test shows that potassium levels are low, your physician may recommend a liquid or effervescent potassium supplement. If the taste or discomfort is unbearable, he may prescribe a pill like **Micro-K.**

Special Precautions: Because too much potassium can be just as dangerous as too little, it is important to have your doctor monitor your serum potassium levels periodically while taking **Micro-K.** This is especially important for anyone with diminished kidney function, a common problem for older people.

Taking the Medicine: **Micro-K** should be taken with food and a full glass of water.

Side Effects and Interactions: There are substantial risks associated with solid potassium formulations. Medications such as **Micro-K** may cause ulceration, bleeding, perforation, or obstruction of the esophagus or digestive tract. Contact your physician immediately if you think a pill has become stuck in your throat or if you experience stomach pain, vomiting, or notice black or tarry stools. Other adverse reactions associated with such potassium supplements include nausea, loss of appetite, and diarrhea. Report any such symptoms promptly.

Micro-K can interact with a number of other medications. Blood pressure drugs such as **Accupril, Altace, Capoten, Vasotec, Prinivil,** or **Zestril** can raise potassium to dangerous levels in combination with **Micro-K**. The same thing could occur with potassium-based salt substitutes and potassium-sparing diuretics such as **Aldactone, Dyazide, Dyrenium, Midamor,** or **Moduretic**. Check with your doctor and pharmacist to make sure **Micro-K** is safe in combination with any other drugs you take.

Micronase

glyburide

Overview: **Micronase** is used together with diet and exercise to control non–insulin-dependent, or Type II, diabetes. This pill seems to stimulate the pancreas to make more insulin. It may also make body tissues more responsive to insulin.

Special Precautions: **Micronase** must not be taken by people who are allergic to sulfa drugs. Your doctor will need frequent blood tests to adjust the dose of **Micronase** when you begin taking it. Illness or a change in your exercise program may also make it necessary to adjust the dose later on.

Taking the Medicine: **Micronase** may be taken with food, especially if it upsets your stomach. The manufacturer suggests that it be taken with breakfast or the first meal of the day.

Side Effects and Interactions: Episodes of dangerously low blood sugar, or hypoglycemia, are a hazard with **Micronase** as with any oral diabetes drug. Be alert for symptoms of fatigue, shakiness, headache, cold sweat, or confusion, because they could signal this hazardous reaction. Be sure to discuss the symptoms and treatment of hypoglycemia with your health care provider.

Other possible side effects of this medication include nausea, heartburn, skin rash, changes in liver enzymes, susceptibility to sunburn, ringing in the ears, and blood changes. Fever, sore throat, and bruising or bleeding could signal a rare but serious reaction that requires immediate attention. Report any symptoms or suspected side effects without delay.

A number of compounds may interact with **Micronase**. Alcohol should be avoided if you are on this drug, because it could cause low blood sugar or uncomfortable skin flushing and breathlessness. Other drugs that could lead to drops in blood sugar include nonsteroidal arthritis medicines such as **Motrin**, blood thinners such as **Coumadin**, aspirin and similar medicines, MAO-inhibitor antidepressants such as **Nardil**, as well as the ulcer drugs **Tagamet** and **Zantac**.

Many blood pressure pills and heart medicines also interact with **Micronase**. So may estrogen (including oral contraceptives), thyroid hormones, niacin used to lower cholesterol, and the seizure medication **Dilantin**. Check with your doctor and pharmacist to find out whether **Micronase** is likely to interact with any other drug you must take.

Motrin

ibuprofen

Overview: **Motrin** is a pain reliever used primarily for arthritis, but also useful in reducing inflammation due to bursitis, tendinitis, sprains, strains, and other painful conditions. It belongs to a class of medications commonly called NSAIDs or nonsteroidal anti-inflammatory drugs, and like the others in its class, may be used to ease menstrual cramps. **Motrin** was one of the first of these arthritis drugs on the market. As **Motrin IB** it is a very popular over-the-counter pain reliever. It is also available generically as ibuprofen.

Special Precautions: People who are allergic to aspirin or other anti-inflammatory agents should avoid **Motrin**. Signs of allergy include breathing difficulties, rash, fever, or a sudden drop in blood pressure. Any of these requires prompt medical attention.

Taking the Medicine: Because **Motrin** can be hard on the digestive tract, it may be taken with food to reduce stomach trouble. This does not guarantee that the drug will be safe for the stomach, however.

Side Effects and Interactions: No matter how you swallow this medicine, the most common side effects of **Motrin** involve the gastrointestinal tract. They include nausea, indigestion, heartburn, cramps, gas, constipation, and diarrhea. Some people may develop ulcers and intestinal bleeding while taking **Motrin**.

Occasionally these problems can occur without obvious symptoms and lead to a life-threatening crisis due to perforation of the stomach lining. Older people appear to be more susceptible to this problem and should be monitored carefully. Warning signs include weight loss, persistent indigestion, a feeling of fullness after moderate meals, dark or tarry stools, anemia, and unusual fatigue. Home stool tests such as **Hemoccult** or **Fleet Detecatest** may provide an early indication of bleeding.

Other side effects to be alert for include headache, ringing in the ears, rash, itching, nervousness, fluid retention, and loss of appetite. Drowsiness, dizziness, light-headedness, and confusion are possible, so do not drive if you become impaired. Less common adverse reactions include insomnia, heart palpitations, hair loss, depression, tiredness, anemia or other blood changes, fever, visual disturbances, meningitis, and sores in the mouth. Report any symptoms to your physician without delay. **Motrin** can affect both the kidney and liver, so periodic blood tests to monitor the function of these organs is important. Some people might become sensitive to sunlight while on **Motrin**, so use an effective sunscreen or stay well covered.

This medication can interact with many other drugs, including aspirin and alcohol. **Motrin** may blunt the effectiveness of many blood pressure medicines, including beta-blockers such as **Corgard** or **Tenormin**, ACE inhibitors such as **Capoten, Vasotec,** or **Zestril,** and diuretics such as **Dyazide** or **Lasix.** It can increase blood levels of the heart drug **Lanoxin** and increase the toxicity of the transplant drug **Sandimmune** and the cancer medicine methotrexate. Because it has the potential to cause GI bleeding, **Motrin** could be dangerous in combination with the blood thinner **Coumadin.** If you must take **Motrin** in conjunction with either the seizure medication **Dilantin** or the manic-depression medicine lithium, your physician should monitor blood levels and effects of these drugs closely. Check with both your doctor and your pharmacist before taking **Motrin** in combination with any other drugs.

Naprosyn

naproxen

Overview: **Naprosyn** is a pain reliever used primarily for arthritis. Like other nonsteroidal anti-inflammatory drugs, or NSAIDs, it may also be prescribed for menstrual cramps, bursitis, tendinitis, sprains, strains, and other painful conditions. **Naprosyn** is virtually identical to **Anaprox,** a popular pain reliever, so these two drugs should never be taken together. It is also available by its generic name, naproxen, and as an over-the-counter pain reliever, **Aleve.**

Special Precautions: People who are allergic to aspirin or other anti-inflammatory agents should avoid **Naprosyn.** Signs of allergy include breathing difficulties, rash, fever, or a sudden drop in blood pressure and require immediate medical attention.

Taking the Medicine: Because **Naprosyn** can be hard on the digestive tract, it may be taken with food to reduce stomach irritation. This offers no guarantee of safety, however.

Side Effects and Interactions: No matter how you swallow this medicine, the most common side effects of **Naprosyn** involve the gastrointestinal tract. They include nausea, indigestion, heartburn, cramps, gas, constipation, and diarrhea.

Some people may develop ulcers and intestinal bleeding while taking **Naprosyn.** Occasionally these problems can occur without obvious symptoms and lead to a life-threatening crisis due to perforation of the stomach lining. Older people appear to be more susceptible to this problem and should be monitored carefully. Warning signs include weight loss, persistent indigestion, a feeling of fullness after moderate meals, dark or tarry stools, anemia, and unusual fatigue. Home stool tests such as **Hemoccult** or **Fleet Detecatest** may provide an early indication of bleeding.

Other side effects to watch for include headache, ringing in the ears, rash, itching, difficulty breathing, and fluid retention. Drowsiness, dizziness, light-headedness, difficulty concentrating, and confusion are possible, so do not drive if you become impaired. Less common adverse reactions include jitteriness, insomnia, heart palpitations, hair loss, depression, tremor, tiredness, visual disturbances, and sores in the mouth. Report any symptoms to your physician promptly.

Naprosyn can affect both the kidney and liver, so periodic blood tests to monitor the function of these organs is important. Some people become sensitive to sunlight while on **Naprosyn**, with a severe burn or rash resulting, so use an effective sunscreen, stay covered, or avoid the sun.

This medication can interact with many other drugs, including aspirin and alcohol. **Naprosyn** may blunt the effectiveness of many blood pressure medicines, including beta-blockers such as **Corgard** or **Tenormin**, ACE inhibitors such as **Capoten, Vasotec,** or **Zestril,** and diuretics such as **Dyazide** or **Lasix**. It can increase blood levels of the heart drug **Lanoxin** and increase the toxicity of the transplant drug **Sandimmune** and the cancer medicine methotrexate. Because it has the potential to cause GI bleeding, **Naprosyn** could be dangerous in combination with the blood thinner **Coumadin**. If you must take **Naprosyn** together with either the seizure medication **Dilantin** or the manic-depression medicine lithium, your physician should monitor blood levels and effects of these drugs closely. Check with both your doctor and your pharmacist before taking **Naprosyn** in combination with any other drugs.

Nitrostat

nitroglycerin sublingual tablets

Overview: **Nitrostat** is prescribed to people who suffer chest pain due to angina. It is used both for prevention and to treat an acute attack. The medication is taken by holding it under the tongue at the first sign of pain or five to ten minutes before doing anything that might precipitate angina.

Special Precautions: **Nitrostat** should be stored in a tightly closed container away from heat, cold, or moisture. It should not be given to anyone who is in the early phase of a heart attack or who has increased pressure inside the head due to injury.

Taking the Medicine: No food, gum, or beverage should be used while **Nitrostat** is dissolving under the tongue. Because **Nitrostat** might make you dizzy, it is best to sit down while using it. If three tablets within 15 minutes do not ease chest pain, call your doctor or get to a hospital emergency room immediately.

Side Effects and Interactions: Headache is not uncommon after using **Ni-**

trostat. If it is very severe or lasts a long time, contact your doctor, because a change in dose may be advisable. Nitroglycerin may also cause flushing of the skin, dizziness or fainting, nausea, rapid heartbeat, weakness, or rash. Report any symptoms, including blurred vision or dry mouth, to your doctor without delay.

Nitrostat may interact with other drugs, including alcohol, to lower blood pressure dangerously. Beta-blockers, calcium channel blockers, and other blood pressure drugs may interact with nitroglycerin. Ergotamine medicines for migraine headaches also interact with this drug. Check with your physician and pharmacist before taking other drugs in combination with **Nitrostat**.

Nolvadex

tamoxifen

Overview: **Nolvadex** is a nonsteroidal agent with potent antiestrogenic properties. The antiestrogenic effects allow it to compete with estrogen for binding sites in target tissues, particularly the breast. **Nolvadex** is prescribed to delay the recurrence of breast cancer following appropriate treatment and to combat metastatic breast cancer as an alternative to radiation or removal of the ovaries.

Special Precautions: **Nolvadex** should not be taken during pregnancy, and any woman taking this medicine should use effective contraception.

Not all breast cancers are sensitive to estrogen, so the doctor will order hormone receptor studies on the tumor tissue to see if it is susceptible to **Nolvadex**.

Changes of the endometrium (lining of the uterus) have been reported in women taking Nolvadex. These include growths (polyps), overgrowth (hyperplasia), and even cancer. Experts believe that the underlying mechanism is related to the estrogenic properties of **Nolvadex**. Any woman on **Nolvadex** who experiences abnormal vaginal bleeding should report it to her doctor immediately.

Nolvadex should be used cautiously in women with abnormal blood counts. Regular blood tests to check both white and red cells and also liver enzymes may be appropriate.

Taking the Medicine: **Nolvadex** is taken twice a day, preferably on an empty stomach. The pills may be taken with food if they cause stomach upset. **Nolvadex** tablets should be protected from heat and light.

Side Effects and Interactions: Without question, the most common side effects of **Nolvadex** are hot flashes and nausea and/or vomiting. Up to one-fourth of the women on this medication may experience them; they are not usually severe enough for women to stop their medicine, however.

Other side effects to be alert for include vaginal bleeding, vaginal discharge, menstrual irregularities, and skin rash. Less commonly **Nolvadex** may produce a temporary flare of bone pain associated with metastatic disease, high calcium levels, swelling of the hands and feet, distaste for food, genital itching, depression, dizziness, headache, and hair thinning or partial hair loss.

Some women have experienced visual changes while taking **Nolvadex**, and periodic eye exams are prudent. There are some cases of serious blood clots in patients on **Nolvadex**. Notify your doctor immediately if you suddenly notice confusion, blurred vision, shortness of breath, weakness, sleepiness, or pain and swelling in the leg or groin, because these might be signs of a clot.

This medication can interact with the blood thinners **Coumadin** and increase bleeding time. If they must be used together, prothrombin time should be monitored carefully. There are hints that phenobarbital and **Parlodel** may alter **Nolvadex** blood levels. This medication can affect thyroid tests, raising T_4 levels without changing thyroid function. This should be taken into account in interpreting the results of a thyroid test. Check with your pharmacist and physician to make sure **Nolvadex** is safe in combination with any other drugs you take.

Ortho-Novum 7/7/7

ethinyl estradiol and norethindrone

Overview: This combination oral contraceptive contains synthetic hormones similar to the female hormones estrogen and progestin. It works primarily by preventing the release of eggs from the ovary.

Ortho-Novum 7/7/7 may be prescribed in either 21- or 28-pill packets. Make sure you discuss the regimen with your health care provider so you understand exactly how to take it. The proportions of norethindrone and ethinyl estradiol vary each week to simulate the natural fluctuations of hormones during a woman's cycle.

Special Precautions: **Ortho-Novum**, like other oral contraceptives, is quite effective. Some women are at greater risk of negative consequences, however. Tell your doctor if you smoke cigarettes, have had phlebitis or other clotting problems, or if you or someone in your family has had uterine or breast cancer. You will also be asked about asthma, diabetes, epilepsy, migraine, depression, and certain other conditions that could be aggravated by oral contraceptives.

Taking the Medicine: **Ortho-Novum** should be swallowed at the same time every day to maintain consistent levels in the body. If you forget one dose, take it as soon as you remember it, and take the next one at the usual time. If you miss more than one dose, start taking your pills again at the usual time as soon as you remember, and use additional contraceptive protection such as spermicidal foam and/or condoms for the rest of that cycle.

Side Effects and Interactions: Unexpected vaginal bleeding may occur during the first cycle or two on **Ortho-Novum**. Notify your physician if you continue to experience bleeding between periods after the second month on this medication.

Serious side effects are rare, but they may include high blood pressure, heart attacks, stroke, blood clots, visual changes, problems with liver or gallbladder, and birth defects. In the unlikely event you become pregnant, do not continue taking **Ortho-Novum.**

Less dangerous reactions include headache, nausea, fluid retention, spotty darkening of the skin, changes in menstrual flow, depression, nervousness, breast tenderness, rash, vaginal infections, and inability to wear contact lenses. Report any symptoms or suspected side effects promptly.

Ortho-Novum interacts with many other medications, especially antibiotics such as penicillin, tetracycline, and related drugs that may reduce its contraceptive protection. This is also a potential hazard with barbiturates like phenobarbital or **Mysoline**, the antifungal medicine griseofulvin, the tuberculosis drug rifampin, and seizure medications such as **Dilantin**.

Antianxiety drugs such as **Halcion, Valium,** or **Xanax**, asthma drugs containing theophylline or aminophylline, oral corticosteroids such as hydrocortisone or prednisone, and caffeine, an ingredient common in many beverages and over-the-counter drugs, may all have more serious adverse effects if they are taken together with birth control pills. Check with your doctor and pharmacist before taking any other medicine in combination with **Ortho-Novum 7/7/7**. Birth control pills can alter results on a number of laboratory tests, so be sure the laboratory and the doctor are aware that you are taking **Ortho-Novum** before any tests are interpreted.

Paxil

paroxetine

Overview: **Paxil**, like the earlier antidepressant **Prozac**, apparently works by enhancing the action of a brain chemical called serotonin. This medication is prescribed to treat major depression, and has been shown to be effective for up to one year. Like **Prozac, Paxil** is less likely to cause typical side effects associated with older medications. Tricyclic antidepressants such as **Elavil, Tofranil, Sinequan,** and **Pamelor** often produce dry mouth, dizziness, weight gain, and a sluggish or lethargic feeling. **Paxil** may not have these effects, and may have a slight stimulant action.

Special Precautions: Some people may need very close monitoring if the doctor prescribes **Paxil**. For people who have had an episode of mania, there is a risk that manic symptoms could be triggered by **Paxil**. Patients who have had seizures also need to be followed carefully, since **Paxil**, like most other antidepressants, may provoke seizures in susceptible individuals.

Because **Paxil** may cause drowsiness or dizziness, people taking this medicine should not drive or use dangerous machines unless an objective evaluation shows they are not impaired. **Paxil** should never be stopped suddenly, since abrupt discontinuation could bring on very unpleasant withdrawal symptoms.

Older people and those with kidney disease or liver problems may need to start on a reduced dose, because they may eliminate **Paxil** less efficiently than otherwise healthy people.

Anyone with a history of suicide attempts must also be extremely vigilant. There have been reports that some people may develop a preoccupation with suicide or violence while taking **Prozac**. It is still not certain whether this is caused by the underlying mental condition or is in some way related to the drug. If **Prozac** were responsible for any of these incidents, there might also be a risk with **Paxil**. Family members must help monitor people on **Paxil** for suicidal thoughts or self-destructive behaviors. The doctor must be notified immediately in such cases.

Taking the Medicine: According to the manufacturer, **Paxil** should be taken once a day, preferably in the morning. It may be taken either with or without food.

Side Effects and Interactions: Side effects associated with **Paxil** include exhaustion, sweating, nausea, decreased appetite, drowsiness, dry mouth, dizziness, insomnia, tremor, problems with ejaculation, and anxiety. Less common adverse reactions include headache, palpitations, constipation, diarrhea, blurred vision, and decreased libido. A wide range of other reactions have been reported but appear to be uncommon. Report any symptoms to your physician promptly.

Paxil can interact with a number of other medications. Anyone taking other antidepressants, especially drugs such as **Nardil** or **Parnate** (MAO inhibitors), should stop such a medicine at least two weeks before starting on **Paxil**. If **Paxil** is taken first, two weeks should elapse before starting on one of these other medicines.

If the amino acid tryptophan ever becomes available in the U.S. again, it should not be taken with **Paxil**, because it may increase the potential for adverse reactions. Tricyclic antidepressants such as **Elavil, Pamelor,** or **Tofranil** could in theory have stronger actions and more pronounced toxicity when they are combined with **Paxil**. This may also occur with certain medications prescribed to regulate heart rhythm. Other compounds that could cause complications in combination with **Paxil** include the blood thinner **Coumadin** and possibly the heart medicine **Lanoxin**. The antiulcer and stomach medicine **Tagamet** may increase **Paxil** levels, while phenobarbital or **Dilantin** can lower them. Check with your pharmacist and physician before taking any other medicines in combination with **Paxil**.

penicillin VK

Beepen-VK	**Pen-Vee K**
Betapen-VK	**Robicillin VK**
Ledercillin VK	**V-Cillin K**
Pen-V	**Veetids**

Overview: Penicillin represents one of the most important drugs ever developed. Its discovery in 1946 permanently changed medicine and set the stage for man's ability to overcome what had previously been life-threatening infections.

Penicillin is effective in fighting infections in many places in the body including the urinary tract, lungs, ears, throat, skin, and genital tract.

Penicillin V potassium is prescribed generically or under a variety of brand names including **Beepen-VK, Betapen-VK, Ledercillin VK, Pen-V, Pen-Vee K, Robicillin VK, V-Cillin K,** and **Veetids**.

Special Precautions: Anyone who is allergic to penicillin-type antibiotics must generally avoid such drugs like the plague. Symptoms such as breathing difficulty, wheezing, sneezing, hives, itching, and skin rash require immediate emergency treatment. Life-threatening anaphylactic shock may produce an inability to breathe and cardiovascular collapse can occur within minutes of exposure. If you are allergic to penicillin and you ever have to go into the hospital, make sure a sign is placed over the bed alerting hospital personnel to penicillin allergy.

Taking the Medicine: Penicillin VK resists acid breakdown in the stomach so it may be taken with food if it upsets your stomach. However, for maximum absorption take this antibiotic on an empty stomach. That usually means at least one hour before meals or two hours after eating.

Side Effects and Interactions: The most common side effects of penicillin involve digestive tract upset. Nausea, vomiting, and diarrhea can be troublesome for some people. A black hairy tongue, rash, sore mouth, and yeast infections of the mouth, anus, or vagina are other potential adverse reactions. Less common but possibly more serious side effects include anemia and blood disorders. Report any symptoms to your physician promptly. Long-term treatment with penicillin-type antibiotics requires periodic monitoring by a health professional.

Penicillin VK may interact with aspirin and certain other arthritis medicines. In addition, oral contraceptives may be less effective in combination with this antibiotic. Check with your pharmacist and physician before taking any other medicine together with penicillin VK.

Pepcid

famotidine

Overview: **Pepcid** is a popular ulcer drug similar in many respects to **Tagamet** or **Zantac.** It works by suppressing the secretion of stomach acid, so it is also used to treat conditions of abnormal acidity as well as helping ulcers clear up rapidly. Doctors sometimes prescribe **Pepcid** as maintenance therapy to keep ulcers from coming back. This drug is also available without prescription as **Pepcid AC.**

Special Precautions: Perhaps because **Pepcid** is so effective at reducing stomach acid concentrations, patients taking this medicine have higher levels of certain microorganisms in their stomachs than would normally survive there. Scientists do not yet know whether these bacteria have negative long-term consequences, but it has been suggested that vitamins C and E might provide a measure of protection.

Taking the Medicine: **Pepcid** may be taken with food or on an empty stomach. If antacids are needed for relief of ulcer pain, they should generally be taken at a different time.

Side Effects and Interactions: Side effects associated with **Pepcid** are uncommon. Some people may experience headache, constipation, diarrhea, and dizziness. Other reactions that have occasionally been reported include insomnia, fever, fatigue, jaundice, nausea, drowsiness, breathing difficulties, hair loss, palpitations, and ringing in the ears. Older patients may experience mental confusion or even hallucinations. Report any symptoms to your physician promptly.

According to the manufacturer, there are no significant drug interactions between **Pepcid** and other medications. Nevertheless, it is theoretically possible that **Pepcid** could diminish the effectiveness of the antifungal agent **Nizoral**. It is probably a good idea to check with your physician or pharmacist to make sure **Pepcid** will be safe in combination with other medications you may be taking.

Polymox

amoxicillin

Overview: **Polymox** closely resembles other penicillin-type antibiotics. This medicine is frequently prescribed because of its broad-spectrum activity against a large number of bacteria. **Polymox** is effective in fighting infections in many parts of the body including the urinary tract, lungs, ears, throat, and genital tract.

Special Precautions: Because **Polymox** is related to penicillin, anyone who is allergic to this class of antibiotics must generally avoid such drugs like the plague. Symptoms such as breathing difficulty, wheezing, sneezing, hives, itching, and skin rash require immediate emergency treatment. Life-threatening anaphylactic shock may produce an inability to breathe, and cardiovascular collapse can occur within minutes of exposure. If you are allergic to penicillin and you ever have to go into the hospital, make sure a sign is placed over the bed alerting hospital personnel to penicillin allergy.

Taking the Medicine: The most effective way to swallow amoxicillin is probably on an empty stomach with a full eight-ounce glass of water. That usually means at least one hour before eating or two hours after food. There is some disagreement among health professionals on this matter, however, and if **Polymox** upsets your stomach it may be taken with meals without losing potency. Ask your pharmacist for a recommendation on how best to take **Polymox**.

Side Effects and Interactions: The most common side effects of amoxicillin involve digestive tract upset. Nausea, vomiting, and diarrhea can be troublesome for some people. Less common but possibly more serious side effects include liver enzyme elevations, anemia, blood disorders, and psychological reactions. Report any such symptoms to your physician promptly. Long-term treatment with **Poly-**

mox or any other penicillin-type antibiotic requires periodic monitoring by a health professional.

Pravachol

pravastatin

Overview: **Pravachol** is prescribed primarily to lower cholesterol. Heart specialists recognize that coronary artery disease is associated with certain risk factors, including high serum cholesterol, bad LDL cholesterol, elevated triglycerides, and reduced levels of protective HDL cholesterol.

Diet, exercise, and weight control are usually considered important first-line preventive approaches. When they are insufficient, drugs such as **Pravachol** may be important in reducing the risk of heart disease. This medication has been found to increase good HDL cholesterol while lowering triglycerides and certain other negative blood fats.

Special Precautions: Anyone with liver problems should probably not take **Pravachol**. Liver enzyme changes have been reported in a small proportion of patients using this medicine, and may indicate serious problems. Liver function should be tested before anyone starts taking **Pravachol** and every month or so for the first year. Periodic tests are needed thereafter.

Because cholesterol is essential for the developing fetus, pregnant women should not take **Pravachol**.

Research on animals has also shown strokelike bleeding in dogs on **Pravachol**, but only at relatively high doses. Whether there is a risk for humans remains to be determined.

It is important to see an ophthalmologist before starting on **Pravachol**. An eye test should also be performed annually to ensure there is no damage to the lens.

Taking the Medicine: The manufacturer recommends that **Pravachol** be taken at bedtime. It may be taken without regard to food.

Side Effects and Interactions: **Pravachol** has relatively few side effects and most people tolerate it well. Some adverse reactions that may occur include nausea, flatulence, constipation, diarrhea, stomachache, fatigue, headache, and skin rash. Less common complications include dizziness, muscle pain, change in the sense of taste, insomnia, and numbness or tingling of the hands or feet. Muscle aches or weakness could be a sign of a serious reaction called rhabdomyolysis or myopathy, and call for a test of kidney function. Kidney failure might be the outcome of untreated myopathy. Report any symptoms to your physician promptly.

The danger of rhabdomyolysis or myopathy is increased when **Mevacor** is combined with certain other drugs. Troleandomycin or erythromycin antibiotics such as **E.E.S., E-Mycin, Erythrocin,** or **PCE** have been involved in several cases. The new antibiotics **Biaxin** and **Zithromax** belong to the same class of drugs, but it is not clear if they have a potential for such an interaction. Because **Pravachol** is in the same class as **Mevacor**, this interaction may pose hazards with **Pravachol** as well.

When **Pravachol** is combined with other cholesterol-lowering medicines such as **Lopid** or niacin, be alert for muscle pain, weakness, and kidney damage, because rhabdomyolysis may be more common in this situation. The transplant drug **Sandimmune** might also increase the risk of this dangerous reaction.

Pravachol may also increase the action of the blood thinner **Coumadin**; pro-thrombin time should be closely monitored. The lipid-lowering drugs **Questran** or **Colestid** may reduce the absorption of **Pravachol** if they are given at the same time. **Tagamet** also appears to interact with **Pravachol.** Check with your physician and pharmacist to make sure **Pravachol** is safe in combination with any other drug you may take.

prednisone

Meticorten

Deltasone   **Orasone**

Overview: Prednisone is available both by generic name and under several brand names. It is a corticosteroid, or hormonelike medication prescribed for a wide variety of conditions. Other cortisone-like medicines that are similar to pred-nisone include prednisolone or **Delta-Cortef**, cortisone or **Cortone**, hydrocortisone or **Cortef**, and triamcinolone, also prescribed as **Aristocort** or **Kenacort**. Much of the information on prednisone is also applicable to these other medications.

It is quite effective in short-term treatment for flare-ups of rheumatoid arthri-tis, bursitis, gout, and other rheumatic conditions; for short-term or long-term treatment of conditions such as lupus (SLE) or polymyositis; for a number of se-vere skin problems; to control incapacitating allergic reactions from hay fever and asthma to poison ivy or drug reactions; and for many eye disorders. It is also indi-cated in certain cancers, blood diseases, respiratory diseases, multiple sclerosis, a severe kidney problem (nephrotic syndrome), some endocrine disorders, and to tide a patient over a critical episode of ulcerative colitis or regional enteritis.

Special Precautions: Prednisone should not be taken when there is a sys-temic fungal infection. Prednisone may reduce the body's resistance to infection and mask the signs of a new infection, including certain laboratory tests for infec-tion.

Long-term use of prednisone may increase the risk of developing cataracts or glaucoma. Regular eye checkups are advisable. In addition, prednisone, like other corticosteroids, increases calcium loss and long-term use may result in weakened bones.

Taking the Medicine: The lowest effective dose should be used. Because dosage regimens vary depending on what condition is being treated, be sure you understand exactly how many pills you should take and when you should take them. For some conditions, early morning (before 8 A.M.) is preferable The doctor may prescribe prednisone to be taken every other day (twice the usual daily dose) rather than every day at the regular dose.

Stopping prednisone abruptly may result in symptoms of inadequate adrenal gland function. To avoid this, you may be instructed to taper off prednisone gradually. This is important, because it may take months for the adrenal gland to return to normal if it is suppressed.

Side Effects and Interactions: At high doses, prednisone can lead to salt and water retention which may raise blood pressure. Blood pressure should be monitored. Susceptible people may experience low potassium or congestive heart failure.

Prednisone may also cause muscle weakness, weakened bones, peptic ulcer, inflamed pancreas or esophagus, menstrual irregularities, and hormonal imbalances, including reduced ability to handle carbohydrates (insulin problems). Rash and itching may be a sign of allergy to prednisone. The skin may also become thin and fragile, with slower wound-healing, redness, and increased sweating.

Side effects involving the nervous system may include mood swings, personality changes, insomnia, euphoria, and depression. Headache, dizziness, and convulsions have also been reported. Children who must take prednisone should be measured on a regular basis to make sure their growth is not affected. Report any symptoms to your physician promptly.

If you are taking any other medicines, check with a physician or pharmacist. Barbiturates, birth control pills, blood thinners such as **Coumadin**, estrogen replacement therapy such as **Premarin**, seizure medicine such as **Dilantin** or **Peganone,** and the tuberculosis treatment rifampin, can all interact seriously with prednisone. Even over-the-counter drugs such as aspirin or **Pepto-Bismol** may be affected.

Premarin

conjugated estrogens

Overview: This natural estrogen formulation is one of the most commonly prescribed medicines in the country. The hormones are purified from pregnant mares' urine.

Estrogen replacement therapy is prescribed primarily to relieve menopausal symptoms such as hot flashes. It has also become a popular measure for preventing osteoporosis and reducing the risk of heart disease. It is approved for treating breast engorgement right after childbirth when a woman does not plan to breast-feed.

Estrogen can also be helpful in various conditions where a woman does not produce enough natural estrogen. Certain cancers in men and women may benefit from estrogen therapy.

Special Precautions: There are a number of situations in which **Premarin** may be inappropriate. Pregnant women should not use this medication, because it could affect the fetus. Women with a history of breast cancer or other malignant disease susceptible to estrogen are generally advised to avoid this hormone. Blood-clotting disorders such as thrombophlebitis are also a reason to be wary of **Premarin**.

Prolonged use of postmenopausal estrogen has been controversial because of questions about cancer. Endometrial carcinoma, or cancer of the uterine lining, is more of a risk for women exposed to estrogen. This adverse reaction may be counteracted by simultaneous administration of progestins. Vaginal bleeding could be an early warning sign of cancer and requires immediate medical attention.

The risk of breast cancer is more uncertain. Studies have provided conflicting results, and more research is needed. Women with a strong family history of breast cancer will want to discuss this issue with their doctor.

Taking the Medicine: It is important to take **Premarin** exactly according to the doctor's instructions, since the dose and timing are different depending on the purpose for which it is being used. Women who have menopausal symptoms but are still having menstrual cycles start taking **Premarin** on the fifth day of menstrual bleeding. They then take one pill daily for three weeks, and no **Premarin** for the following week. Doctors often prescribe a progestin compound in addition for women who have not had a hysterectomy. Make sure you understand the schedule of when to take **Premarin** and when to take the progestin.

Side Effects and Interactions: **Premarin** has a number of potential side effects, including breakthrough menstrual bleeding, breast tenderness, bloating, nausea, vomiting, stomach pain, headache, gallbladder problems, liver tumors, depression, jaundice, and high blood pressure. Some women experience an increase in blood sugar and may go on to develop diabetes. The skin may become more sensitive to sunburn, so it is wise to use sunscreen or wear protective clothing (including sunglasses) if you will be out in the sun.

Some kinds of vaginal infections may be more common in women using estrogen. *Candida,* or yeast overgrowth, may be a problem. Other adverse reactions include a change in weight, fluid retention, alteration in sex drive, hair loss, and change in the curvature of the cornea. This may make contact lenses inappropriate.

Your doctor should be notified immediately of any of the following symptoms: pain in the calf or groin, sudden shortness of breath or sharp chest pain, sudden severe headache, blurred vision or speech, weakness or numbness in an arm or leg, yellow skin or eyes, or severe abdominal pain. Let your doctor know if you suspect you may have become pregnant, if you feel seriously depressed, if you notice lumps in your breast, or if vaginal bleeding is abnormal.

Premarin may interact with several other medications, such as the antiepileptics **Dilantin** or **Mesantoin**, the tuberculosis drug rifampin, or cortisone and other steroids. The activity of the anticoagulant **Coumadin** and that of certain antidepressants may be altered. Adequate calcium and vitamins B_6 and folic acid are important. Check with your doctor and pharmacist before taking any other medicine while taking **Premarin**.

Prilosec

omeprazole

Overview: **Prilosec** is the first of a new class of powerful drugs that combat ulcers by blocking the final step in acid secretion. This so-called proton pump inhibitor is prescribed for the treatment of duodenal ulcer and for conditions of abnormal acidity such as serious heartburn (GERD) or the rare Zollinger-Ellison syndrome. It has a very quick onset and is extremely effective in reducing stomach acid.

Special Precautions: Animal studies have shown that **Prilosec** is associated with a dose-related increase in stomach cancers. It is not known whether this risk also applies to humans. In addition, because it is so effective at reducing stomach acid concentrations, patients taking this medicine have higher levels of certain microorganisms in their stomachs than would normally survive there. Scientists do not yet know whether these bacteria have negative long-term consequences. Regular supplementation with vitamins C and E might in theory provide protection against nitrosamines produced by the bacteria.

People with liver disease have more trouble metabolizing **Prilosec**. Older people also remove the drug from circulation more slowly.

Taking the Medicine: **Prilosec** should be taken before meals. These delayed-release capsules should not be opened, crushed, or chewed, because that might expose them to stomach acid. The medication can be inactivated by acid. Antacids may be taken with **Prilosec** if they are needed.

Side Effects and Interactions: **Prilosec** is generally well tolerated. However, headache, diarrhea, stomachache, muscle weakness, and rash have been reported. Other adverse reactions that have been reported less commonly include constipation, cough, fatigue, sore throat, and vomiting. Report any symptoms or suspected reactions to your physician promptly.

Prilosec slows the elimination of several drugs that must be processed by the liver, including the anxiety medicine **Valium**, the antiepileptic **Dilantin,** and the blood thinner **Coumadin.** Blood levels of these drugs may rise and side effects become a problem. If you take both **Prilosec** and **Coumadin**, tell your doctor right away if you experience any unusual bruising, bleeding, reddish urine, or blackened stools. **Prilosec** is also reported to alter blood levels of the immunosuppressant **Sandimmune** or the antialcohol drug **Antabuse.**

Many other prescription drugs require acidity for absorption. **Prilosec** can interfere with such medicines, which include **Nizoral**, ampicillin, and iron supplements, among others. Extra supplementation with vitamin B_{12} may be a good idea. Be sure to check with your pharmacist and physician about potential interactions before taking any other medication in combination with **Prilosec**.

Prinivil

lisinopril

Overview: **Prinivil** is one of the more recent entries in a class of drugs called ACE (angiotensin-converting enzyme) inhibitors. The development of this group of medications almost reads like a medical mystery. It all started with the venom of a poisonous Brazilian snake. The deadly jararaca caused severe hemorrhaging. An extract from the venom was found to affect the kidney and ultimately blood pressure regulation. This led to the creation of enzyme blockers, including **Capoten, Vasotec,** and **Prinivil,** which are revolutionizing the treatment of hypertension and congestive heart failure. **Prinivil** is prescribed to lower blood pressure.

Special Precautions: The very first dose of **Prinivil** you take may cause dizziness, especially for older people. Be especially careful until your body adjusts.

When you first start taking **Prinivil**, be alert for a rare but serious reaction. Some people have experienced swelling of the face, lips, tongue, and throat, which can make breathing difficult if not impossible. This requires immediate emergency treatment.

Taking the Medicine: **Prinivil** may be taken with food or on an empty stomach. It should be swallowed at the same time every day to maintain consistent levels in the body. Do not stop taking **Prinivil** suddenly, because this could lead to complications.

Side Effects and Interactions: People with kidney problems must be monitored extremely carefully, because **Prinivil** can make kidney function worse. Even normal people should have their physician monitor the kidneys periodically.

Prinivil can cause a number of less serious but uncomfortable side effects. Be alert for an annoying dry cough, skin rash, headache, tiredness, chest pain, nausea, vomiting, diarrhea, muscle cramps, low blood pressure, nasal congestion, heart rhythm disturbances, and sexual difficulties. Report any symptoms or suspected side effects without delay.

There are a number of compounds that can interact with **Prinivil**. In general it is important to avoid potassium supplements, including low-sodium salt substitutes. Diuretics such as **Dyazide, Aldactazide,** and **Moduretic,** which preserve potassium, can also cause dangerous elevations in potassium.

Other drugs that can interact with **Prinivil** include other diuretics, the arthritis medicine **Indocin,** and the manic-depression drug lithium. Check with your doctor and pharmacist to make sure **Prinivil** is safe in combination with any other drugs you take.

Procardia XL

nifedipine (sustained release)

Overview: **Procardia XL** belongs to a class of medicines called calcium channel blockers. **Procardia** was the first of these to be used in the United States. Because of their safety and effectiveness, calcium channel blockers have helped revolutionize the treatment of angina and high blood pressure. Unlike certain other drugs in this class, **Procardia XL** is not approved for treating irregular heart rhythms. This sustained-release **Procardia** has been approved only for treatment of high blood pressure. Controversy surrounds the short-acting version of this drug (see page 34).

Preliminary research suggests some calcium channel blockers may be able to prevent migraine headaches, ease nighttime leg cramps, relieve asthma brought on by exercise, and perhaps reduce atherosclerosis. **Procardia** is under investigation for its effect on asthma, preterm labor, and Raynaud's disease.

Special Precautions: **Procardia XL** lowers blood pressure more in elderly people than in middle-aged or younger patients. Occasionally, people react to this drug with low blood pressure, which may show up as light-headedness and dizziness. To avoid falling, these patients should rise slowly and make sure they are holding on to a support.

Taking the Medicine: **Procardia XL** needs to be taken only once daily. It should be swallowed whole, and not chewed or crushed. Check with your pharmacist for specific instructions. Do not worry if you see a tablet in your stool; this is normal and does not indicate the drug is passing through unabsorbed. **Procardia XL** should not be taken with grapefruit juice because the interaction could make side effects more likely.

Do not stop taking **Procardia XL** suddenly, because this could lead to complications. Your doctor will tell you how to taper off gradually if you no longer need this medication.

Side Effects and Interactions: **Procardia XL** is usually well tolerated with few side effects. Flushing or a feeling of heat, headache, loss of strength, or nausea may also occur. Another reaction to be alert for is fluid retention leading to swelling of the legs, feet, or hands.

Any unusual bruising or bleeding should be reported to your doctor, as should irregular heartbeat, shortness of breath, nausea, dizziness, or constipation. Other side effects may include heart palpitations, muscle cramps, diarrhea, gas, nasal congestion, cough, rash, nervousness, sexual difficulties, dry mouth, blurred vision, and trouble sleeping. People with liver disease should use **Procardia XL** only under close medical supervision, because careful monitoring is necessary. It is wise to report any symptoms or suspected side effects to your physician promptly.

Procardia XL can interact with a number of other drugs, including several that are used to treat high blood pressure or heart conditions, the asthma medicine theophylline, and the ulcer drug **Tagamet**. If you took a beta-blocker such as **Corgard, Inderal,** or **Tenormin** before starting on **Procardia XL**, your beta-blocker medicine should be tapered off gradually. Aspirin in combination with **Procardia** could increase susceptibility to bleeding. Asthma medicine and tuberculosis medicine could also present difficulties. Check with your doctor and pharmacist to make sure **Procardia XL** is safe in combination with any other drugs you may be given.

Propoxyphene N with APAP

propoxyphene napsylate and acetaminophen

Overview: This pain reliever is a combination of propoxyphene napsylate and acetaminophen. It is sometimes prescribed under the brand name **Darvocet-N.**

Propoxyphene is a mild synthetic analgesic. In combination with acetaminophen, it offers relief for mild to moderate pain, such as that caused by a bad toothache or the aftermath of minor surgery.

Special Precautions: Some people react to propoxyphene with nausea or vomiting. Taking it with food may reduce stomach upset. Nausea, dizziness and other common reactions may be less troublesome if you lie down for a while.

Taking the Medicine: This medicine is less likely to upset your stomach if you take it with food. Ask the doctor how often you should take it and if it needs to be taken on a regular schedule or only when the pain starts to bother you.

Side Effects and Interactions: Like any narcotic, propoxyphene may make you drowsy. Do not drive or attempt any activity that requires coordination and judgment. Older people may be more susceptible to this reaction. Light-headedness or dizziness could make walking dangerous. Standing up suddenly could make you feel faint.

Other side effects to be aware of include headache, euphoria, abdominal pain, sweating, and constipation. Some people experience shortness of breath, especially if they have asthma. Other less common reactions include skin rash, disorientation, dry mouth, visual problems, and urinary difficulties. Report any such symptoms to your physician promptly.

Long-term use of this combination pain-reliever has drawbacks. Like any narcotic, it may be habit-forming if you take it regularly in large doses. Do not increase the dose on your own in a quest to achieve greater pain relief. But don't play the hero by skipping doses during an acute crisis. Pain is more easily managed if it can be nipped in the bud instead of trying to play catch-up when it has gotten out of control.

Acetaminophen and propoxyphene may both cause liver problems in large doses or over long periods. Liver function should be monitored. Because kidney damage is also a potential risk, your physician should evaluate your need for this combination pain reliever periodically.

If you are taking any other medicines, check with a physician or pharmacist. Alcohol as well as many over-the-counter and prescription drugs can add to the sedative effect of this analgesic. Antihistamines, antianxiety agents, antidepressants, and sleeping pills require extra caution. Anticonvulsants and blood thinners such as **Coumadin** may become more dangerous for patients who are also taking propoxyphene with APAP.

Propulsid

cisapride

Overview: **Propulsid** promotes good muscle tone in the gastrointestinal tract and in so doing facilitates the proper movement of food through the system. It is prescribed for nighttime heartburn due to acid splashback from the stomach to the esophagus through the ring of muscle known as the lower esophageal sphincter. Instead of combating the symptoms of heartburn by neutralizing or reducing the acid produced in the stomach, **Propulsid** tightens the sphincter to help keep the acid in the stomach where it belongs.

Special Precautions: **Propulsid** should not be taken when there is gastrointestinal bleeding, obstruction of the bowel, or a possible perforation. Increasing digestive tract movement in such cases could be dangerous.

Although Propulsid doesn't slow reflexes or impair judgment on its own, it may increase the impairment experienced by a person taking an antianxiety medicine such as **Valium** or **Xanax**. If **Propulsid** must be taken together with a benzodiazepine, a prudent person will avoid driving or operating dangerous machinery.

Taking the Medicine: **Propulsid** is taken four times a day, at least 15 minutes before meals and at bedtime. Store the pills away from moisture at room temperature (between 59 and 86 degrees Fahrenheit).

Side Effects and Interactions: Reported side effects of **Propulsid** include headache, diarrhea, stomachache, constipation, flatulence, runny nose, and vision disturbances. Other reactions, such as insomnia or drowsiness, vaginitis, dry mouth, palpitations, tremor, and migraine, are less common. Many other effects were reported rarely during clinical trials, and some potential side effects of this relatively new drug may not yet have been recorded. Report any symptoms to your physician promptly.

Because **Propulsid** is prescribed for heartburn, other medicines that work to reduce acid secretion may be prescribed at the same time. Both **Tagamet** and **Zantac** are absorbed more rapidly when given with **Propulsid**. **Tagamet** also increases the blood levels of **Propulsid**. Other stomach medicines such as **Donnatal** or **Pro-Banthine** would work against **Propulsid** and shouldn't be combined with it.

Besides increasing sphincter pressure, **Propulsid** hastens stomach-emptying. This is generally beneficial but it could interfere with proper absorption of other medicines taken together with **Propulsid**. Blood levels of such medicines may need to be monitored more frequently. **Propulsid** increases the action of blood thinners such as **Coumadin**. Blood-clotting time should be checked carefully both when patients on anticoagulants start taking **Propulsid** and when they stop. Alcohol and sedative drugs such as **Halcion, Restoril, Ativan,** or **Xanax** produce more impair-ment in a person who is also taking **Propulsid**. Because **Propulsid** is a relatively new medication, there may be other drug interactions that have not yet been iden-tified. Do not take any other medication without first asking your physician and pharmacist to check on the potential for interaction with **Propulsid**.

Proscar

finasteride

Overview: **Proscar** is a unique compound that counters some of the negative effects of testosterone in the body. It blocks an enzyme that converts testosterone to a more potent hormone called 5-alpha-dihydrotestosterone (DHT for short). This testosterone derivative is apparently responsible in most cases for the gradual enlargement of the prostate gland that occurs as a man ages. It may also have a role to play in male pattern baldness. **Proscar** is prescribed to treat the symptoms of be-nign prostatic hypertrophy (BPH—noncancerous enlargement of the prostate gland). Although prostate tissue actually shrinks in most men who take **Proscar**, only about half or possibly fewer will get good relief from symptoms such as diffi-cult urination. A man must take **Proscar** for 6 months before the benefits of the medicine can be assessed.

Special Precautions: DHT is crucial for the normal development of a male fetus and is important in early male sexual development. **Proscar** should never be administered to children or women for this reason. The manufacturer warns that pregnant women should not handle crushed **Proscar** tablets or be exposed to the semen of a patient on **Proscar** to avoid possible harm to a male infant.

Because **Proscar** is relatively new, the long-term experience with it is limited. Periodic physical examination of the prostate is recommended for men on **Proscar**.

Taking the Medicine: **Proscar** is taken once a day with or without meals. It should be stored at temperatures below 86 degrees Fahrenheit in a tightly closed container.

Side Effects and Interactions: **Proscar** is usually very well tolerated and side effects are uncommon. A few men have experienced impotence, lower sex drive, or less ejaculate. Report any symptoms to your physician.

No significant drug interactions have shown up in the medical literature. As doctors and patients acquire more experience with **Proscar**, however, that may change. Check with your doctor and pharmacist to make sure **Proscar** is safe in combination with any other drugs you take.

Proventil Aerosol

albuterol

Overview: **Proventil** is the most commonly prescribed asthma inhaler in this country. Although this medicine is also available in tablet form for oral use, the aerosol formulation is less likely to cause general side effects and is more frequently prescribed.

Proventil Aerosol is prescribed for the prevention as well as the treatment of asthma attacks. It may also be used 15 minutes before vigorous activity to prevent exercise-induced asthma.

Special Precautions: Although **Proventil** is very effective, care must be taken not to overuse it. Because of a relatively short duration of action—4 to 6 hours—people may be tempted to use their inhaler too frequently. This could lead to complications.

Taking the Medicine: **Proventil Aerosol** needs to be kept at room temperature—that is, between 59 and 86 degrees Fahrenheit. If the aerosol is used at a different temperature, it may not provide an accurate dose.

Use of inhalers is not so easy as it may seem. Make sure your physician provides detailed instructions and demonstrates how to inhale the aerosol so that the medicine ends up in the lungs and not in the back of the throat.

Side Effects and Interactions: One advantage of inhaled asthma medicine is that relatively little is absorbed into the body to cause unpleasant side effects. However, inhaled **Proventil** can cause palpitations or rapid heartbeat in some people. Individuals with preexisting heart conditions, diabetes, seizures, or an overactive thyroid gland should use such medicine with great caution, if at all.

Other side effects include nausea, tremor, nervousness, increased blood pressure, heartburn, and dizziness. There are rare reports of rash, itching, and allergic reactions that interfere with breathing. In addition, the active ingredient in **Proventil** can precipitate angina, insomnia, headache, unusual taste, and irritation of the throat. Report any symptoms to your physician promptly.

Proventil can interact with several other medications. Do not use a similar kind of bronchodilating inhaler such as **Ventolin, Berotec, Brethaire, Alupent, Metaprel,** or **Tornalate** simultaneously with **Proventil**. Certain antidepressants may also be dangerous in combination with this asthma drug, and beta-blocker medications may counteract the effectiveness of **Proventil**. Check with your pharmacist and physician before using any other medication in combination with this inhaler.

Provera

medroxyprogesterone

Overview: **Provera** is derived from a natural female hormone, progesterone. It is prescribed to bring on menstrual periods or treat abnormal uterine bleeding.

Although other uses have not yet been approved by the Food and Drug Administration, **Provera** is probably prescribed most often to menopausal women in conjunction with estrogen hormones such as **Premarin**. Estrogens increase the risk of uterine cancer, and **Provera** may help offset this danger. Doctors also sometimes prescribe this progestin for severe sleeping disturbances characterized by breathing difficulties,

Special Precautions: Some people should probably not take **Provera**. Those with a history of thrombophlebitis or other blood-clotting problems are at increased risk. Patients with liver disease, breast cancer, a history of miscarriage, stroke, seizures, or undiagnosed vaginal bleeding should probably not receive **Provera** unless there are extenuating circumstances. This drug should generally be avoided during pregnancy.

Other conditions that require caution include diabetes, asthma, heart problems, migraine headaches, kidney disease, and psychological depression. A controversy exists over the potential carcinogenicity of medroxyprogesterone. Some animal studies have shown an increased risk of breast cancer.

Taking the Medicine: **Provera** may be taken with food, especially if it upsets your digestive tract.

Side Effects and Interactions: Side effects associated with **Provera** include breast tenderness, psychological depression, headache, bloating, acne, breakthrough vaginal bleeding and changes in menstrual flow, fluid retention, changes in weight, reduced libido, excess facial hair and loss of scalp hair, and rash.

Other adverse reactions include insomnia, increased susceptibility to sunburn, increased cholesterol, jaundice, freckling of the skin, dizziness, fatigue, backache, and the development of blood clots in the legs, lungs, and brain. Report any symptoms to your physician promptly. Pain, swelling, and redness in the calves, sudden shortness of breath or chest pain, sudden severe headache or vomiting, fainting, or numbness in an arm or leg should all trigger an immediate call to the doctor or a trip to the emergency room.

Provera interacts with certain other medications. The tuberculosis medicine rifampin, and **Cytadren**, a drug used for Cushing's syndrome, may interfere with **Provera**. Check with your pharmacist and physician before using any other medication in combination with this drug.

Prozac

fluoxetine

Overview: **Prozac** was the first of a new generation of antidepressants to come on the market. It works by enhancing the action of a brain chemical called serotonin. In a few short years this drug has become so popular that, in addition to becoming the most prescribed antidepressant on the physicians' hit parade of drugs, it has become a household name. **Prozac** has been featured on the covers of newsmagazines and has even been the subject of a best-selling book (*Listening to Prozac*).

This success comes largely because **Prozac** is less likely to cause typical side effects associated with older medications. Tricyclic antidepressants such as **Elavil,**

Tofranil, Sinequan, and **Pamelor** can produce dry mouth, constipation, dizziness, weight gain, and a sluggish or lethargic feeling. **Prozac** does not. If anything, it has a slight stimulant action.

Prozac is used in the treatment of depression; it is also approved for treating obsessive-compulsive disorder (OCD). Psychiatrists continue to experiment with the use of this medication for eating disorders and other problems.

Special Precautions: Some people may need very close monitoring if the doctor prescribes **Prozac**. Because this drug may cause anxiety, nervousness, and insomnia in a substantial number of people, those with a predisposition to such conditions need to alert their physicians if such symptoms are aggravated by **Prozac**.

Patients with kidney disease, diabetes, liver problems, or a history of seizures also require careful monitoring while they are taking **Prozac**.

People with a history of suicide attempts must also be extremely vigilant. There have been reports that some people may develop a preoccupation with suicide or violence while taking **Prozac**. It is still not certain whether this is caused by the underlying mental condition or is in some way related to the drug. Family members must help monitor people on **Prozac** for suicidal thoughts or self-destructive behaviors. The doctor must be notified immediately in such cases.

Taking the Medicine: According to the manufacturer, you may take **Prozac** with or without food. If it upsets your stomach you may find that swallowing **Prozac** with meals may be helpful.

Side Effects and Interactions: Side effects associated with **Prozac** include headache, nervousness, agitation, insomnia, tremor, fatigue, rash, light-headedness, drowsiness, dizziness, depersonalization, nausea, upset stomach, diarrhea, loss of appetite, stomach pain, sweating, and dry mouth.

Somewhat less common adverse reactions include impaired concentration and memory, weird dreams, lowered libido, loss or delay of orgasm, abnormal ejaculation, dry skin, constipation, hair loss, and itching. Report any symptoms to your physician promptly.

Uncommon, but very serious side effects to be alert for, are rash with flulike symptoms such as chills, fever, or sore throat, anemia, breathing problems, severe allergy, or seizures.

Prozac interacts with a number of other medications. Anyone taking other antidepressants, especially drugs such as **Nardil** or **Parnate** (MAO inhibitors) should stop such a medicine at least two weeks before starting on **Prozac**. If **Prozac** was taken first, five weeks should elapse before starting on one of these other medicines, because **Prozac** can last in the body a long time.

Tricyclic antidepressants such as **Elavil** or **Tofranil,** and even **Anafranil** for obsessive-compulsive disorder, may have stronger actions and more pronounced toxicity when they are combined with **Prozac**. If such a combination is prescribed, the physician should monitor blood levels of the medications. The same is true of the antipsychotic drug **Haldol**.

If the amino acid tryptophan ever becomes available in this country again, it should not be taken with **Prozac,** because it may increase the potential for adverse reactions. Other compounds that could cause complications in combination with **Prozac** include the bipolar-disorder treatment lithium, the anticoagulant **Coumadin,** the heart drug **Lanoxin,** and the antianxiety agent **Valium** (or similar medications such as **Dalmane, Halcion,** or **Klonopin**). Check with your pharmacist and physician before taking any other medicines.

Relafen

nabumetone

Overview: **Relafen** belongs to a class of medications commonly called NSAIDs, or nonsteroidal anti-inflammatory drugs. It is prescribed for both short-term and long-term treatment of osteoarthritis and rheumatoid arthritis.

Pain relief begins relatively quickly, but the full benefits of **Relafen**'s ability to fight inflammation may take a week or two to set in. **Relafen** is converted by the liver into the compound that actually provides relief.

Special Precautions: People who are allergic to aspirin, ibuprofen, or other anti-inflammatory agents should avoid **Relafen** as well. Signs of allergy include breathing difficulties, rash, fever, or a sudden drop in blood pressure, and require immediate medical attention.

Taking the Medicine: **Relafen** may be taken with or without food, once or twice a day. Taking **Relafen** with food may help reduce possible stomach irritation. This will increase the peak concentration in the bloodstream by approximately one-third and may speed the onset of pain relief slightly. Taking an NSAID with food does not guarantee that the drug will be safe for the stomach.

Relafen should be stored at room temperature between 59 and 86 degrees Fahrenheit in a tightly closed, light-resistant container.

Side Effects and Interactions: Unquestionably the most common side effects of **Relafen** involve the gastrointestinal tract. They include diarrhea, indigestion, and stomachache. Constipation, gas, and nausea are not unusual. Some people may develop ulcers and intestinal bleeding while taking any NSAID. Although **Relafen** may be somewhat less likely to cause such complications, the risk remains. Occasionally these problems can occur without obvious symptoms, and lead to a life-threatening crisis due to perforation of the stomach lining.

Older people appear to be more susceptible to this problem and should be monitored carefully. Warning signs include weight loss, persistent indigestion, a feeling of fullness after moderate meals, dark or tarry stools, anemia, and unusual fatigue. Home stool tests such as **Hemoccult** or **Fleet Detecatest** may provide an early indication of bleeding.

Other side effects to be alert for include dizziness, headache, fatigue, rash, itching, fluid retention, and ringing in the ears. Less common complications include dry or sore mouth, vomiting, increased sweating, drowsiness, insomnia, and nervousness. Do not drive if you become impaired due to insomnia or sleepiness. Report any symptoms to your physician promptly.

Relafen can affect both the kidney and liver, so periodic blood tests to monitor the function of these organs are important for anyone on this drug long-term.

This medication may interact adversely with certain other drugs. In clinical trials it was used successfully with gold, penicillamine, and corticosteroids in treating rheumatoid arthritis, but this therapy should be supervised by an experienced physician. A person taking a blood thinner such as **Coumadin** may become more vulnerable to a dangerous bleeding ulcer. Aspirin interferes with the effectiveness of other NSAIDs for reducing inflammation, although it is not clear whether this is true of **Relafen**.

Most NSAIDs can make methotrexate (**Folex** and **Rheumatrex**), lithium (**Eskalith, Lithobid**, etc.), and **Lanoxin** far more toxic and this possibility should be considered for **Relafen**. When **Relafen** is combined with **Sandimmune** the risk of kidney damage may be increased. **Relafen** is still a relatively new drug and more interactions may become apparent as clinical experience accumulates. Ask your doctor and pharmacist to check whether **Relafen** interacts with any other drugs you take.

Retin-A

tretinoin

Overview: This acne medication is available in cream, gel, and liquid formulations in various strengths. It is very effective in cases of mild or moderate acne, and that is the only condition for which the FDA has approved its use. However, doctors also prescribe **Retin-A** to smooth the fine wrinkling and discoloration of skin that has been damaged by years of sun exposure, and it is under study for use in treating precancerous skin lesions. It has been used experimentally to treat several kinds of skin cancer as well as certain forms of psoriasis and other rare skin conditions.

Special Precautions: Although there has been no evidence of danger to the fetus, pregnant women are advised not to use this medication unless a doctor tells them it is necessary.

Retin-A may increase the skin's susceptibility to sunburn, so it is best to avoid sunbathing or tanning lamps. Many sunscreens can interact with **Retin-A** to inactivate it, so they should not be applied at the same time. Putting sunscreen on in the morning if **Retin-A** was applied at bedtime should not pose a problem.

Taking the Medicine: **Retin-A** is usually applied to clean, dry skin once a day, at bedtime. It should be kept away from the eyes, the corners of the mouth, and the angles of the nose. Putting the medicine on damp skin may cause irritation, so at least 30 minutes should be allowed between washing the face and applying the medication. If the skin becomes red and starts to flake, hurt or blister, it is prudent to stop using **Retin-A** for a few days or switch to a lower concentration.

When using **Retin-A** to treat wrinkles, dermatologists recommend using the highest concentration that can be managed. After two or three years of daily use, it may be possible to maintain the benefits using **Retin-A** twice a week.

Side Effects and Interactions: The most common side effect of **Retin-A** is skin irritation. This is made worse by exposure to wind, cold, or other irritating chemicals, including abrasive or drying cleansers, products containing alcohol or astringents, and many over-the-counter acne preparations. Some people have reported temporary changes in skin color where **Retin-A** was applied. Notify your physician if you develop any unexpected symptoms.

Risperdal

risperidone

Overview: **Risperdal** is the first in its class, a new kind of medicine prescribed to treat psychotic disorders. Clinical studies show that it is effective against the symptoms of schizophrenia such as hallucinations, suspiciousness, and disorganized thought. It also appears to be helpful against other schizophrenic symptoms, including apathy and social withdrawal, that don't respond well to other medications. **Risperdal** may be effective for certain patients who haven't responded well to other antipsychotic drugs. Some experts believe that **Risperdal** is better than the older and more conventional schizophrenia drug **Haldol**, and it has a different side-effect profile.

Special Precautions: Because **Risperdal** is metabolized through the liver and kidneys, people with kidney disease or liver problems need to have their dose of **Risperdal** adjusted carefully. Older people, who often have reduced kidney or liver function, may also require lower doses.

Since **Risperdal**, like other drugs that affect the nervous system, might slow reflexes or impair judgment, people taking it should be advised not to drive or operate dangerous equipment unless they can determine that they are unimpaired.

Antipsychotic drugs may in some cases trigger a life-threatening reaction in which body temperature rises, muscles become rigid, heart rhythm and blood pressure changes, and the person loses consciousness. This is a medical emergency, and a person on any schizophrenia medicine who develops some of these symptoms should be treated immediately.

Long-term use of conventional antipsychotic drugs can lead to the development of involuntary repetitive movements such as jerks, tics, twitches, chewing, or tongue-thrusting. Called *tardive dyskinesia,* this side effect is among the most unpleasant drawbacks of chronic treatment for schizophrenia. It is hoped that holding **Risperdal** doses to 6 mg daily or less will reduce the risk of tardive dyskinesia. Because the drug is so new, however, long-term experience with it is limited.

Taking the Medicine: **Risperdal** should be taken twice a day and may be taken with or without meals.

Side Effects and Interactions: Some people starting on **Risperdal** may find that they feel dizzy or faint if they stand up suddenly. They should take care to avoid falling when they first get up. **Risperdal** may cause anxiety, drowsiness, dizziness, constipation, nausea, indigestion, runny nose, rash, rapid heartbeat, and uncontrollable muscle movements,

Other adverse reactions to be alert for include sleeping longer and dreaming more, visual problems, sensitivity to sunlight leading to sunburn, fatigue, weight gain, diarrhea, constipation, sexual difficulties, difficult urination, heavy menstrual periods, dry vagina, and reduced salivation. Report any symptoms to your physician promptly.

Risperdal may interact with other medications, but most of the potential interactions have not yet been carefully studied. Alcohol should be avoided by patients taking this drug. Blood pressure medicines may increase the trouble with feeling faint upon standing up (orthostatic hypotension). **Risperdal** may counteract the benefits of the Parkinson's disease drug, levodopa. The antiseizure drug **Tegretol** may speed removal of **Risperdal** from the body, possibly reducing its concentration below the desired level. The antischizophrenic medicine **Clozaril** can reduce the body's ability to eliminate **Risperdal** and may lead to increased blood levels. Many medications processed by the same liver enzyme as **Risperdal** have a potential for interaction, but the medicine is still so new that there are few if any reports as of this writing. Check with your doctor and pharmacist to make sure **Risperdal** is safe in combination with any other drugs you take.

Seldane

terfenadine

Overview: **Seldane** was the first of a new generation of allergy medicines called histamine (H_1) receptor antagonists. This nonsedating antihistamine was first introduced in Europe in 1981. It was approved in the United States in 1985 and quickly took the market by storm.

Prior to **Seldane**, virtually all oral antihistamines caused some degree of sedation. This made driving or operating machinery dangerous. Since many allergy sufferers felt spaced out on such drugs, they often questioned whether the treatment was worse than the sniffles and sneezes it was supposed to relieve. When **Seldane** became available, the medicine provided many people symptom-management without reducing alertness or coordination. And unlike other allergy medicine, **Seldane** did not appear to interact with sedatives.

Special Precautions: Although **Seldane** is available over the counter in many countries, including Canada, Switzerland, England, Germany, and Belgium, some people develop irregular heart rhythms and abnormal electrocardiograms while on **Seldane.** This hazard seems particularly pertinent at higher doses or in combination with certain other medications. (See "*Side Effects and Interactions,*" below.) Do not exceed the prescribed dose of Seldane, and report any symptoms such as dizziness or faintness, chest discomfort, or palpitations. Be aware, however, that there may be no warning symptoms other than changes on an ECG (electrocardiogram). Patients with preexisting heart or liver problems or those with unusually low levels of potassium or calcium in the body may be more susceptible to this danger.

Taking the Medicine: The usual dose is one tablet taken twice daily. The manufacturer makes no recommendation about whether this medicine should be taken with food or on an empty stomach. Because many antihistamines, including **Seldane**, can cause digestive tract upset, it is often recommended that they be taken with food to lessen this problem. Do not take **Seldane** with grapefruit juice. Grapefruit and grapefruit juice, like **Nizoral** or erythromycin, affect the liver enzyme that processes **Seldane**. In theory, this combination might lead to dangerously high levels of **Seldane**, and possibly heart rhythm disturbances.

Side Effects and Interactions: Side effects with **Seldane** are relatively rare, but people occasionally report dry mouth, nausea, vomiting, headache, jitteriness, hair loss, increased appetite, fatigue, cough, and sore throat. Although less sedating than most other antihistamines, some individuals do experience drowsiness or tiredness while taking **Seldane.** Report any symptoms or suspected side effects to your physician promptly.

Heart rhythm changes, including torsade de pointes, have been reported in people also taking the antifungal medicines **Nizoral** or **Sporanox** or antibiotics including **Biaxin,** erythromycin, and troleandomycin. Other drugs, such as **Luvox** (fluvoxamine), that affect the same liver enzyme (cytochrome P450 3A4) may also turn out to be hazardous in combination with **Seldane.** ECGs that show prolonged QT intervals or irregular heartbeats may be the only warning that **Seldane** levels are too high. Let your doctor know immediately if you experience chest discomfort, shortness of breath, fainting, or dizziness while taking **Seldane** in combination with another medication.

Other drugs that prolong the QT interval might turn out to be dangerous in connection with **Seldane**, although we don't know of any cases. These include the cholesterol medicine **Lorelco,** the schizophrenia drugs **Haldol** and **Mellaril,** and a number of heart medicines such as **Betapace, Cardioquin, Norpace,** or **Quinidex** (quinidine). Ask your doctor to monitor closely if you require such a combination.

Synthroid

levothyroxine

Overview: Thyroid hormones come in a variety of formulations and brand names. **Synthroid** is the most commonly prescribed of all the thyroid supplements. That is because the dose is more reliable than natural products made of dried thyroid glands. **Synthroid** is long-acting and comes in a wide variety of doses that allow for individualized treatment.

When people develop a sluggish thyroid gland they often feel tired and weak. They may become constipated, sensitive to cold, or anemic. They may also suffer with dry skin and hair, thick brittle fingernails, and have shortness of breath when they exercise. Some people report clumsiness, weight gain, or puffy eyes.

Thyroid problems are diagnosed with blood tests. The best is one that measures thyroid-stimulating hormone, or TSH. This test also helps determine the proper dose of thyroid hormone for treatment.

Special Precautions: Too much **Synthroid** can make a person more susceptible to osteoporosis or weakened bones. You may wish to discuss with your doctor whether you need tests to monitor bone density. Thyroid replacement is usually needed for the rest of one's life, and stopping the medicine suddenly could precipitate symptoms of inactive thyroid. Don't discontinue **Synthroid** without your doctor's supervision.

Taking the Medicine: The usual recommendation is to take **Synthroid** before breakfast. Although this hormone is probably best taken on an empty stomach, it is more important to take it at the same time every day to maintain a constant level in your body. Do not take this medication with iron pills, as they can interfere with proper absorption.

Side Effects and Interactions: Side effects of thyroid replacement therapy are rare if the dose is appropriate. Specialists recommend beginning treatment with a low dose and gradually increasing it until symptoms of underactive thyroid disappear and the TSH blood test is normal. This may initially require blood tests every four to six weeks and good communication with the doctor.

Signs of overdose include insomnia, heart palpitations, jitteriness, rapid heartbeat, increased sweating, higher blood pressure, changes in appetite, and reduced menstrual flow. Other adverse reactions of excessive thyroid levels include tremor, headache, heart disease, diarrhea, and weight loss. Report any such symptoms to your physician promptly.

A number of medications may interact with **Synthroid** or alter the tests that detect thyroid problems. People taking estrogen, asthma medicines, decongestants (including those found in over-the-counter cold or flu remedies), antidepressants, certain cholesterol-lowering drugs, blood thinners such as **Coumadin,** or heart medicine such as digoxin should check with a physician or pharmacist. And never stop taking **Synthroid** without first checking with your health care provider.

Tagamet

cimetidine

Overview: **Tagamet** was the first of a new class of ulcer drugs, called "H_2 antagonists." It works by suppressing the secretion of stomach acid, so it is also used to treat conditions of abnormal acidity such as serious heartburn, as well as helping ulcers clear up rapidly. Doctors sometimes prescribe **Tagamet** as maintenance therapy to keep ulcers from coming back. **Tagamet HB** is now available over the counter to treat indigestion.

Special Precautions: Perhaps because **Tagamet** is so effective at reducing stomach acid concentrations, patients taking this medicine have higher levels of certain microorganisms in their stomachs than would normally survive there. Scientists do not yet know whether these bacteria have negative long-term consequences. Regular supplementation with vitamins C and E might in theory provide protection against possible adverse consequences.

People with liver or kidney trouble may not be able to tolerate the usual dose of **Tagamet**. Ask your doctor to monitor you as you begin this medicine.

Taking the Medicine: **Tagamet** may be taken with food, especially if it upsets your stomach. If antacids are needed for relief of ulcer pain, they should generally be taken at a different time.

Side Effects and Interactions: Side effects associated with **Tagamet** are not common. However, headache, drowsiness, dizziness, and diarrhea have been reported. Older patients may experience mental confusion or even hallucinations. Other adverse reactions that have been reported include impotence, breast enlargement in men, rash, hair loss, changes in heart rhythm, liver problems, and blood alterations. Report any symptoms to your physician promptly.

Tagamet can interact with many other drugs. The blood thinner **Coumadin** may become far more potent in the presence of **Tagamet** and can lead to dangerous bleeding. Tell your doctor right away if you experience any unusual bruising, bleeding, reddish urine or blackened stools. **Tagamet** may also increase blood levels of the asthma drug theophylline, possibly to dangerous levels.

Other prescription drugs that may be more dangerous with **Tagamet** include anticonvulsants such as **Dilantin** or **Tegretol**, the antifungal medicine **Nizoral,** and certain drugs prescribed to control irregular heart rhythms (moricizine, procainamide, quinidine). Certain others don't mix well, either, including such antianxiety agents as **Valium**, some beta-blocker blood pressure drugs, antidepressants such as **Pamelor**, and oral diabetes medicines.

Nonprescription drugs that interact with **Tagamet** include antacids, alcohol, caffeine, and cigarettes. Caffeine may have more impact on people taking this medicine, while cigarette smoking may tend to counteract its antiulcer benefits. Check with your pharmacist and physician before taking any other medication in combination with **Tagamet**.

Tegretol

carbamazepine

Overview: **Tegretol** is prescribed for the control of a variety of seizure disorders. It is also used as a special kind of pain reliever for trigeminal neuralgia, which produces severe facial pain. Although the Food and Drug Administration has not approved **Tegretol** for other uses, doctors sometimes prescribe it for a variety of psychiatric disorders, alcohol withdrawal, and restless leg syndrome.

Special Precautions: Some people should not take **Tegretol.** Elderly patients may be especially susceptible to side effects of confusion, agitation, or even psychosis. People with glaucoma, heart disease, kidney problems, liver damage, lupus, or a history of blood disorders should take **Tegretol** only under close medical supervision, if at all.

This medicine can produce a dangerous anemia or blood disorder that can be life-threatening. Periodic blood tests, particularly during the first two months, are crucial to reduce the risk of this hazard.

Pregnant women should use **Tegretol** only after careful evaluation and discussions with an obstetrician. Anticonvulsants in general have the potential to cause birth defects.

Taking the Medicine: **Tegretol** is best absorbed when it is taken with meals. This should also reduce the likelihood of stomach upset. To maintain its effectiveness, this medicine should be stored in a tightly closed container away from heat and humidity. Stopping it abruptly could lead to seizures and should be avoided.

Side Effects and Interactions: Side effects associated with **Tegretol** include dizziness, drowsiness, incoordination, unsteadiness, mood changes, nausea, vomiting, stomachache, and loss of appetite. Other adverse reactions to be alert for include both diarrhea and constipation, rash, itching, urinary difficulties, headache, fatigue, blurred vision, ringing in the ears, numbness and tingling of the hands and feet, swollen legs and feet, heart failure, blood pressure problems, fainting, sexual problems, dehydration, unexplained sore throat with fever and chills, mouth ulcers, and aching joints and muscles.

Blood tests are needed to detect kidney failure, liver enzyme elevations, and blood disorders. Report any symptoms to your physician immediately.

A large number of over-the-counter and prescription medications may interact with **Tegretol** in a dangerous way. Some drugs, such as **Biaxin,** erythromycin, **Darvon** or **Darvocet,** can make **Tegretol** much more toxic, with dangerous blood levels building up surprisingly quickly. Other anticonvulsants interact with **Tegretol** in complicated ways and may even reduce its effectiveness. In addition, **Tegretol** can interfere with the benefits of many other compounds.

Just a few of the many drugs that interact with **Tegretol** include several different kinds of antidepressants, the blood thinner **Coumadin,** the ulcer drug **Tagamet,** the heart and blood pressure medicines **Cardizem, Calan,** and **Verelan,** and certain antibiotics such as tetracycline, **Vibramycin,** and **INH.** Other medications that may cause problems include the asthma drug theophylline, the antipsychotic agent **Haldol,** the immunosuppressant **Sandimmune,** the hormone **Danocrine,** and even flu vaccine and activated charcoal. Do not take any other medication without first checking with your physician and pharmacist.

Tenormin

atenolol

Overview: **Tenormin** is known as a beta-blocker. That means the drug works in part by blunting the action of adrenaline, the body's natural fight-or-flight chemical. People normally respond to stressful situations with a rapid pulse, a pounding heart, and an increase in blood pressure. **Tenormin** helps block such reactions.

This medicine is normally prescribed for high blood pressure, chest pain caused by angina, or heart attack. Although the FDA has not specifically approved its use for other purposes, doctors sometimes prescribe **Tenormin** to treat irregular heart rhythms and performance anxiety such as stage fright. It has also been used to help prevent migraine headaches. The dose will vary depending upon the condition being treated.

Special Precautions: Some people must be very careful if they take beta-blockers. Asthmatics and patients with other respiratory problems are especially vulnerable as these drugs can make breathing worse. **Tenormin** is a little better than other beta-blockers in this regard, but monitor your breathing carefully. People with heart failure must also be extremely cautious if prescribed beta-blockers, because the medicine could occasionally lead to cardiac complications.

Taking the Medicine: **Tenormin** can be taken at mealtime or on an empty stomach. If you find this medicine causes digestive tract upset, it may be better tolerated when taken with food. Because of its relatively long action in the body, **Tenormin** offers the convenience of once-daily dosing. Don't take calcium supplements or antacids at the same time as **Tenormin,** because they may reduce its absorption. Never stop taking **Tenormin** suddenly. Your doctor must phase you off gradually to prevent serious heart problems.

Side Effects and Interactions: **Tenormin** can cause a number of side effects. They include slow heart rate, cold hands and feet, tiredness, nightmares, blurred vision, sexual difficulties, nerve tingling, dizziness, nausea, stomachache, gas, diarrhea, indigestion, rash, arthritis, and muscle pain. This medicine may also have a negative effect on cholesterol and other blood fats, so a lipid test before treatment and periodically thereafter would be prudent.

Although **Tenormin** is a little less likely to affect the nervous system than certain other drugs in this class, be alert for the beta-blocker blahs. Symptoms of psychological depression, fatigue, decreased concentration, memory loss, and mood swings may come on slowly and insidiously. Notify your physician promptly of any adverse reactions, especially breathing difficulties, fluid retention in the legs, or a night cough. These drugs may make treatment of diabetes and thyroid disorders more complicated. Check with your physician about special precautions.

Tenormin can interact with a number of other compounds, including the blood pressure medicine **Catapres** (clonidine). This drug should never be suddenly discontinued by a person on **Tenormin** or any other beta-blocker, because the sudden increase in blood pressure could be life-threatening. A potentially fatal increase in blood pressure may also occur when epinephrine is injected into someone taking a beta-blocker such as **Tenormin**. Epinephrine is often included with a local anesthetic injected for dental work or minor surgery, or may be given if someone has a serious allergic reaction that closes airways. A host of other drugs interacting with **Tenormin** include ampicillin and medicines used to treat anxiety, asthma, blood pressure, and heart problems. Arthritis medicine and aspirin may reduce the effectiveness of some beta-blockers. Drugs used to treat migraines, tuberculosis, and high cholesterol do not mix well with beta-blockers. Check with your doctor and pharmacist to make sure **Tenormin** is safe in combination with any other drugs you may take.

Theo-Dur

theophylline

Overview: **Theo-Dur** is a commonly prescribed oral asthma medication that helps open the airways. **Theo-Dur** is an extended-release formulation that enables patients to control breathing symptoms with one or two daily doses. Smokers and children may need more frequent doses. The doctor's instructions on dose and timing should be followed carefully.

Special Precautions: Some people should not take **Theo-Dur**. They include those with peptic ulcers and anyone with a history of seizures. Those with liver problems, heart disease or high blood pressure should be monitored closely if they take **Theo-Dur**.

An acute asthmatic attack in which a person is having difficulty breathing will not respond adequately to **Theo-Dur** and requires immediate medical attention. The patient should be taken for emergency treatment.

Taking the Medicine: There is some question about the best way to swallow **Theo-Dur**. Do not chew or crush the capsule. The manufacturer suggests that a high-fat breakfast does not interfere with absorption. Because theophylline may upset your stomach, you may wish to take this medicine with food to try and reduce digestive tract disturbances. With **Theo-Dur Sprinkle**, the contents of the capsule may be sprinkled on applesauce or other soft food to make it easier for a child or elderly person to swallow. The food should not be chewed.

Side Effects and Interactions: Side effects of theophylline include nausea, vomiting, loss of appetite, stomach pain, diarrhea, headaches, insomnia, restlessness, nervousness, muscle twitching, heart palpitations, increased urination, hair loss, rash, and increased blood sugar. Less common but more serious adverse reactions include heart rhythm disturbances. Seizures, vomiting blood, and dehydration can be symptoms of overdose. Report any complications to your physician promptly. A blood test is extremely helpful in monitoring treatment and determining proper dose. Blood levels should not be higher than 20 micrograms per milliliter.

Theo-Dur interacts with many other drugs, including caffeine. Large amounts of coffee or cola can exacerbate side effects of theophylline. Be aware that some nonprescription pain relievers may also contain caffeine, and exercise appropriate caution.

Although people with asthma may be more susceptible to respiratory tract infections, quinolone antibiotics such as **Cipro, Noroxin,** or **Penetrex** may be dangerous in combination with **Theo-Dur.** They may raise blood levels of the drug gradually and insidiously to the point where serious adverse reactions such as convulsions or heart rhythm changes may occur. A similar and equally dangerous interaction is possible with **Tagamet,** the ulcer medicine.

Other drugs that may cause increased **Theo-Dur** toxicity include antibiotics such as erythromycin or TAO, the antiseizure medicine **Tegretol,** and certain beta-blockers (**Blocadren, Cartrol, Inderal, Levatol, Timoptic** and **Visken**). (People with asthma should avoid beta-blockers in the first place, because they often make breathing worse.) Medications that require extra caution due to potential interactions with **Theo-Dur** include oral contraceptives, calcium blockers such as **Calan** or **Cardizem,** the heart drug **Mexitil,** anticonvulsants such as **Dilantin** or barbiturates, and tuberculosis medicines. It's a good idea to check with your pharmacist and physician before using any other medication in combination with **Theo-Dur.**

thyroid hormones

Cytomel

Euthroid

Levo-T

Levothroid

Levoxine

Proloid

Synthroid

Overview: Thyroid hormones come in a variety of formulations and brand names. Natural products made of dried thyroid glands from beef and pork are sold as **Armour Thyroid, Thyroid Strong,** and **Thyroid USP.** They are generally quite inexpensive, but dosage levels may vary. That is why endocrinologists usually prescribe synthetic products such as **Synthroid** or **Levothroid.**

When people develop a sluggish thyroid gland they often feel tired and weak. They may become constipated, sensitive to cold, or anemic. They may also suffer with dry skin and hair, thick brittle fingernails, and have shortness of breath when they exercise. Some people report clumsiness, weight gain, or puffy eyes. Thyroid problems are diagnosed with blood tests. The best is one that measures thyroid-stimulating hormone, or TSH. This test also helps determine the proper dose of thyroid hormone for treatment.

Special Precautions: Too much thyroid hormone can make a person more susceptible to osteoporosis or weakened bones. You may wish to discuss with your doctor whether you need tests to monitor bone density. Thyroid replacement is usually needed for the rest of one's life, and stopping the medicine suddenly could precipitate symptoms of inactive thyroid. Don't discontinue any thyroid hormone without your doctor's supervision. It is usually best to stick with one formulation rather than switching from one brand to another frequently.

Taking the Medicine: The usual recommendation is to take thyroid hormone before breakfast. Although this hormone is probably best taken on an empty stomach, it is more important to take it at the same time every day to maintain a constant level in your body. Do not take this medication with iron pills, because they can interfere with proper absorption.

Side Effects and Interactions: Side effects of thyroid replacement therapy are rare if the dose is appropriate. Specialists recommend beginning treatment with a low dose and gradually increasing it until symptoms of underactive thyroid disappear and the TSH blood test is normal. This may initially require blood tests every four to six weeks and good communication with the doctor.

Too much thyroid hormone can lead to complications such as osteoporosis and heart disease. Signs of overdose include insomnia, heart palpitations, jitteriness, rapid heartbeat, increased sweating, higher blood pressure, changes in appetite, and reduced menstrual flow. Other adverse reactions of excessive thyroid levels include tremor, headache, diarrhea, and weight loss. Report any such symptoms to your physician promptly.

A number of medications may interact with thyroid hormone or alter the tests that detect thyroid problems. People taking estrogen, asthma medicines, decongestants (including those found in over-the-counter cold or flu remedies), antidepressants, certain cholesterol-lowering drugs, blood thinners such as **Coumadin**, or heart medicine such as digoxin should check with a physician or pharmacist. And never stop taking thyroid hormone without first checking with your health care provider.

Timoptic

timolol

Overview: **Timoptic** eyedrops are very effective at lowering pressure within the eye and have helped provide an important advance in the treatment of some types of glaucoma. The active ingredient, timolol, is known as a beta-blocker. **Timoptic** is normally prescribed alone or with other glaucoma medications to reduce the pressure within the eye.

Special Precautions: Some people should avoid beta-blockers such as **Timoptic** or take them only with great caution. Asthmatics and patients with other respiratory problems are especially vulnerable, because these drugs can make breathing worse. People with heart failure should also alert the ophthalmologist, because beta-blockers may lead to cardiac complications. These eyedrops can also affect blood lipid levels in a negative manner. A consultation between the eye doctor and the one treating lung or heart problems may be in order.

Taking the Medicine: Timoptic is less likely than oral timolol (**Blocadren**) to affect the entire body. Nevertheless, some people absorb this medicine through the eye and into the body as a whole.

Absorption can be reduced somewhat with proper application. It helps to pull the lower eyelid away from the eye to make a pouch, look upward, and put the drop in the pouch without touching the dropper to the eye. As soon as the drops are in, the eyelid should be closed gently for 1 to 2 minutes and pressure applied with a finger to the inside corner of the eye.

Do not stop using **Timoptic** on your own. Your physician will give you special instructions if you need to discontinue these eyedrops or change to another one.

Side Effects and Interactions: Timoptic can cause eye irritation and some visual disturbances. It may also provoke headache, dizziness, slow heart rate, heart rhythm disturbances, chest pain, drowsiness, muscle weakness, sexual difficulties, nausea, diarrhea, muscle weakness, rash, hair loss, and trouble breathing.

Although **Timoptic** is less likely to affect the nervous system than oral beta-blockers, be alert for the beta-blocker blahs. Symptoms of psychological depression, fatigue, confusion, and memory loss may come on slowly and insidiously. Notify your physician promptly of any adverse reactions, especially breathing difficulties, fluid retention in the legs, or a night cough.

Timoptic may interact with surgical anesthetics and increase the risk of heart problems in surgery. Check with the doctor ahead of time to see if you should phase off these eyedrops gradually before you enter the operating room.

This drug may also interact with a number of other compounds, including several that are used to treat blood pressure or heart problems. MAO inhibitors for depression (**Nardil** and **Parnate**) should not be taken with oral timolol and may pose problems with **Timoptic**. **Dilantin** and digoxin may also cause trouble. Oral contraceptives, estrogen replacement therapy, and medicines for arthritis, asthma, migraine headaches, diabetes, and thyroid problems have potential interactions with these eyedrops. Check with your doctor and pharmacist to make sure **Timoptic** is safe in combination with any other drugs you may take.

Toprol XL

metoprolol

Overview: **Toprol XL** belongs to the group of drugs known as beta-blockers. That means it works partly by blunting the action of adrenaline, the body's natural fight-or-flight chemical. People normally respond to stressful situations with a rapid pulse, a pounding heart, and an increase in blood pressure. **Toprol XL** helps block such reactions.

This medicine is normally prescribed for hypertension, chest pain caused by angina, and prevention of a second heart attack. Although the FDA has not specifically approved its use for other purposes, doctors have prescribed **Toprol XL** to treat irregular heart rhythms, tremor, and aggressive behavior and to prevent migraine headaches. The dose will vary depending upon the condition being treated.

Special Precautions: Some people must be very careful if they take beta-blockers. Asthmatics and patients with other respiratory problems are especially vulnerable, as these drugs can make breathing more difficult. **Toprol XL** is a little better than other beta-blockers in this regard, but monitor your breathing carefully. People with heart failure must also be extremely cautious if prescribed beta-blockers because the medicine could lead to cardiac complications.

Taking the Medicine: **Toprol XL** can be taken on an empty stomach, though it is best absorbed when swallowed at mealtime. Food may also reduce the risk of digestive tract upset. To maintain a constant level of the medicine in your bloodstream, try to maintain a regular regimen, taking **Toprol XL** at roughly the same times each day.

Side Effects and Interactions: **Toprol XL** can cause a number of side effects. These include slow heart rate, cold hands and feet, insomnia, nightmares, blurred vision, sexual difficulties, nerve tingling, dizziness, nausea, stomachache, gas, diarrhea, indigestion, rash, arthritis, and muscle pain. This medicine may also have a negative effect on cholesterol and other blood fats, so a lipid test before treatment and periodically thereafter would be prudent.

Toprol XL is a little more likely to affect the nervous system than certain other drugs in this class. Be alert for the beta-blocker blues. Symptoms of psychological depression, fatigue, decreased concentration, memory loss, and mood swings may come on slowly and insidiously. Notify your physician promptly of any adverse reactions, especially breathing difficulties, fluid retention in the legs, or a night cough.

Never stop taking any beta-blocker medication abruptly unless you are under very close medical supervision. Angina or a heart attack could occur. These drugs may also make treatment of diabetes and thyroid disorders more complicated. Your physician will need to monitor such conditions closely.

Toprol XL can interact with a number of other medicines. Antacids containing aluminum or calcium can reduce absorption and interfere with the effectiveness of **Toprol XL**, as can many arthritis drugs and aspirin. Cholesterol-lowering medications like **Cholybar, Questran** or **Colestid,** and penicillin-type antibiotics, might have the same effect on this beta-blocker. The ulcer medicines **Tagamet** and **Zantac** may increase the effects of **Toprol XL**, however.

Other blood pressure medicines such as **Apresoline** or calcium channel blockers like **Calan** or **Procardia** could interact with **Toprol XL** so that the blood pressure–lowering power of each drug is enhanced. **Minipress** is more likely to cause fainting problems when combined with **Toprol XL**. Be aware that over-the-counter asthma medicines containing epinephrine, the blood thinner **Coumadin,** or ergotamine-containing migraine drugs like **Cafergot,** could all interact badly with **Toprol XL**. Check with your doctor and pharmacist before taking any other drugs to make sure you are aware of the risks the combination may carry.

Toradol

ketorolac tromethamine

Overview: **Toradol** is a pain reliever in the class of medications commonly called NSAIDs, or nonsteroidal anti-inflammatory drugs. Unlike most of the other medicines in this category, which include over-the-counter analgesics such as aspirin, ibuprofen (**Advil, Motrin IB**, etc.), and naproxen (**Aleve**), as well as prescription arthritis pills (**Lodine, Naprosyn, Relafen**, etc.), **Toradol** is used for the short-term relief of pain from trauma or surgery. It should not be used over weeks or months for arthritis relief, nor is it appropriate for preoperative treatment or pain relief during labor and delivery. It is available both as an intramuscular injection for hospital use and as a pill. According to the manufacturer, it is as effective as some commonly prescribed narcotic pain relievers. It does not have narcotic activity.

Special Precautions: People who have had an allergic reaction to **Toradol** and those who are allergic to aspirin or other anti-inflammatory agents should not take this drug. Signs of allergy include breathing difficulties, rash, fever, or a sudden drop in blood pressure, and require immediate medical attention.

Older people may be more vulnerable to **Toradol** side effects and may require a lower dose.

Taking the Medicine: **Toradol** injections are given either on a regular schedule or an "as needed" (*p.r.n.*) basis. **Toradol** tablets are given once every 4 to 6 hours as needed on a short-term basis. Because **Toradol** can be hard on the digestive tract, it may be taken with food or an antacid. A high-fat meal may delay absorption and reduce the peak concentration slightly, with no effect on the overall absorption of this medicine. Taking **Toradol** with food does not guarantee that the drug will be safe for the stomach.

Side Effects and Interactions: Among the most common side effects of **Toradol** are those affecting the digestive tract. They include stomach pain, nausea, indigestion, diarrhea, and mouth irritation. Some people may develop ulcers and intestinal bleeding, particularly if **Toradol** is taken for a longer period. Occasionally these problems can occur without obvious symptoms and lead to a life-threatening crisis due to perforation of the stomach lining.

Older people appear to be more susceptible to this problem and should be monitored carefully. Warning signs include weight loss, persistent indigestion, a feeling of fullness after moderate meals, dark or tarry stools, anemia, and unusual fatigue. Home stool tests such as **Hemoccult** or **Fleet Detecatest** may provide an early indication of bleeding.

Other side effects to be alert for include headache, fluid retention, high blood pressure, rash, itching, gas, constipation, and dizziness. Do not drive or operate dangerous equipment if you become impaired by insomnia, vertigo, fainting, or euphoria. Less common adverse reactions include flushing, palpitations, changes in appetite, difficulty breathing, and flank pain related to kidney problems. Report any symptoms to your physician promptly.

Toradol can affect both the kidney and liver, so the doctor should monitor their function while you take this medicine.

This medication may interact with other drugs, including aspirin. A person taking a blood thinner such as **Coumadin,** or being given heparin, may become more vulnerable to a dangerous bleeding ulcer and should be closely monitored on this combination. **Lasix, Benemid,** and certain muscle relaxants used in surgery interact with **Toradol.** Most NSAIDs can make methotrexate (**Folex, Mexate, Rheumatrex**), lithium (**Eskalith, Lithobid,** etc.), and **Lanoxin** far more toxic. It is not known if **Toradol** also interacts with these drugs or with the immunosuppressant drug **Sandimmune.** Check with your pharmacist and physician to make sure **Toradol** is safe in combination with any other drugs you take.

Trental

pentoxifylline

Overview: This medicine makes blood flow more easily through blood capillaries. It improves red blood-cell flexibility so these oxygen-carrying cells can squeeze through small vessels or those that are almost blocked. **Trental** is used to treat a leg condition called intermittent claudication, which causes pain upon walking.

Although the FDA has not approved **Trental** for any other use, doctors sometimes prescribe this medicine for complications of diabetes, sickle-cell anemia, Raynaud's syndrome, hearing problems, mountain sickness, stroke, and other conditions in which blood flow to the brain is compromised.

Special Precautions: People who are especially sensitive to caffeine or the closely related asthma drug theophylline may not be able to tolerate **Trental.** The doctor should proceed cautiously when prescribing **Trental** for someone with kidney disease or arteriosclerosis.

Taking the Medicine: Although food may slow the absorption of **Trental**, it does not reduce the total amount of medicine absorbed into the body. If this drug upsets your stomach it should be taken with meals.

Side Effects and Interactions: Side effects associated with **Trental** are relatively infrequent. Those that have been reported include dizziness, flushing, stomach upset, flatulence, belching, bloating, loss of appetite, nausea, indigestion, and vomiting. Other adverse reactions to be aware of are headache, blurred vision, constipation, excessive salivation, tremor, confusion, anxiety, nasal congestion, chest pain, brittle fingernails, rash, itching, bad taste in the mouth, swelling, difficulty breathing, thirst, and dry mouth. Report any symptoms to your physician promptly.

Trental does not interact with many other medications. There have been, however, reports that it may affect blood-clotting time, especially in combination with blood thinners such as **Coumadin**. This could lead to hemorrhaging unless blood is carefully monitored by a test called a prothrombin time. Blood pressure should also be determined periodically, particularly if you must take antihypertensive medications. Check with your physician and pharmacist to make sure **Trental** is safe in combination with any other medicines you may take.

Tri-Levlen 28

ethinyl estradiol and levonorgestrel

Overview: This combination oral contraceptive contains compounds similar to the female hormones estrogen and progestin. It works primarily by preventing the release of eggs from the ovary. Each packet contains 28 pills with four different levels of hormones.

Oral contraceptives also offer some additional benefits beyond the prevention of pregnancy. They can make the menstrual cycle more regular and decrease the likelihood of painful menstruation and of ovarian cysts. In addition, they reduce the risk of cancer of the uterus or the ovaries over the long term.

Special Precautions: **Tri-Levlen 28**, like other oral contraceptives, is quite effective. Some women are at greater risk of negative consequences, however. Tell your doctor if you smoke cigarettes, have had phlebitis or other clotting problems, or if you or someone in your family has had uterine or breast cancer. You will also be asked about asthma, diabetes, epilepsy, migraine, depression, and certain other conditions that could be aggravated by oral contraceptives. Tests for thyroid function and blood sugar may be altered by oral contraceptives.

Taking the Medicine: Each **Tri-Levlen** tablet should be swallowed at the same time every day to maintain consistent levels in the body. The manufacturer recommends it be taken after supper or at bedtime. They should be taken in the order indicated on the package: first brown, then white, then yellow, and finally green. The light green ones to be taken during the last week of the cycle contain no active ingredients, allowing for normal menstruation.

If you forget one dose, take it as soon as you remember it, and take the next one at the usual time. If you miss two doses, take both as soon as you remember and take the next at the usual time. If you have missed two or more pills, use additional contraceptive protection such as spermicidal foam or condoms for a week after getting back on schedule.

Side Effects and Interactions: Unexpected vaginal bleeding may occur during the first month or two on **Tri-Levlen**. Notify your physician if you continue to experience bleeding between periods after the second month on this medication.

Serious side effects are rare, but they may include high blood pressure, heart attacks, stroke, blood clots, visual changes, and problems with liver or gallbladder. Do not continue taking **Tri-Levlen** if you become pregnant. Less dangerous reactions include nausea, vomiting, fluid retention, headache, darkening of the skin across the face, changes in menstrual flow, depression, nervousness, breast tenderness, rash, inability to wear contact lenses, and susceptibility to vaginal infections. Report any symptoms or suspected side effects promptly.

Some women become more susceptible to sunburn while taking **Tri-Levlen**. Use a good sunscreen and sunglasses to protect yourself.

Tri-Levlen interacts with many other medications. Antibiotics such as penicillin, tetracycline, and related drugs may reduce contraceptive protection. This is also a potential hazard with barbiturates such as phenobarbital or **Mysoline**, the antifungal medicine griseofulvin, the tuberculosis drug rifampin, and seizure medications such as **Dilantin**.

Antianxiety drugs such as **Halcion, Valium,** or **Xanax**, asthma drugs containing theophylline or aminophylline, the beta-blocker **Lopressor,** oral corticosteroids like hydrocortisone or prednisone, and caffeine, an ingredient common in many beverages and over-the-counter drugs, may all have more serious adverse effects if they are taken together with birth control pills. So may antidepressants or the OCD medicine **Anafranil**. Check with your doctor and pharmacist before taking any other medicine in combination with **Tri-Levlen 28**.

Triphasil-28

ethinyl estradiol and levonorgestrel

Overview: This combination oral contraceptive contains compounds similar to the female hormones estrogen and progestin. It works primarily by preventing the release of eggs from the ovary. Each packet contains 28 pills with four different levels of hormones.

Oral contraceptives also offer some additional benefits beyond the prevention of pregnancy. They can make the menstrual cycle more regular and decrease the likelihood of painful menstruation and of ovarian cysts. In addition, they reduce the risk of cancer of the uterus or the ovaries over the long term.

Special Precautions: Triphasil-28, like other oral contraceptives, is quite effective. Some women are at greater risk of negative consequences, however. Tell your doctor if you smoke cigarettes, have had phlebitis or other clotting problems, or if you or someone in your family has had uterine or breast cancer. You will also be asked about asthma, diabetes, epilepsy, migraine, depression, and certain other conditions that could be aggravated by oral contraceptives. Tests for thyroid function and blood sugar may be altered by oral contraceptives.

Taking the Medicine: Each **Triphasil-28** tablet should be swallowed at the same time every day to maintain consistent levels in the body. The manufacturer recommends it be taken after supper or at bedtime. They should be taken in the order indicated on the package: first brown, then white, then yellow, and finally green. The light green ones to be taken during the last week of the cycle contain no active ingredients, allowing for normal menstruation.

If you forget one dose, take it as soon as you remember it, and take the next one at the usual time. If you miss two doses, take both as soon as you remember and take the next at the usual time. If you have missed two or more pills, use additional contraceptive protection such as spermicidal foam or condoms for a week after getting back on schedule.

Side Effects and Interactions: Unexpected vaginal bleeding may occur during the first month or two on **Triphasil**. Notify your physician if you continue to experience bleeding between periods after the second month on this medication.

Serious side effects are rare, but they may include high blood pressure, heart attacks, stroke, blood clots, visual changes, and problems with liver or gallbladder. Do not continue taking **Triphasil-28** if you become pregnant. Less dangerous reactions include nausea, vomiting, fluid retention, headache, darkening of the skin across the face, changes in menstrual flow, depression, nervousness, breast tenderness, rash, inability to wear contact lenses, and susceptibility to vaginal infections. Report any symptoms or suspected side effects promptly.

Some women become more susceptible to sunburn while taking **Triphasil-28**. Use a good sunscreen and sunglasses to protect yourself.

Triphasil interacts with many other medications. Antibiotics such as penicillin, tetracycline, and related drugs may reduce contraceptive protection. This is also a potential hazard with barbiturates such as phenobarbital or **Mysoline**, the antifungal medicine griseofulvin, the tuberculosis drug rifampin, and seizure medications such as **Dilantin**.

Antianxiety drugs such as **Halcion, Valium,** or **Xanax**, asthma drugs containing theophylline or aminophylline, the beta-blocker **Toprol XL**, oral corticosteroids such as hydrocortisone or prednisone, and caffeine, an ingredient common in many beverages and over-the-counter drugs, may all have more serious adverse effects if they are taken together with birth control pills. So may antidepressants or the OCD medicine **Anafranil**. Check with your doctor and pharmacist before taking any other medicine in combination with **Triphasil-28**.

Tylenol with Codeine

acetaminophen with codeine

Overview: Acetaminophen and codeine is an excellent analgesic combination for mild to moderate pain relief. It can ease the discomfort of a bad toothache or the aftermath of minor surgery, as well as a wide array of other situations that call for pain management. One of the most commonly prescribed brand-name preparations is **Tylenol with Codeine**. It is also available as **Margesic** and **Phenaphen with Codeine**. The number on the formula represents the amount of codeine the formula contains. No. 1 has 7.5 mg of codeine; No. 2, 15 mg; No. 3, 30 mg; and No. 4 contains 60 mg of codeine.

Special Precautions: Like any narcotic, codeine may make you drowsy. Do not drive or attempt any activity that requires coordination and judgment. Older people may be more susceptible to this reaction. Light-headedness or dizziness could make walking dangerous. Never stand up suddenly, because it may make you feel faint.

Long-term use of acetaminophen and codeine has drawbacks since codeine may be habit-forming if you take it regularly. Do not increase the dose on your own in a quest to achieve greater pain relief. But don't play the hero by skipping doses during an acute crisis. Pain is more easily managed if it can be dealt with immediately instead of after it has gotten out of control.

Taking the Medicine: Some people react to codeine with nausea or vomiting. Taking it with food may reduce stomach upset. Nausea, dizziness, and other common reactions may be less troublesome if you lie down for a while.

Side Effects and Interactions: Other than dizziness, drowsiness and nausea, side effects may include constipation, loss of appetite, headache, sweating, and euphoria. Some people experience shortness of breath, especially if they have asthma. Other less common reactions include an allergic rash, disorientation, dry mouth, and urinary difficulties. Report any such symptoms to your physician promptly.

Acetaminophen may cause liver or kidney problems in large doses or over long periods. Your physician should evaluate your need for this combination pain reliever periodically.

If you are taking any other medicines, check with a physician or pharmacist about compatibility. Alcohol as well as many over-the-counter and prescription drugs can add to the sedative effect of this analgesic and should be avoided. Antihistamines, antianxiety agents, and sleeping pills require extra caution. Both tricyclic and MAO inhibitor–type antidepressants may interact with this analgesic to cause greater toxicity.

Vasotec

enalapril

Overview: **Vasotec** is one of the most successful blood pressure medicines on the market. It belongs to a class of drugs called ACE (angiotensin-converting enzyme) inhibitors, which includes **Accupril, Capoten, Prinivil,** and **Zestril,** among others.

The development of this group of medications reads almost like a medical mystery. It all started with the venom of a poisonous Brazilian snake, the deadly jararaca. Its bite causes severe hemorrhaging, but an extract from the venom was found to affect the kidney and ultimately blood pressure regulation. This led to the creation of enzyme blockers found in **Capoten** and later **Vasotec,** and certain other medicines that are revolutionizing the treatment of hypertension and congestive heart failure.

Special Precautions: The very first dose of **Vasotec** you take may cause dizziness, especially in older people. Be especially careful until your body adjusts.

When you first start taking **Vasotec**, be alert for a rare but serious reaction. Some people have experienced swelling of the face, lips, tongue and throat, which can make breathing difficult if not impossible. This requires immediate emergency treatment.

Another uncommon but dangerous reaction is a drop in infection-fighting white blood cells. If you develop chills, fever, sore throat, and mouth sores contact your physician promptly. Blood tests are required to detect this problem. This risk is greater for patients with certain predisposing conditions such as lupus, scleroderma, or kidney problems.

Vasotec should not be taken by pregnant women in their second or third trimester unless there is no alternative. It may damage the fetus.

Taking the Medicine: **Vasotec** may be taken with meals or on an empty stomach. Absorption of the drug into the bloodstream is not affected by food but may be reduced by antacids, which should be taken at least 2 hours apart from **Vasotec.** Do not stop taking **Vasotec** suddenly, as this could lead to complications.

Side Effects and Interactions: **Vasotec** can cause a number of uncomfortable side effects. Be alert for a skin rash, itching, sweating, an annoying dry cough, fast or irregular heartbeats, chest pain, nausea, diarrhea, muscle cramps, vomiting, insomnia, fatigue, dizziness, nervousness, and headache. Report any symptoms or suspected side effects without delay.

People with kidney problems must be monitored extremely carefully, because **Vasotec** can make kidney function worse. The doctor will check the urine to see if it contains protein. It's wise for everyone on **Vasotec** to have their physicians monitor the kidneys periodically.

There are a number of compounds that can interact with **Vasotec**. In general it is important to avoid potassium supplements, including low-sodium salt substitutes. Diuretics such as **Dyazide, Aldactazide,** and **Moduretic,** which preserve potassium, can also cause dangerous elevations in potassium.

Other drugs that can interact adversely with **Vasotec** include lithium, aspirin, and the arthritis medicine **Indocin.** The gout medicine **Zyloprim** and the transplant drug **Sandimmune** may present special hazards in combination with **Vasotec.** Check with your doctor and pharmacist to make sure **Vasotec** is safe in combination with any other drugs you take.

Veetids

penicillin VK

Overview: Penicillin represents one of the most important drugs ever developed. Its discovery in 1946 permanently changed medicine and set the stage for man's ability to overcome what had previously been life-threatening infections. Penicillin is effective in fighting infections in many places in the body including the urinary tract, lungs, ears, throat, skin, and genital tract.

Special Precautions: Anyone who is allergic to penicillin-type antibiotics must generally avoid such drugs like the plague. Symptoms such as breathing difficulty, wheezing, sneezing, hives, itching, and skin rash require immediate emergency treatment. Life-threatening anaphylactic shock may produce an inability to breathe and cardiovascular collapse, and can occur within minutes of exposure. If you have experienced an allergic reaction to this drug and you ever have to go into the hospital, make sure a sign is placed over the bed alerting hospital personnel to penicillin allergy.

Taking the Medicine: **Veetids** resists acid breakdown in the stomach so it may be taken with food if it upsets your stomach. However, for maximum absorption take this antibiotic on an empty stomach. That usually means at least one hour before meals or two hours after eating. Do not stop taking this drug until you finish the prescription unless your doctor directs you otherwise. Stopping after a few days could make a recurrence of the infection harder to treat.

Side Effects and Interactions: The most common side effects of **Veetids** involve digestive tract upset. Nausea, vomiting, and diarrhea can be troublesome for some people. A black hairy tongue, rash, sore mouth, and yeast infections of the mouth, anus, or vagina are other potential adverse reactions. Less common but possibly more serious side effects include anemia and blood disorders. Report any symptoms to your physician promptly. Long-term treatment with penicillin-type antibiotics requires periodic monitoring by a health professional.

Veetids may interact with a number of other antibiotics. In addition, oral contraceptives may be less effective in combination with this antibiotic. Check with your pharmacist and physician before taking any other medicine together with **Veetids**.

Ventolin Inhaler

albuterol

Overview: **Ventolin** is one of the more commonly prescribed asthma inhalers in this country. Although this medicine is also available in tablet form for oral use, the aerosol formulation is less likely to cause general side effects. **Ventolin Inhaler** is prescribed for the prevention as well as the treatment of asthma attacks. It may also be used 15 minutes before vigorous activity to prevent exercise-induced asthma.

Special Precautions: Although **Ventolin** is very effective, care must be taken not to overuse it. Because of a relatively short duration of action of 4 to 6 hours, people may tempted to use their inhaler too frequently. This could lead to complications, including increased breathing difficulties or heart problems. Individuals with preexisting heart conditions, diabetes, seizures, prostate problems, or an overactive thyroid gland should use **Ventolin** only under close supervision, if at all.

Ventolin Inhaler needs to be kept at room temperature—that is, between 59 and 86 degrees Fahrenheit. If the aerosol is used at a different temperature, it may not provide an accurate dose.

Taking the Medicine: Use of inhalers is not as easy as it may seem. Make sure your physician provides detailed instructions and demonstrates how to inhale the aerosol so that the medicine ends up in the lungs and not in the back of the throat. Never try to use the inhaler when you have food, beverage, chewing gum, or anything else in your mouth.

Side Effects and Interactions: One advantage of inhaled asthma medicine is that relatively little is absorbed into the body to cause unpleasant side effects. However, inhaled **Ventolin** can cause palpitations or rapid heartbeat in some people.

Other possible side effects include nausea, tremor, nervousness, increased blood pressure, heartburn, and dizziness. There are rare reports of rash, itching, and allergic reactions that interfere with breathing. In addition, the active ingredient in **Ventolin** can precipitate angina, insomnia, headache, unusual taste, and irritation of the throat. Report any symptoms to your physician promptly.

Ventolin can interact with several other medications. Do not use a similar kind of bronchodilating inhaler such as **Berotec, Brethaire, Alupent, Metaprel, Proventil,** or **Tornalate** simultaneously with **Ventolin.** Certain antidepressants may also be dangerous in combination with this asthma drug. Thyroid medication and antihistamines do not mix well with **Ventolin,** and beta-blocker medications may counteract its effectiveness. Check with your pharmacist and physician before using any other medication in combination with this inhaler.

Vicodin

hydrocodone with acetaminophen

Overview: **Vicodin** is the most popular brand name for a narcotic pain reliever containing hydrocodone and acetaminophen. Hydrocodone is a semisynthetic analgesic similar in most respects to codeine. Acetaminophen is a widely used and effective pain reliever available alone in such nonprescription products as **Anacin-3** or **Tylenol.**

This combination offers excellent relief for moderate to fairly severe pain. **Vi-**

codin tablets also contain a sulfite and should be avoided by people who are sensitive to these preservatives.

Special Precautions: Long-term use of hydrocodone and acetaminophen has drawbacks. Hydrocodone, like other narcotics, may be habit-forming if you take it regularly. Do not increase the dose on your own in a quest to achieve greater pain relief. But don't play the hero by skipping doses during an acute crisis. Pain is more easily managed if it can be dealt with immediately instead of after it has gotten out of control.

Acetaminophen may cause liver or kidney problems in large doses or over long periods. Your physician should evaluate your need for this combination pain reliever periodically.

Taking the Medicine: Some people react to hydrocodone with nausea or vomiting. Taking **Vicodin** with food may reduce stomach upset. Nausea, dizziness, and other common reactions may be less troublesome if you lie down for a while.

Side Effects and Interactions: Like any narcotic, hydrocodone may make you drowsy. Do not drive or attempt any activity that requires coordination and judgment. Older people may be more susceptible to this reaction. Light-headedness or dizziness could make walking dangerous. Never stand up suddenly, as it may make you feel faint.

Other side effects to be aware of include weakness, euphoria, loss of appetite, sweating, and constipation. Some people experience shortness of breath, especially if they have asthma. Other less common reactions include an allergic rash, disorientation, dry mouth, and urinary difficulties. Report any such symptoms to your physician promptly.

If you are taking any other medicines, check with a physician or pharmacist before adding **Vicodin**. Alcohol as well as many over-the-counter or prescription medications can add to the sedative effect of this analgesic. Antihistamines, antianxiety agents, antidepressants, and sleeping pills require extra caution.

Voltaren

diclofenac sodium

Overview: **Voltaren** is a pain reliever used for arthritis. It belongs to a class of medications commonly called NSAIDs or nonsteroidal anti-inflammatory drugs. Other medicines in this category include over-the-counter analgesics such as aspirin, ibuprofen (**Advil, Motrin IB**, etc.), and naproxen (**Aleve**) as well as prescription arthritis pills such as **Lodine, Naprosyn,** or **Relafen.**

Special Precautions: People who are allergic to aspirin or other anti-inflammatory agents should avoid **Voltaren**. Signs of allergy include breathing difficulties, rash, fever, or a sudden drop in blood pressure, and require immediate medical attention.

Taking the Medicine: Because **Voltaren** can be hard on the digestive tract, it may be taken with food to reduce stomach trouble. This does not, however, guarantee that the drug will be safe for the stomach.

Side Effects and Interactions: Unquestionably the most common side effects of **Voltaren** involve the gastrointestinal tract. They include nausea, indigestion, heartburn, cramps, gas, constipation, and diarrhea. Some people may develop ulcers and intestinal bleeding while taking **Voltaren**. Occasionally these problems can occur without obvious symptoms and lead to a life-threatening crisis due to perforation of the stomach lining.

Older people appear to be more susceptible to this problem and should be monitored carefully. Warning signs include weight loss, persistent indigestion, a feeling of fullness after moderate meals, dark or tarry stools, anemia, and unusual fatigue. Home stool tests such as **Hemoccult** or **Fleet Detecatest** may provide an early indication of bleeding.

Other side effects to be alert for include headache, ringing in the ears, rash, itching, and fluid retention. Drowsiness, dizziness, light-headedness, difficulty concentrating, and confusion are possible, so do not drive if you become impaired. Less common adverse reactions include jitteriness, insomnia, difficulty breathing, hair loss, depression, changes in appetite, hearing loss, visual disturbances, sores in the mouth, and heart palpitations. Report any symptoms to your physician promptly.

Voltaren can affect both the kidney and liver, so periodic blood tests to monitor the function of these organs are important. Some people become sensitive to sunlight while on **Voltaren**, so use an effective sunscreen, stay covered, or avoid the sun.

This medication can interact with many other drugs including aspirin, alcohol, certain blood pressure pills, and the ulcer medicine **Pepcid**. A person taking a blood thinner such as **Coumadin** may become more vulnerable to a dangerous bleeding ulcer. All the NSAIDs, including **Voltaren**, can make methotrexate (**Folex, Mexate, Rheumatrex**), lithium (**Eskalith, Lithobid**, etc.), and the heart drug **Lanoxin** far more toxic. When **Voltaren** is combined with the immunosuppressant drug **Sandimmune** the risk of kidney damage is increased. Check with your pharmacist and physician to make sure **Voltaren** is safe in combination with any other drugs you take.

Xanax

alprazolam

Overview: **Xanax** is the most frequently prescribed antianxiety agent in the country. It is similar in certain respects to **Valium**. Once called minor tranquilizers or sedatives, such drugs are prescribed to calm jittery nerves and relieve excessive tension. **Xanax** is also prescribed for anxiety associated with depression and for panic attacks.

This drug belongs to a class of medications called benzodiazepines. **Xanax** is a little more rapid in action than many other such compounds and its calming effect lasts for a relatively short period of time.

Special Precautions: Do not drive, operate machinery, or undertake any activity that requires close attention while you are taking **Xanax.** This medicine may make narrow-angle glaucoma worse and should not be taken by people diagnosed with this condition.

Regular reliance on **Xanax** for many months may lead to dependence. Sudden discontinuation of the drug could trigger withdrawal symptoms including convulsions, nervousness, agitation, difficulty concentrating, insomnia, fatigue, headache, and tremor. Never stop taking **Xanax** without medical supervision, because the medication may have to be phased out gradually over a period of weeks or months.

Taking the Medicine: **Xanax** can be taken with food, especially if it upsets your stomach. Do not drink alcohol or use any other sedative while on this drug, because the combination may lead to dizziness, drowsiness, lack of coordination, or confusion. If you are also taking antacids, take them at least one hour before or after taking **Xanax**.

Side Effects and Interactions: Side effects associated with **Xanax** include sedation, dizziness, unsteadiness, fatigue, and confusion. These may fade after a few days or weeks. Other possible reactions include dry mouth, visual problems, menstrual irregularities, slurred speech, increased salivation, rash, itching, change in appetite, altered sex drive, urinary difficulties, and reduced blood pressure. Report any symptoms to your physician promptly.

Many drugs can interact with **Xanax**, including over-the-counter antihistamines, prescription antidepressants, the asthma drug theophylline, and the ulcer medicine **Tagamet**. Anticonvulsants such as **Dilantin** and the heart medicine **Lanoxin** do not mix well. Check with your pharmacist and physician to make sure **Xanax** is safe in combination with any other medicines you take.

Zantac

ranitidine

Overview: **Zantac** is a popular treatment for ulcers that helps them clear up rapidly. It works in part by suppressing the secretion of stomach acid, so it is also used to treat conditions of excess secretion and the severe heartburn called reflux esophagitis. Doctors also prescribe **Zantac** as maintenance therapy to keep ulcers from coming back.

Special Precautions: Perhaps because **Zantac** is so effective at reducing stomach acid concentrations, patients taking this medicine have higher levels of certain microorganisms in their stomachs than would normally survive there. Scientists do not yet know whether these bacteria have negative long-term consequences, but it appears that vitamins C and E might provide some measure of protection.

Taking the Medicine: **Zantac** may be taken with food, especially if it upsets your stomach. If antacids are needed for relief of ulcer pain, they should generally be taken at a different time.

Zantac tablets should be kept away from heat, cold, light, and moisture. The container should be capped very tightly.

Side Effects and Interactions: Side effects associated with **Zantac** are uncommon. Some people experience constipation, nausea, diarrhea, stomach upset, and headache. Dizziness, insomnia or drowsiness, and mental confusion have been reported occasionally. Very ill or elderly people appear to be more susceptible to these problems.

Other adverse reactions include rash, hair loss, changes in heart rhythm, elevated liver enzymes, joint pain, and anemia or other blood problems. Report any symptoms to your physician promptly.

Zantac appears less likely to interact with other medications than its predecessor, **Tagamet**. Nevertheless, people who take drugs such as the antifungal drug **Nizoral**, blood-thinning medications such as **Coumadin**, antianxiety agents, and oral diabetes medicines may need altered dosing regimens and other special precautions. The possibility that this medication may interact with alcohol to produce higher blood-alcohol levels remains controversial. Check with your pharmacist and physician before taking any other medication in combination with **Zantac**.

Zestril

lisinopril

Overview: **Zestril** is one of the more recent entries in a class of drugs called ACE (angiotensin-converting enzyme) inhibitors. The development of this group of medications reads almost like a medical mystery, starting with the venom of a poisonous Brazilian snake. The bite of the deadly jararaca causes severe hemorrhaging. An extract from the venom was found to affect the kidney and ultimately blood pressure regulation through the conversion of angiotensin from one form to another. This led to the creation of enzyme blockers including **Capoten, Vasotec,** and **Zestril,** which are revolutionizing the treatment of hypertension and congestive heart failure. **Zestril** is prescribed to lower blood pressure.

Special Precautions: The very first dose of **Zestril** you take may cause dizziness, especially for older people. Be especially careful until your body adjusts.

When you first start taking **Zestril**, be alert for a rare but serious reaction. Some people have experienced swelling of the face, lips, tongue, and throat, which can make breathing difficult if not impossible. This requires immediate emergency treatment.

Another uncommon but dangerous reaction is a drop in infection-fighting white blood cells. If you develop chills, fever, sore throat, and mouth sores contact your physician promptly. Blood tests are required to detect this problem. This risk is greater for patients with certain predisposing conditions such as lupus, scleroderma, or kidney problems.

Zestril should not be taken by pregnant women in their second or third trimester unless there is no alternative. It may damage the fetus.

Taking the Medicine: **Zestril** may be taken with food or on an empty stomach. It should be swallowed at the same time every day to maintain consistent levels in the body. Don't swallow **Zestril** within two hours of taking an antacid, though.

Do not stop taking **Zestril** suddenly, because this could lead to complications. If you must discontinue the drug, your physician will instruct you in tapering off gradually.

Side Effects and Interactions: People with kidney problems must be monitored extremely carefully, because **Zestril** can make kidney function worse. Even healthy people should have their physician monitor the kidneys periodically.

Zestril can cause a number of less serious but uncomfortable side effects. Be alert for skin rash, headache, tiredness, an annoying dry cough, chest pain, nausea, vomiting, diarrhea, muscle cramps, low blood pressure, nasal congestion, heart rhythm disturbances, and sexual difficulties. Report any symptoms or suspected side effects without delay.

There are a number of compounds that can interact with **Zestril**. In general it is important to avoid potassium supplements, including low-sodium salt substitutes. Diuretics such as **Dyazide, Aldactazide,** and **Moduretic,** which preserve potassium, can also cause dangerous elevations in potassium.

Other drugs that can interact with **Zestril** include other diuretics, the arthritis medicine **Indocin,** the gout medicine **Zyloprim,** and lithium (**Eskalith, Lithobid,** etc.). Check with your doctor and pharmacist to make sure **Zestril** is safe in combination with any other drugs you take.

Zocor

simvastatin

Overview: **Zocor** is prescribed primarily to lower cholesterol. Heart specialists recognize that coronary artery disease is associated with certain risk factors, including high serum cholesterol, bad LDL cholesterol, elevated triglycerides, and reduced levels of protective HDL cholesterol.

Diet, exercise, and weight control are usually considered important first-line preventive approaches. When they are insufficient, drugs such as **Zocor** may be important in reducing the risk of heart disease. This medication has been found to reduce LDL cholesterol and triglycerides while raising HDL a variable amount.

Special Precautions: Anyone with liver problems should probably not take **Zocor.** Liver enzyme changes have been reported in a small proportion of patients using this medicine, and may indicate serious problems. Liver function should be tested before anyone starts taking **Zocor** and every month or so for the first year. Periodic tests are needed thereafter.

Because cholesterol is essential for the developing fetus, pregnant women should not take **Zocor.**

Research on animals has also shown optic-nerve problems and strokelike bleeding in dogs on **Zocor,** but only at relatively high doses. Whether there is a risk for humans remains to be determined.

It is wise to see an ophthalmologist before starting on **Zocor.** An eye test should also be performed annually to make there is no damage to the lens.

Taking the Medicine: The manufacturer recommends that **Zocor** be taken at bedtime. It may be taken without or with meals.

Side Effects and Interactions: **Zocor** has relatively few side effects and most people tolerate it well. Some adverse reactions that may occur include stomachache, constipation, flatulence, diarrhea, nausea, headache, fatigue, and skin rash. Less common complications include dizziness, muscle pain, change in the sense of taste, insomnia, and numbness or tingling of the hands or feet. Muscle aches or weakness could be a sign of a serious reaction called rhabdomyolysis or myopathy, and call for a test of kidney function. Kidney failure might be the outcome of untreated myopathy. Report any symptoms to your physician promptly.

The danger of rhabdomyolysis or myopathy is increased when **Mevacor** is combined with certain other drugs. Troleandomycin or erythromycin antibiotics such as **E.E.S., E-Mycin, Erythrocin,** or **PCE** have been involved in several cases. The new antibiotics **Biaxin** and **Zithromax** belong to the same class of drugs, but it is not clear if they have a potential for such an interaction. Because **Zocor** is in the same class as **Mevacor,** this interaction may pose hazards with **Zocor** as well.

When **Zocor** is combined with other cholesterol-lowering medicines such as **Lopid** or niacin, be alert for muscle pain, weakness, and kidney damage, because rhabdomyolysis may be more common in this situation. The transplant drug **Sandimmune** also appears to increase the risk of this dangerous reaction.

Zocor may also increase the action of the blood thinner **Coumadin;** prothrombin time should be closely monitored. **Lanoxin** levels should also be monitored in people taking both medications. Check with your physician and pharmacist to make sure **Zocor** is safe in combination with any other drug you may take.

Zoloft

sertraline

Overview: **Zoloft,** like the earlier antidepressant **Prozac,** apparently works by enhancing the action of a brain chemical called serotonin. This medication is prescribed to treat major depression. Long-term efficacy beyond four months has not been studied.

Like **Prozac, Zoloft** is less likely to cause typical side effects associated with older medications. Tricyclic antidepressants such as **Elavil, Tofranil, Sinequan,** and **Pamelor** often produce dry mouth, dizziness, weight gain, and a sluggish or lethargic feeling. **Zoloft** may have a slight stimulant action, with the usual bothersome reactions being less prevalent.

Special Precautions: Some people may need very close monitoring if the doctor prescribes **Zoloft.** For people who have had an episode of mania, there is a risk that manic symptoms could be triggered by **Zoloft.** In rare cases, **Zoloft** has led to significant weight loss. This may be a problem for an underweight person.

Because **Zoloft** may cause drowsiness or dizziness, people taking this medicine should not drive or use dangerous machines unless an objective evaluation shows they are not impaired.

People with liver problems or kidney disease may need to start on a reduced dose, because they may eliminate **Zoloft** less efficiently than otherwise healthy people.

Anyone with a history of suicide attempts must also be extremely vigilant. There have been reports that some people may develop a preoccupation with suicide or violence while taking **Prozac.** It is still not certain whether this is caused by the underlying mental condition or is in some way related to the drug. If **Prozac** were responsible for any of these incidents, there might also be a risk with **Zoloft.** Family members should help monitor people on **Zoloft** for suicidal thoughts or self-destructive behaviors. The doctor must be notified immediately in such cases.

Taking the Medicine: **Zoloft** should be taken once a day, either in the morning or the evening. Food has only a small impact on **Zoloft** overall, but blood levels of the drug reach a higher maximum concentration sooner when **Zoloft** is taken with a meal.

Side Effects and Interactions: Side effects associated with **Zoloft** include nausea, diarrhea, indigestion, tremor, dizziness, insomnia, drowsiness, sweating, dry mouth, and sexual difficulties (particularly ejaculation disturbances). Other adverse reactions include agitation, loss of appetite, headache, confusion, fatigue, constipation, blurred vision, and hot flushes. A wide range of other reactions have been reported but appear to be uncommon. Report any symptoms to your physician promptly.

Zoloft may interact with a number of other medications. Anyone taking other antidepressants, especially drugs such as the MAO inhibitors **Nardil** or **Parnate,** should stop such a medicine at least two weeks before starting on **Zoloft.** If **Zoloft** is taken first, two weeks should elapse before starting on one of these other medicines.

Zoloft can slow elimination of oral diabetes drugs. It is unclear what impact this interaction may have, but it would be wise for diabetics to monitor their blood sugar closely when they start or stop **Zoloft,** because it may increase the potential for adverse reactions. If a person needs both **Zoloft** and lithium for the treatment of manic depression, lithium blood levels should be followed carefully. Other compounds that could cause complications in combination with **Zoloft** include the blood thinner **Coumadin** and possibly the heart drug **Lanoxin**. Check with your pharmacist and physician before taking any other medicines, including nonprescription drugs, in combination with **Zoloft**.

Zovirax

acyclovir

Overview: This antiviral medicine has revolutionized the way the medical profession treats viruses. Prior to **Zovirax,** many researchers believed that it would be impossible to develop safe and effective virus treatments. This medicine proved that such compounds are practical.

Zovirax is used to treat genital herpes and zoster infections, or shingles. Although it is not a cure, it can speed healing and can be used to prevent recurrences of genital sores. Another potential use may be the treatment of chicken pox. Studies are under way to determine the drug's effectiveness.

Special Precautions: If **Zovirax** is being used to treat genital herpes it is best to avoid intercourse when active sores are apparent. Because virus can be shed even in the absence of lesions, it makes sense for the male partner to use a condom.

Taking the Medicine: **Zovirax** can be taken with meals or on an empty stomach. The dose for shingles is substantially higher than that for genital herpes. A new 800 mg–strength pill was developed especially for zoster infections and must be taken five times a day. This is far more convenient than the 20-pill-per-day regimen previously necessary with the 200-mg strength.

Side Effects and Interactions: Side effects of **Zovirax** are rare. Most people will not even notice they are taking a medicine. People with kidney problems, however, will require carefully medical supervision and monitoring. Adverse reactions to be aware of include nausea, vomiting, diarrhea, itching, rash, dizziness, headache, liver enzyme elevations, lethargy, tremors, confusion, nervousness, or seizures. Report any symptoms to your physician promptly.

Drug interactions with **Zovirax** are uncommon. However, people taking the anticancer medicines methotrexate or interferon must use this drug with caution and only under careful medical supervision. There may be problems in combining **Zovirax** with AZT (**Retrovir**). Check with your physician or pharmacist to make sure **Zovirax** is safe in combination with any other drug you may take.

Index

Please note that entries in boldface indicate brand names; page numbers in boldface indicate drug profiles; and page numbers in italics indicate tables.

ABOUT THE AUTHORS

Joe Graedon

Pharmacologist Joe Graedon is a best-selling author, nationally syndicated newspaper columnist, host of an award-winning internationally syndicated radio talk show, and lecturer at the University of North Carolina School of Pharmacy. He is president of Graedon Enterprises, Inc., a corporation providing pharmaceutical and health care information services.

Joe Graedon received his B.S. from Pennsylvania State University in 1967 and went on to do research on mental illness, sleep, and basic brain physiology at the new Jersey Neuropsychiatric Institute in Princeton. In 1971 he received his M.S. in pharmacology from the University of Michigan. He then accompanied his medical anthropologist wife Teresa to Mexico, where he taught clinical pharmacology to second-year medical students at the Benito Juárez University of Oaxaca. While in Mexico, he started work on *The People's Pharmacy* (New York: St. Martin's Press, 1976; revised 1985), a popular book on medicines that would eventually go on to become a *New York Times* number one best-seller.

Joe's other books, coauthored with Dr. Terry Graedon, include *The People's Pharmacy-2* (New York: Avon, 1980), *The New People's Pharmacy #3: Drug Breakthroughs of the '80s* (New York: Bantam, 1985), *Totally New and Revised The People's Pharmacy* (New York: St. Martin's Press, 1985), *50+: The Graedons' People's Pharmacy for Older Adults* (New York: Bantam, 1988), *Graedons' Best Medicine: From Herbal Remedies to High-Tech ℞ Breakthroughs* (New York: Bantam, 1991) and *The People's Guide to Deadly Drug Interactions* (New York: St. Martin's Press, 1995). *No Deadly Drug* (New York: Pocket Books, 1992), coauthored with Dr. Tom Ferguson, is Joe Graedon's first novel. Joe and Terry also coauthored with Dr. Ferguson *The Aspirin Handbook: A User's Guide to the Breakthrough Drug of the '90s* (New York: Bantam, 1993). The total number of the Graedons' books in print well exceeds two million.

Joe has lectured at Duke University School of Nursing, the University of California School of Pharmacy (UCSF), and the University of North Carolina School of Pharmacy. He served as a consultant to the **Federal Trade Commission** from 1978 to 1983, and was on the Advisory Board for the **Drug Studies Unit** at UCSF from 1983 to 1989. He is a member of the **Board of Visitors** of the School of Pharmacy at the University of North Carolina, Chapel Hill. He is a member of the **American Association for the Advancement of Science,** the **Society for Neuroscience,** the **New York Academy of Science,** and the **Mystery Writers of America.** For more than a decade Joe and Terry contributed a regular column on self-medication for the journal *Medical Self Care.* Joe is an editorial advisor to *Men's Health Newsletter.* Joe and Terry's newspaper column, **"The People's Pharmacy,"** is syndicated nationally by King Features. *The People's Pharmacy* radio show won a Silver Award from the Corporation for Public Broadcasting in 1992. It is syndicated to more than 500 radio stations in the United States and 134 countries on public radio, the In Touch Radio Reading Service, and the U.S. Armed Forces Radio and Television Network.

Joe's features on health and pharmaceuticals have been syndicated nationally to public television stations via Intraregional Program Service member exchange. He is considered the country's leading drug expert for consumers. He has been a guest expert on *Donahue, 20/20, Geraldo, Oprah!, Sally Jessy Raphael, Live with Regis and Kathie Lee, Today, Good Morning America, CBS Morning News, Sonia Live, The Home Show, Everyday with Joan Lunden, The Larry King Show,* and *The Tonight Show with Johnny Carson.* He lives in Durham, North Carolina, with his wife and coauthor, Teresa, and their two children. Joe speaks frequently on issues of pharmaceuticals, nutrition, and self-care.

Teresa Graedon

Medical anthropologist Teresa Graedon is a best-selling author, syndicated newspaper columnist, and cohost of an award-winning internationally syndicated radio talk show. Teresa Graedon received her A.B. from Bryn Mawr College in 1969, graduating magna cum laude with a major in anthropology. She attended graduate school at the University of Michigan, receiving her A.M. in 1971. She received a fellowship from the Institute for Environmental Quality (1972–1975), which enabled her to pursue doctoral research on health and nutritional status in a migrant community in Oaxaca, Mexico. Her doctorate was awarded in 1976.

Teresa taught at Duke University School of Nursing with an adjunct appointment in the Department of Anthropology from 1975 to 1979. Since that time she has taught courses periodically in medical anthropology and international health at Duke University. From 1982 to 1983 she pursued postdoctoral training in medical anthropology at the University of California, San Francisco.

Dr. Graedon has coauthored with Joe Graedon the following books: *The People's Pharmacy-2* (New York: Avon, 1980), *The New People's Pharmacy #3: Drug Breakthroughs of the '80s* (New York: Bantam, 1985), *Totally New and Revised The People's Pharmacy* (New York: St. Martin's Press, 1985), *50+: The Graedons' People's Pharmacy for Older Adults* (New York: Bantam, 1988) *Graedons' Best Medicine: From Herbal Remedies to High-Tech ℞ Breakthroughs* (New York: Bantam, 1991). *The Aspirin Handbook: A User's Guide to the Breakthrough Drug of the '90s* (New York: Bantam Books, 1993), and *The People's Guide to Deadly Drug Interactions* (New York: St. Martin's Press, 1995). The total number of the Graedons' books in print well exceeds two million.

Teresa is a member of the **Society for Applied Anthropology,** the **American Anthropological Association,** the **Society for Medical Anthropology,** and the

American Public Health Association. The newspaper column she writes with Joe, **"The People's Pharmacy,"** is syndicated nationally by King Features. In 1992 *The People's Pharmacy* radio show won a Silver Award from the Corporation for Public Broadcasting. It is syndicated nationally by MIR Productions, Inc., and is heard on more than 500 radio stations in the United States and 134 countries on public radio, the In Touch Radio Reading Service, and the U.S. Armed Forces Radio and Television Network.

AFTERWORD

The People's Pharmacy has grown from one book, started on a manual typewriter in a small Mexican village in 1971, to a series of books (ten at last count, including one novel). We never imagined in our wildest dreams that we would get to be on national television and would have our own internationally syndicated talk-radio show. And who could have anticipated a syndicated newspaper column? We never had a single journalism course.

Underlying everything we do is the goal of empowerment. We strive to inform and help people become active health-care consumers. Over the years we have received hundreds of thousands of letters from people who shared their tragedies and triumphs. We invite you to write with your story or question. We also welcome home remedies. We cannot promise to answer each communication (we average over a thousand letters a week). But we will attempt to include the most poignant and relevant in our next publication. Thanks for reading *The People's Pharmacy*. Remember, information is your best protection!

Address your cards and letters to:

Joe and Terry Graedon
The People's Pharmacy
c/o St. Martin's Press
175 Fifth Avenue
New York, NY 10010